T0383811

HEALTH PROMOTION IN MIDWIFERY

The fourth edition of *Health Promotion in Midwifery* explores the principles of health promotion within the practical context of midwifery. It clearly outlines and discusses the midwife's role in health promotion, linking theory, and practice.

This thoroughly updated new edition considers recent changes and developments in midwifery practice and public health. It explores essential topics such as infant feeding, smoking, mental health, behaviour change, models for health promotion, violence and abuse, and sexual health promotion and includes seven entirely new chapters. These new additions reflect the need to improve inequalities in care for service users from a range of backgrounds such as for clients from racially diverse communities, clients from the LGBT+ communities, and migrant and displaced clients. Further chapters, such as those looking at public health in a global world, vaccinations in pregnancy, and self-care for midwives, meet needs highlighted by the recent pandemic and its aftermath.

Text boxes throughout ensure the text is accessible and user-friendly, and case studies and summaries put the material in a practical context. Further reading sections encourage readers to further research and reflect on their own practice. This textbook is essential reading for all midwives, student midwives, health visitors, and other health care professionals in maternity care education and practice.

Jan Bowden is an experienced lecturer in midwifery at the Florence Nightingale Faculty of Nursing, Midwifery and Palliative Care, King's College London, and an external examiner. She is passionate about the role of the midwife in public health and health promotion, contraception, and sexual health, including abortion, FGM, and women's health. She is currently involved in a project to develop the academic literacy skills of midwifery students.

Sam Bassett is the head of the Department of Education and lead midwife for education at King's College London. As an experienced midwife, her specialist areas of interest are maternal medical complexities, midwifery emergencies, and maternal high-dependency care. Clinical midwifery practice remains central to Sam's work, and she continues to contribute nationally to the development of key guidelines/publications, instruct on courses such as NLS, and represent midwifery on courses such as mMOET.

FOURTH EDITION

HEALTH PROMOTION IN MIDWIFERY
PRINCIPLES AND PRACTICE

Edited by
Jan Bowden and Sam Bassett

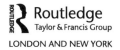

Routledge
Taylor & Francis Group

LONDON AND NEW YORK

Designed cover image: Sarah Johnson has generated this text in part with DALL·E, OpenAI's large-scale image-generation model. Upon generating draft images, the author reviewed, edited, and revised the image to their own liking and takes ultimate responsibility for the content of this publication.

Fourth edition published 2025
by Routledge
4 Park Square, Milton Park, Abingdon, Oxon, OX14 4RN

and by Routledge
605 Third Avenue, New York, NY 10158

Routledge is an imprint of the Taylor & Francis Group, an informa business

© 2025 Jan Bowden and Sam Bassett

First edition published by Arnold 1997
Second edition published by Arnold 2006
Third edition published by Taylor & Francis 2017

British Library Cataloguing-in-Publication Data
A catalogue record for this book is available from the British Library

Library of Congress Cataloging-in-Publication Data
Names: Bowden, Jan, editor. | Bassett, Sam, editor.
Title: Health promotion in midwifery: principles and practice/edited by Jan Bowden and Sam Bassett.
Description: Fourth edition. | Abingdon, Oxon; New York, NY: Routledge, 2025. |
Includes bibliographical references and index.
Identifiers: LCCN 2024029391 (print) | LCCN 2024029392 (ebook) | ISBN 9781032395166 (hardback) |
ISBN 9781032394657 (paperback) | ISBN 9781003350071 (ebook)
Classification: LCC RG950 .H37 2025 (print) | LCC RG950 (ebook) | DDC 618.2—dc23/eng/20240708
LC record available at https://lccn.loc.gov/2024029391
LC ebook record available at https://lccn.loc.gov/2024029392

ISBN: 978-1-032-39516-6 (hbk)
ISBN: 978-1-032-39465-7 (pbk)
ISBN: 978-1-003-35007-1 (ebk)

DOI: 10.4324/9781003350071

Typeset in Palatino LT Std
by codeMantra

Access the Support Material: www.routledge.com/9781032394657

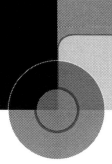

Contents

Contents

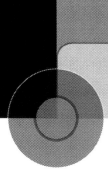

About the Editors

Jan Bowden is an experienced lecturer in midwifery at the Florence Nightingale Faculty of Nursing, Midwifery and Palliative Care, King's College London, and an external examiner. She is passionate about the role of the midwife in public health and health promotion, contraception, and sexual health, including abortion, FGM, and women's health. She is currently involved in a project to develop the academic literacy skills of midwifery students.

Sam Bassett is the Head of the Midwifery department and Lead Midwife for education at King's College. As an experienced midwife, her specialist areas of interest are maternal medical complexities, midwifery emergencies, and maternal high-dependency care. Clinical midwifery practice remains central to Sam's work and she continues to contribute nationally to the development of key guidelines/publications, instruct on courses such as NLS, and represent midwifery on courses such as mMOET.

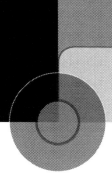

About the Contributors

Teresa Arias is a senior lecturer in midwifery education and a senior fellow of the Higher Education Academy at the Florence Nightingale Faculty of Nursing, Midwifery and Palliative Care, King's College London. Her clinical background includes Caseload and Independent Midwifery which served to enhance her commitment to person-centred midwifery care. Teresa's passion is in working with midwifery students to develop skills to enhance the relational continuity of midwifery care.

Rose Beaumont qualified as a midwife in 2014 from the University of Bradford with a first-class honors BSc in midwifery. She worked at a large London hospital whilst completing her MSc in global health at King's College London, where she also worked as a member of the midwifery teaching team. She currently works as a lecturer in midwifery at the University of Leeds and has a special interest in global health, maternal mental health, and perinatal suicide.

Kenda Crozier is a professor of midwifery and the head of the School of Nursing and Midwifery at Queens University Belfast. Previously, she was the dean of School of Health Sciences, University of East Anglia, She balances a research and education portfolio to include leadership, advanced practice, sustainable midwifery care models, technology use in practice, and maternal mental health and well-being. She is a visiting professor at Naresuan University, Thailand, and the University of Sharjah, United Arab Emirates.

Charlotte Dewar has an MSc in public health. She is a fellow of the Higher Education Academy and is a midwifery lecturer at the University of York. Her areas of special interest include health promotion in midwifery, physiological childbirth, and bereavement care.

Amanda Firth is senior lecturer in midwifery and researcher at the University of Huddersfield. Her areas of research expertise include perinatal mental health, forced migration, and addressing health inequalities, particularly those associated with race, ethnicity and language barriers.

Lucy Flatley has a BA (Hons) in midwifery practice and a master's in public health. She is a transformation lead midwife, York and Scarborough Teaching Hospitals, NHS Foundation Trust. She has worked in many areas of midwifery, including in a midwifery continuity of carer team and as a midwifery lecturer. She is passionate about co-production with women and families to improve maternity services. Public health is an area of expertise with regard to the role of the midwife in improving public health and reducing health inequalities both globally and locally.

Kelda Folliard is a clinical academic midwife and a professional midwifery advocate working at Norfolk and Norwich University Hospital and the University of East Anglia. Her current clinical work is in specialist midwifery support of women and birthing people with mental health challenges and social complexity. Her doctoral research explored the lived experience of perinatal anxiety, and her areas of expertise and interest include maternal mental health and midwives' professional development.

Maria Garcia De Frutos is a senior midwifery lecturer at City University of London with a strong public health expertise. She has over 20 years of nursing and midwifery experience, both within health systems and third-sector organisations. In addition to her strong clinical background, she gained an MSc in public health at the LSHTM. Her interests relate to social and reproductive justice, reducing health inequalities, women with complex socio-political needs, migrant needs, migrants and displaced populations.

Verona Hall is an experienced midwife and nurse with over 35 years in healthcare. Currently, she is a lecturer at Middlesex University and is known for her creative teaching and use of simulation technology. Verona advocates for diversity and inclusion in the healthcare field and supports the belief that everyone should have equal access to high-quality care.

Grace Howard is a midwifery lecturer, Florence Nightingale Faculty of Nursing, Midwifery and Palliative Care, King's College London. Her special areas of interest include equity, diversity and inclusion, cultural safety, and mental health.

Sarah Johnson is a dedicated senior midwifery lecturer and BFI lead at the University of Central Lancashire. She empowers future midwives while advocating for inclusive education and healthcare. With 15 years of clinical experience, she promotes compassionate care and transformative leadership in infant feeding. Sarah's award-winning dedication to inclusivity is shaped by her personal experience of dyslexia and ADHD, diagnosed later in life; she serves as a neurodivergent role model in education and midwifery.

Charlotte Anne Kenyon is a senior lecturer in midwifery at the University of Huddersfield, UK. She has a wide range of experience in clinical settings and a keen interest in both educational and professional regulations. Her interests are in supporting women's choices, facilitating safe birth, and integrating complementary therapies into conventional maternity care to promote physiological birth and positive experiences for women. She also leads the teaching of systematic examination of the newborn and works from a lens of promoting the mother/baby dyad.

Sarah Kipps trained as a nurse at St Thomas Hospital in 1988. She worked in gynaecology clinics until 1995 when she left to work in community clinics, initially in community contraception and then in integrated sexual health. She has led projects relating to young people and vulnerable women, taught in schools, and lectured in reproductive sexual health at King's College London. She currently works for 'Your Healthcare', Surbiton, as a senior contraceptive and sexual health nurse.

Zeni Koutsi is a midwife lecturer with over 23 years of midwifery experience in the UK and Greece. She was originally trained in Greece and practised midwifery mainly in the UK. She has an MSc (University of Nottingham) and a PGCE (King's College London). She is a fellow of the Higher Education Authority. She has been the co-lead of the South-East England BFI Network. Her special interests are infant feeding, maternal medicine, global health, and supporting diaspora midwives.

Chelsea Leadley is an associate lecturer in psychology at the University of York. She is a mixed methods researcher examining the complex relationships between online behaviour and mental health. She currently specialises in emotional disclosures and help-seeking on social media and has a background in forensic psychology and suicide note content.

Elsa Montgomery is a senior lecturer in midwifery at the Florence Nightingale Faculty of Nursing, Midwifery and Palliative Care, King's College London. Her main area of expertise is trauma-informed maternity care for women and birthing people who have experienced child sexual abuse.

Alessandra Morelli is a senior research midwife at Oxford University Hospitals and the University of Oxford, and an associate midwifery lecturer at Oxford Brookes University. As a member of UK-MED, she responds to humanitarian crises, recently lending her expertise in Türkiye and Libya. With a BSc in midwifery from La Sapienza, University of Rome, Alessandra ventured to the UK for clinical and research roles, furthering her education with an MSc in global health from King's College London.

Ian P S Noonan is a consultant nurse for mental health at Calderdale & Huddersfield NHS Foundation Trust, UK, and an honorary senior lecturer at the University of Huddersfield. He is a principal fellow of the Higher Education Academy and a fellow of the Royal Society for Public Health. His research includes self-harm cessation, interventions to reduce suicide on railways, and arts and humanities in health education.

Hannah Rayment-Jones is a midwife and a senior research fellow at the Department of Women and Children's Health, King's College London. Her research focuses on maternal and child health inequalities and has been largely informed by her clinical experience and strong interest in equity and social justice. Her current advanced NIHR fellowship focuses on the long-term health and social outcomes of women and children with no recourse to public funds and irregular migrant status.

Ruth Sanders is a midwifery lecturer at the University of East Anglia. She is currently undertaking a professional doctorate in health and social care. She sits on the Royal College of Midwives Editorial Board and the Cavell Advisory Panel, and she is a professional midwifery advocate. She has been involved with developing advanced clinical practice in midwifery nationally, and her areas of expertise include decision-making, health communication, pain management, and creative reflection.

Claire Singh is a lecturer in midwifery at the Florence Nightingale Faculty of Nursing, Midwifery and Palliative Care, King's College London, and she is a programme lead for the three-year midwifery undergraduate programme. She has a special interest in optimising birth for women and birthing people and equity of maternity care provision. Prior to working in education, she worked extensively in clinical research delivery within reproductive health and childbirth within the NHS.

Tomasina Stacey is a senior lecturer in midwifery and maternal health research at the Florence Nightingale Faculty of Nursing, Midwifery and Palliative Care, King's College London. Her research focusses on exploring modifiable risks for stillbirth and developing public health interventions to improve perinatal outcomes. She has previously worked as a consultant midwife in public health.

Octavia Wiseman is a midwife at King's College Hospital and a research fellow at City, University of London. She has worked on a range of studies focused on midwifery-led models of care, including the REACH Pregnancy Circles trial and an evaluation of the implementation of Continuity of Carer for NHSE. She teaches and writes about issues facing pregnant migrants to the UK and is currently developing parent education in six languages for South-East London LMNS.

Rebecca Whybrow is a lecturer in midwifery at King's College London. As an experienced midwife, educator, and researcher, she specialises in public policy, clinician and patient decision-making, complex pregnancies, and intrapartum care. Rebecca was previously senior maternity safety advisor at the Department of Health and Social Care where she contributed to the development of the women's health strategy. Rebecca was a NICE committee member for 'Intrapartum care for women with existing medical conditions and their babies'.

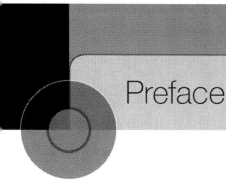

Preface

Public health and health promotion continue to be a crucial part of Global Health Care policy. Its aims are to reduce health inequalities and develop and implement health improvements that will allow generational changes to health. The WHO global strategic directions for midwives 2021–2025 clearly identify the contribution that midwives can make in achieving universal health coverage. Midwives can avert 80% of all maternal deaths, stillbirths, and neonatal deaths as well as impact over 50 other health-related outcomes including sexual and reproductive health, immunisations, breastfeeding, smoking cessation, HIV, obesity in pregnancy, and improvements to mental health, especially postpartum depression.

Our role in public health and health promotion is making a vital difference to the women and birthing people in our care. It is not a new role for us; almost everything we do as midwives impacts the health promotion of those in our care. However, it is being undertaken against a backdrop of rapidly changing challenges following the COVID-19 pandemic, the current global economic downturn, natural disasters, and war. Leading to changes in the midwifery workforce, our working practices and service provisions, while still striving in our aim of meeting the health needs of those accessing midwifery services.

The principles of health promotion are important to underpin good midwifery health promotion practice. This book aims to bring together these concepts in a way that we hope are user-friendly and accessible and encourages all midwives to look at their health promotion and wider public health roles. This fourth edition has allowed us to welcome a bevy of new chapter writers who are passionate and knowledgeable about their topic areas as well as Sam Bassett as the new co-editor. Each chapter has been revised, and new chapters have been developed to meet emerging challenges in clinical practice such as global health, the challenges of health promotion in racially diverse communities, and midwifery self-care and resilience. This book is intended to be realistic and practical in its suggestions for the promotion of health in midwifery practice and for the provision of holistic care that is woman and birthing people focused.

For further reading and resources of each chapter, please see the support material at www.routledge.com/9781032394657

Jan Bowden and Sam Bassett

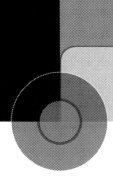

Acknowledgements

We would like to acknowledge the chapter authors who decided to step away and not join us on the fourth edition fun bus. You helped lay the foundations for the second and third editions of this book, and this new fourth edition stands on those foundations. So, thank you to Heather Finlay, Penny Charles, Fabiana Lorencatto, James Harris, Eddie West-Burnham, Louise Long (Armstrong), Mary Malone, Sheila O' Connor, Janette O'Toole, and Emily Nellist.

I personally would like to acknowledge my 'partner in crime' Vicky Manning who was co-editor for the first two editions as well as a chapter author. It has been very strange not to be working with her this time. I have missed her ability to gently cut my overly wordy sentences, to clear my brain when I had a mind blank – I am not a natural writer – and to put perspective on the bumps that appear on the road when writing and editing a book.

So, THANK YOU for the memories made during the second and third editions and I hope you can see I have learnt from your wise words and counsel.

I would also like to acknowledge and thank Sam Bassett, who despite the workload from hell agreed to come on board as co-editor. It's been a pleasure to work alongside you and to all the new chapter authors who have joined with their professional expertise and knowledge allowing us to extend the range of topic areas in this fourth edition. THANK YOU!

We would also like to thank our families and friends, who have, in their own distinctive styles, found ways both big and small to encourage and support us and provided much-needed light-heartedness. Thanks also to Grace McInnes, Amy Thompson, and Madii Cherry-Moreton from Routledge for their help and advice and for giving us the chance to do this new edition.

We would also like to thank Sarah Johnston (one of the authors of Chapter 12) for her help in developing the images for the cover and Robin (aged 3) who helped with the final decision as to which image to go for.

A special acknowledgement to our two fourth edition babies – Ines and Sylvie – welcome to the world and thank you for letting your mums get their chapters in on time and making the editors very happy.

Jan Bowden and Sam Bassett
King's College London

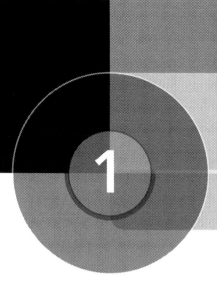

Global Health and Midwifery

ROSE BEAUMONT, LUCY FLATLEY, AND ALESSANDRA MORELLI

WHAT IS GLOBAL HEALTH?

Global health is focused on improving health and achieving health equity for all people worldwide – meaning working towards the absence of avoidable, unfair, or remediable differences among groups of people. Many health issues and concerns transcend national boundaries and require collaboration between countries to address them

Squires (2018)

Global health is an emerging field of healthcare and health practice with an ever-evolving direction and definition (Taylor, 2018). What is clear is that global health is fundamentally similar to public health, aiming to achieve better health outcomes through collaborative intervention, research, and education by understanding the factors that impact on health inequalities and health challenges (Duke Global Health Institute, 2023). The foundations of global health are public health and medicine (Chen et al., 2020). Global health is where the cause and remedy of a public health, medicine, and health issue require either a multi-nation or global response (Taylor, 2018). The World Health Organization (WHO) founded in 1948 is an agency of the United Nations whose sole work is to develop and collaborate on global health issues, to improve universal health coverage by connecting nations, partners, and people (WHO, 2023a).

DOI: 10.4324/9781003350071-1

COVID-19 exposed many weaknesses within local, national, and global health systems and highlighted the potential global impact of Public Health and Health Promotion and a need for a more collaborative global approach (WHO2021a). COVID-19 also highlighted the disproportionate impacts of inequality on determinants of health, and despite developments in global health gains in the last few decades, it exposed the multiple threats we face in health. Globalisation and increasing migration mean that local and national health systems must adapt to be more global as health issues transcend national boundaries (Squires, 2018). Changes to human travel and behaviour, increased risk of future pandemics, and threats of humanitarian crisis impact the health security of the world, making this a pivotal time to start considering health on a more global scale while also considering the changing needs of the UK population due to globalisation. Midwifery care must adapt and evolve to include global health, and this chapter will explore how global health links to midwifery care and public health and promotion in the UK context.

Within this chapter, maternal mortality will be explored, as well as the Millennium Development Goals (MDGs) and the Sustainable Development Goals. Global and UK maternal mortality will then be discussed. This chapter will also consider solutions for reducing maternal mortality bringing in discussions on health inequalities and summarise by discussing recommendations for midwifery practice in the UK.

BACKGROUND: THE GLOBAL HEALTH PICTURE

Since the inception of the WHO in 1948, the United Nations (UN) has created international policy to incorporate global health targets, those that are particularly important to midwifery practice and care are targets to reduce global maternal and neonatal mortality rates as well as policy to improve gender inequality and neonatal outcomes and health (WHO, 2023a).

When discussing global health, we will often refer to them as 'low'-, 'low-middle'-, ' upper-middle'-, and 'high'-income countries – this classification is described and classified by the World Bank (see Table 1.1). Every year the classification is updated and based on the country's economy and gross national income per capita in US dollars (Hamadeh et al., 2022). It will be of no surprise that the majority of upper middle- and high-income countries are in North America, Europe, and the Pacific, while sub-Saharan Africa and South Asia are predominantly made up of low- and low-middle-income countries. Low- and low-middle-income countries tend to have weaker health systems and poorer health outcomes, in terms of life expectancy and maternal and neonatal mortality, so it is important to understand these terms when considering global health.

Table 1.1 World Bank country classifications by income level: 2022–2023

Group	1 July 2022 rating
Low income	<$1,085
Lower-middle income	$1,086–4255
Upper-middle income	$4,256–13,205
High income	$13,205

Source: Hamadeh et al. (2022).

GLOBAL MATERNAL MORTALITY

The WHO (n.d.) defined maternal mortality as:

> The annual number of female deaths from any cause related to or aggravated by pregnancy or its management (excluding accidental or incidental causes) during pregnancy and childbirth or within 42 days of termination of pregnancy, irrespective of the duration and site of the pregnancy

Maternal deaths can be direct and indirect:

Direct obstetric deaths (or direct maternal deaths) are those maternal deaths "resulting from obstetric complications of the pregnant state (pregnancy, labour and puerperium), and from interventions, omissions, incorrect treatment, or from a chain of events resulting from any of the above" (WHO, n.d.). Deaths due to obstetric haemorrhage or hypertensive disorders in pregnancy, for example, or those due to complications of anaesthesia or caesarean section are classified as direct maternal deaths.

Indirect obstetric deaths (or indirect maternal deaths) are those *maternal deaths* "resulting from previous existing disease or disease that developed during pregnancy and not due to direct obstetric causes but were aggravated by the physiologic effects of pregnancy" (WHO, n.d.). For example, deaths due to aggravation (by pregnancy) of an existing cardiac or renal disease are considered indirect maternal deaths.

It is estimated that 95% of maternal deaths occur in developing countries (WHO, 2023b). There is no clear definition of a developing country; however, the Oxford Dictionary defines it as a low-income country which may be undergoing industrialisation (Oxford University Press, 2023). When countries are defined as low or middle income, this is when income is used to define development of a country (UN, 2014). The distribution of maternal mortality rates reflects global inequalities women experience due to socioeconomic status and access and proximity to healthcare (WHO, 2023a). In 2020, nearly 800 women died each day, which is approximately a woman every two minutes. Because inequalities in maternal mortality rates persist worldwide, sub-Saharan Africa still accounted for the majority (70%) of all maternal deaths in 2020 (WHO, 2023b). By contrast, Australia and New Zealand have the lowest global maternal mortality rates at 4 per 100,000 (WHO, 2023b). The maternal mortality rate in sub-Saharan Africa is 136 times higher than in Australia and New Zealand (WHO, 2023b).

There are several factors, often interconnected, that contribute to maternal mortality worldwide. It is well-known that social determinants of health, such as income, housing conditions, education and ethnicity, and low prioritisation of women and girls' rights, put some women at greater risk of dying (WHO, 2023b). In the last few years, the increased impact of air pollution and climate change on poor reproductive, maternal, and perinatal health outcomes has also been recognised (Roos et al., 2021; Chersich et al., 2022). Another important factor impacting maternal mortality includes humanitarian crisis because of conflicts, disease outbreaks, or natural disasters, which is likely to cause disruption to the health system and the care that women and their babies can receive.

Lastly, it is important to mention the "Three delays model" (Thaddeus & Maine, 1994), looking at three factors that can substantially increase a woman's chance of dying – see Table 1.2.

Table 1.2 Three delays model

Delay in seeking care: a delay in seeking care (or never making this decision) for reasons such as perception of inadequate care at the nearest healthcare facility, sociocultural factors, financial, and opportunity costs.

Delay in reaching the healthcare facility: when the decision of seeking care is decisively made, factors such as transportation and distance can be a barrier to reach the healthcare facility.

Delay in receiving care: when women finally reach the healthcare facility, there might be a delay in receiving care from healthcare professionals when needed. When they finally receive care, it might not be of good quality or evidence based.

Source: Adapted from Thaddeus and Maine (1994).

LEARNING ACTIVITY

Review Thaddeus and Maine's (1994) three delays model and apply this to global health and reflect on how it can impact on your practice.

In terms of improving maternal and neonatal outcomes, the importance of midwives has been increasingly recognised worldwide. Nove et al. (2021) reported that a substantial increase in universal coverage of intervention delivered by midwives could avoid more than a third of maternal, neonatal deaths, and stillbirths, equating to 4.3 million deaths averted per year by 2035. On reviewing the Millennium Development Goals Report (UN, 2015), it comes as no surprise that regions such as Southern and Eastern Asia have achieved the greatest reduction in maternal mortality, having increased the number of births attended by a skilled midwife. Yet, there is a global shortfall of 900,000 midwives affecting especially low- and middle-income countries (International Confederation of Midwives [ICM], 2021); however, this shortage is also beginning to hit more economically developed countries such as the UK (Royal College of Midwives, 2022).

REDUCING MATERNAL MORTALITY: FROM THE MILLENNIUM DEVELOPMENT GOALS TO THE SUSTAINABLE DEVELOPMENT GOALS

In September 2000, United Nations Member States adopted the MDGs, eight goals (see Table 1.3), to develop a global partnership for development by 2015 (UN, 2015). The MDGs 4 and 5 particularly focused on reducing child mortality and improving maternal health.

One of the most successful reductions in maternal mortality was achieved by the Maldives, where the maternal mortality ratio declined from 677 in 1990 to 68 deaths per 100,000 live births in 2016 (United Nations Population Fund, 2016). This was possible because of investments and policies aimed specifically towards maternal and child health. This resulted in a rapid increase in the number of midwives, the establishment of in-depth review processes investigating specific causes of maternal deaths, and interventions and policies towards nutrition, aiming at reducing

Table 1.3 The millennium development goals, 2000

Goal 1	To eradicate extreme poverty and hunger
Goal 2	To promote universal primary education
Goal 3	To promote gender equality and empower women
Goal 4	To reduce child mortality
Goal 5	To improve maternal health
Goal 6	To combat HIV/AIDs, malaria and other diseases
Goal 7	To ensure environmental sustainability
Goal 8	To develop a global partnership for development

deficiencies that are a key contributor to conditions such as anaemia and neural tube defects (Our World in Data, 2020).

In 2016, the UN adopted a renewed call for action, The Sustainable Development Goals (SDGs), with the aim of ending poverty, inequalities, and promoting good health while also protecting the environment by 2030 (UN, 2023). While there are 17 goals, there are only 8 relevant to improving the lives of all people, including pregnant women and their babies. SDG 3 'Good Health and Wellbeing' specifically calls for a reduction of maternal mortality ratio to less than 70 per 100,000 live births, and to reduce neonatal mortality to less than 12 per 1,000 live births and under-5 mortality to less than 25 per 1,000 live births. It also highlights universal access to sexual and reproductive healthcare services (UN, 2023). In addition, SDG 5 'Gender Equality' aims to end discrimination and violence against girls and women, and elimination of harmful practices such as female genital cutting.

While substantial progress was made during the MDGs era in reducing maternal mortality, during the first five years of the SDGs, the pace of reduction has slowed down. Reasons for this flatlined reduction in maternal mortality are the COVID-19 pandemic, rising poverty, and worsening humanitarian crises that have increased pressures on health systems that were already struggling (WHO, 2023c).

The WHO plays an important role in public health and health promotion worldwide. Their main function is to lead multiple stakeholders towards common goals and to establish, monitor, and enforce norms and standards to promote health worldwide (Ruger & Yach, 2009). The WHO has led several initiatives over the past 75 years to improve and promote health for all, while also monitoring health outcomes at the country level. An example of these is the Ending Preventable Maternal Mortality (EPMM) initiative, launched by WHO and the United Nations Population Fund (UNFPA) in 2021, which consists of five targets and milestones to be achieved by 2025 to try and meet the SDGs:

- 90% pregnant women to attend four or more antenatal care visits.
- 90% births to be attended by skilled health personnel.
- 80% women to access postnatal care within two days of giving birth.
- 60% of women to have access to emergency obstetric care within two hours of travel time.
- 65% of women to be able to make informed and empowered decisions regarding sexual relations, contraceptive use, and their reproductive health.

(WHO, 2021b)

Significant progress in reducing maternal mortality rates has been made over the last 20 years with rates decreasing by 34.3% from 2000 to 2020; however, this has stagnated in recent years (WHO, 2023b). A recent call to action in the Lancet Global Health discusses these increases and the inequalities between countries and calls for the global health community to act on this and more accurate data on maternal health outcomes (Khalil et al., 2023). If figures continue to follow the most recent trend, the SDGs will not be met. Countries will have to ensure that the healthcare system is strong and stable enough as maternal and neonatal health outcomes affect progress in healthcare globally. The stagnation in the decline in maternal mortality rate is multifactorial; however, there are a number of causes cited by WHO (2023b):

- Obstetric emergencies
- Infectious and non-communicable diseases
- Wider determinants of health.
- Impact of the three delays model
- Harmful gender norms, biases, and inequalities affecting access to appropriate reproductive healthcare.
- External factors including humanitarian crises.

MATERNAL MORTALITY IN THE UK

The most recent figures reporting on maternal death from 2019 to 2021 show an increase in maternal deaths although this was not of statistical significance (National Perinatal Epidemiology Unit [NPEU], 2023). When deaths due to COVID-19 were not included in these figures, there was a non-statistically significant decrease (NPEU, 2023). Between 2019 and 2021, COVID-19 was the leading cause of maternal death in the UK. There is not sufficient data to understand the impact of the pandemic on maternal mortality rates globally (Khalil et al., 2023). Cardiac disease was the second leading cause of maternal mortality. Research has shown that out of eight European countries, the UK had the second-highest maternal mortality rate, and this was significantly higher than Norway and Denmark in particular (Diguisto et al., 2022).

The most recent MBRRACE report (Knight et al., 2022) highlighted the continued significant ethnic inequalities that exist in the UK and the impact these have on maternal mortality. Systematic racism, bias, and health inequalities affect the care provision. Disparities in outcomes for Black and Asian women are more significant in the most recent figures although there is not a statistically significant increase (NPEU, 2022). The trend with disparity in ethnicity and maternal mortality is similar to the UK in several European countries, including Denmark, France, Italy, and the Netherlands (Diguisto et al., 2022). However, it is important to note that not all countries report and record ethnicity in the same way. If we consider the three delays model, much of this can be applied to the factors found in recent MBRRACE reports. This needs to be considered in any policy and planning moving forward, and we must consider as midwives the barriers created for women and birthing people, particularly from racially diverse and other marginalised groups. (See Chapter 5 for further exploration on racial diversity.)

A range of factors are associated with maternal mortality. There are large disparities in maternal mortality by deprivation (Knight et al., 2022). Other contributing factors related to health inequalities in addition to ethnicity are obesity, smoking and substance misuse, maternal age, and engagement with antenatal care (Nair et al., 2015; 2016).

The confidential enquiry into maternal deaths in the UK is an important method of monitoring maternal deaths in the UK, and many countries do not have reporting systems and data collection of this level. Nevertheless, UK maternal mortality rates are of concern and require action. Reducing health inequalities is key to achieving this and policies such as the NHS long-term plan (NHS confederation, 2019) and Core20PLUS5 (NHS England, 2021) are key to supporting these aims.

LEARNING ACTIVITY

The Core20PLUS5 recommends achieving the national aim 'Maternity: ensuring continuity of care for 75% of women from BAME communities and from the most deprived groups' (NHS England, 2021). See links below

NHS England » Core20PLUS5 (adults) – an approach to reducing healthcare inequalities

core20plus5-online-engage-survey-supporting-document-v1.pdf (england.nhs.uk)

- Why have these recommendations been made, what is the evidence base?
- What are the current challenges in midwifery practice to achieve this aim?
- Make three suggestions for how these challenges can be overcome.

THE EVOLVING GLOBAL HEALTH PICTURE: HEALTH INEQUALITIES IN THE UK AND GLOBAL HEALTH IN LOCAL PRACTICE

The COVID-19 pandemic clearly highlighted the need for globalisation, as the world coped with the same challenges in a variety of ways; it demonstrated the need for global learning to improve healthcare and develop skills such as resourcefulness, intercultural skills, resilience, and team building (Evans, 2022).

The pandemic has also had a significant impact on health and wellbeing, globally and within local practice. Health inequalities and weak healthcare systems and processes were exposed particularly the disproportionate effects felt by those from racially diverse and deprived communities (Ham, 2020). The most recent MBRRACE report (Knight et al., 2022) and reports such as the Five X More report (Peter & Wheeler, 2022), the Invisible Report (Gohir, 2022), and The Birthrights Inquiry (2022) all highlight the systematic racism, bias, and inequalities that exist in midwifery care. As the health needs of the UK population is ever changing, these reports and the COVID-19 pandemic have shone a spotlight on the lack of progress on many health outcomes including life expectancy, maternal and neonatal mortality, and mental illness in comparison to other high-income countries, in particular how these issues affect those from racially diverse and deprived communities the most (Mckee et al., 2021).

Surviving childbirth alone should not be the aim of global maternal health policy and marker of success but the promotion of health and wellbeing must also be a priority to improve women and children's health worldwide (WHO, 2021b). In recent years, there have been significant influences on global health which have directly impacted on gains in improving women and children's health; COVID-19 and increasing numbers of humanitarian crises such as war, climate change, and natural disasters have seen a stall on progress made under the MDGs. The global shortage of midwives must be addressed too in order to ensure that universal coverage to midwifery care is also available. There are multiple factors that impact global health in local practice. Globalisation over the last century, increasing humanitarian crisis, and the increased impact of climate change have led to increasing rates of migration. This impacts service provision and needs, as well as the consideration of those navigating a new healthcare system. The MBRRACE report (Knight et al., 2022), as previously discussed, also highlights the huge disparities in maternal death in the UK and the inequalities that exist. If we consider the three delays model, and how this may impact on communities and marginalised groups more – it is an important consideration in the local practice to how we minimise these delays.

Displaced and migrant clients are a particularly vulnerable group (see Chapter 19 for more exploration on displaced and migrant clients) and an impact factor when considering global health in local practice. The three delays model can be applied when considering the barriers faced by this group when accessing maternity care.

LEARNING ACTIVITY

Khadija is a recent migrant from Somalia, she arrived in the UK approximately 10 weeks ago and is currently around 26 weeks pregnant. She is unaware that you need to register with a GP and has not had any antenatal care. She arrives unannounced at the hospital as this is how she would have sought care at home.

1. What barriers to accessing care has Khadija faced?
2. What issues and barriers may Khadija continue to face accessing care?

WHAT DOES THIS MEAN FOR MIDWIFERY PRACTICE IN THE UK?

This chapter has discussed midwifery in the global context, introducing global health and maternal mortality. Midwifery in the UK is also facing a number of challenges and requires the implementation of policies to reduce health inequalities and maternal mortality rates for racially diverse women and those who live in deprivation.

Robust policies to reduce health inequalities are needed to reduce maternal mortality in the UK including embedding NHS England equality and equity guidance (NHS England, 2021a) and ensuring racial disparities are eliminated. Personalised care is the underpinning principle to ensure women receive holistic care individual to their needs (Cumberlege, 2016). Proportionate universalism is also paramount to reducing health inequalities in maternity care by providing increased support to those who are experiencing deprivation (NHS England, 2021a). Proportionate universalism means public health interventions taking socio-economic status and individual circumstances into account (Public Health England, 2014). The policy will improve everyone's outcomes but those who are the most disadvantaged will see the most significant benefit in terms of health outcomes (Public Health England, 2014). This can be applied to Midwifery Continuity of Carer, evidence suggests this improves health for all women (Sandall et al., 2016) but a targeted approach for women who are racially diverse and those who are experiencing deprivation or wider determinants of health is likely to have more impact. When implementing new policies in maternity services co-production with service users is key, working with the Maternity and Neonatal Voices Partnerships and ensuring there is diverse representation will ensure the woman's voice is at the centre of services (Maternity Voices Partnership, 2022).

Supporting and retaining the midwifery workforce is required; employing the principles in the improving staff retention guidance (NHS Employers, 2022) and employing specialist midwives to support this work are key. This will help ensure NHS trusts have the building blocks established to enable further rollout of midwifery continuity of carer (NHS England, 2021b) and achieve the CORE20plus5 principles (NHS England, 2021a). Being culturally competent and safe is also paramount for midwives, and there have been a number of calls for all staff to receive this training including from Birthrights (2022).

An understanding of the global context of maternal mortality and the SDGs as well as being aware of contemporary global challenges is important in midwifery. The future midwifery standards (NMC, 2019) highlight the important point that, wherever women are in the world during the childbirth, continuum needs will be similar, and thus, the midwife's role is paramount. We live in a globalised society, and therefore, events that happen across the globe impact midwifery practice in the UK. Simultaneously, if there is conflict in a country or a humanitarian crisis, this will likely impact maternal and neonatal outcomes.

REFELECTION ACTIVITY

Reflect on your own practice area and consider the following:

- Why does global health matter in midwifery practice in the UK context?
- How can you develop your practice to support clients at the greatest risk of the impact of global health?

SUMMARY

- Maternal mortality rates vary across the globe with most moralities occurring in developing countries. There are a number of reasons attributed to this, including the wider determinants of health and a range of ways in which accessing and receiving timely care is delayed for women during the childbirth continuum.
- While substantial progress was made during the MDGs era in reducing maternal mortality, during the first five years of the SDGs the pace of reduction has slowed down. The reasons for this are multifactorial and the Lancet Global Health has called for global action regarding this.
- Maternal and neonatal outcomes are often an indicator of a country's development thus emphasising the importance of the role of midwifery globally to achieving the SDGs and improving maternal and neonatal outcomes.
- Maternal mortality rates in the UK have risen over the last few years. There are also significant disparities; women who are racially diverse and those who are experiencing deprivation are significantly more likely to die.
- Worldwide and national focus on reducing health inequalities is required to tackle maternal mortality rates both globally and in the UK.

REFERENCES

Birthrights. (2022). *Systemic Racism, Not Broken Bodies.* https://www.birthrights.org.uk/wp-content/uploads/2022/05/Birthrights-inquiry-systemic-racism_exec-summary_May-22-web.pdf

Chen, X., Li, H., Lucero-Prisno, D. E., Abdullah, A. S., Huang, J., Laurence, C., Liang, X., Ma, Z., Mao, Z., Ren, R., Wu, S., Wang, N., Wang, P., Wang, T., Yan, H., & Zou, Y. (2020). What is global health? Key concepts and clarification of misperceptions. *Global Health Research and Policy*, 5(14), 1–8. https://doi.org/10.1186/s41256-020-00142-7

Chersich, M., Scorgie, F., Filippi, V., Lüchters, S., Huggett, A., Sibanda, E. L., Parker, C., Lakhoo, D. P., Maimela, G., Rees, H., Solarin, I., Harden, L. M., Hetem, R. S., & Mavhu, W. (2022). Increasing global temperatures threaten gains in maternal and newborn health in Africa: A review of impacts and an adaptation framework. *International Journal of Gynecology & Obstetrics*, 160(2), 421–429. https://doi.org/10.1002/ijgo.14381

Cumberlege, J. (2016). *Better Births.* NHS England. https://www.england.nhs.uk/wp-content/uploads/2016/02/national-maternity-review-report.pdf

Duke Global Health Institute. (2023). *What Is Global Health?* Duke Global Health Institute. https://globalhealth.duke.edu/what-global-health#top

Diguisto, C., Saucedo, M., Kallianidis, A. F., Bloemenkamp, K. W., Bødker, B., Buoncristiano, M., Donati, S., Gissler, M., Johansen, M., Knight, M., Korbel', M., Krištúfková, A., Nyfløt, L. T., & Deneux-Tharaux, C. (2022). Maternal mortality in eight European countries with enhanced surveillance systems: Descriptive population based study. *BMJ*, 379, e070621. https://doi.org/10.1136/bmj-2022-070621

Evans, N. (2022, February 18). Why is global learning so vital. *Health Education England.* https://www.hee.nhs.uk/news-blogs-events/blogs/%E2%80%98why-global-learning-so-vital%E2%80%99

Gohir, S. (2022). Invisible: Maternity experiences of Muslim women from racialised minority communities: A summary report. Birth Companions. https://hubble-live-assets.s3.eu-west-1.amazonaws.com/birth-companions/file_asset/file/509/MWN_maternity_summary_report_WEB_2022.pdf

Ham, C. (2020). The challenges facing the NHS in England in 2021. *BMJ*, 371, m4973. https://doi.org/10.1136/bmj.m4973

Hamadeh. N., Van Rompaey. C., Metreau. E., & Eapen. S. G. (2022). New World Bank country classifications by income level: 2022–2023. World Bank Data Blogs. https://blogs.worldbank.org/opendata/new-world-bank-country-classifications-income-level-2022-2023

International Confederation of Midwives (ICM). (2021). *New report sounds the alarm on global shortage of 900,000 midwives.* State of the World's Midwifery 2021 | International Confederation of Midwives. https://www.internationalmidwives.org

Khalil, A., Samara, A., O'Brien, P., Coutinho, C. M., Quintana, S. M., & Ladhani, S. (2023). A call to action: The global failure to effectively tackle maternal mortality rates. *The Lancet Global Health*, 11(8), e1165–e1167. https://doi.org/10.1016/s2214-109x(23)00247-4

Knight, M., Bunch, K., Patel, R., Shakespeare, J., Kotnis, R., Kenyon, S., & Kurinczuk, J. J. (2022). *Saving Lives, Improving Mothers' Care: Core Report: Lessons Learned to Inform Maternity Care from the UK and Ireland Confidential Enquiries into Maternal Deaths and Morbidity 2018–20.* MBRRACE-UK. MBRRACE-UK_Maternal_MAIN_Report_2022_UPDATE.pdf (ox.ac.uk)

Maternity Voices Partnership (MVP). (2022). 2022 MVP Toolkit. Retrieved from https://nationalmaternityvoices.org.uk/mvp-toolkit/1-introduction/1-3-equity/

McKee, M., Gugushvili, A., Koltai, J., & Stuckler, D. (2021). Are populist leaders creating the conditions for the spread of COVID-19? Comment on "A scoping review of populist radical right parties' influence on welfare policy and its implications for population health in Europe". *International Journal of Health Policy and Management*, 10(8), 511–515. https://doi.org/10.34172/ijhpm.2020.124

Nair, M., Knight, M., & Kurinczuk, J. (2016). Risk factors and newborn outcomes associated with maternal deaths in the UK from 2009 to 2013: A national case–control study. *BJOG: An International Journal of Obstetrics and Gynaecology*, 123(10), 1654–1662. https://doi.org/10.1111/1471-0528.13978

Nair, M., Kurinczuk, J., Brocklehurst, P., Sellers, S., Lewis, G., & Knight, M. (2015). Factors associated with maternal death from direct pregnancy complications: A UK national case–control study. *BJOG: An International Journal of Obstetrics and Gynaecology*, 122(5), 653–662. https://doi.org/10.1111/1471-0528.13279

National Perinatal Epidemiology Unit (NPEU). (2023). Maternal mortality 2019–2021. https://www.npeu.ox.ac.uk/mbrrace-uk/data-brief/maternal-mortality-2019-2021#maternal-mortality-rates-uk-2019-2021

NHS Confederation. (2019). The NHS long term plan. https://www.longtermplan.nhs.uk/

NHS England. (2021). *Core20PLUS5 an Approach to Reducing Health Inequalities.* Supporting document to enable the completion of the engage online survey on Core20PLUS5 Version 1, 1 November 2021. https://www.england.nhs.uk/about/equality/equality-hub/national-healthcare-inequalities-improvement-programme/core20plus5/

NHS England. (2021a, September). *Equity and Equality Guidance for Local Maternity Systems.* https://www.england.nhs.uk/publication/equity-and-equality-guidance-for-local-maternity-systems/

NHS England. (2021b). *Delivering Midwifery Continuity of Carer at Full Scale. Guidance on Planning, Implementation and Monitoring 2021/22 Version 1, October 2021.* Retrieved from https://www.england.nhs.uk/publication/delivering-midwifery-continuity-of-carer-at-full-scale-guidance-21-22/

NHS Employers. (2022). *Improving Staff Retention Handbook.* NHS Employers resources. https://www.nhsemployers.org/publications/improving-staff-retention

Nove, A., Friberg, I. K., De Bernis, L., McConville, F., Moran, A. C., Najjemba, M., Hoope-Bender, P. T., Tracy, S., & Homer, C. (2021). Potential impact of midwives in preventing and reducing maternal and neonatal mortality and stillbirths: A Lives Saved Tool modelling study. *The Lancet Global Health*, 9(1), e24–e32. https://doi.org/10.1016/s2214-109x(20)30397-1

Nursing and Midwifery Council. (2019). *Standards of Proficiency for Midwives.* standards-of-proficiency-for-midwives.pdf (nmc.org.uk)

Our World in Data. (2020). Exemplars in global health: Which countries are most successful in preventing maternal deaths? https://ourworldindata.org/exemplars-maternal-mortality#:~:text=Globally%2C%20the%20Maldives%20achieved%20the,births%20%E2%80%93%20a%20very%20impressive%20achievement

Oxford University Press. (2023). Overview: Developing countries. https://www.oxfordreference.com/display/10.1093/oi/authority.20110803095714191

Peter, M., & Wheeler, R. (2022). The Black maternity experiences survey. *Five X more.* https://fivexmore.org/blackmereport

Public Health England. (2014). *Local Action on Health Inequalities: Tackling Health Inequalities Through Action on the Social Determinants of Health: Lessons from Experience* (Healthy Equity Briefing). UCL Institute of Health Equity.

Roos, N., Kovats, S., Hajat, S., Filippi, V., Chersich, M., Luchters, S., Scorgie, F., Nakstad, B., & Stephansson, O. (2021). Maternal and newborn health risks of climate change: A call for awareness and global action. *Acta Obstetricia et Gynecologica Scandinavica*, 100(4), 566–570. https://doi.org/10.1111/aogs.14124

Royal College of Midwives (RCM). (2022). Midwife numbers now lower than at the last general election says RCM. *RCM Media Releases.* https://www.rcm.org.uk/media-releases/2022/may/midwife-numbers-now-lower-than-at-the-last-general-election-says-rcm/

Ruger, J. P., & Yach, D. (2009). The global role of the World Health Organization. *Global Health Governance: The Scholarly Journal for the New Health Security Paradigm*, 2(2), 1.

Sandall, J., Soltani, H., Gates, S., Shennan, A., & Devane, D. (2016). Midwife-led continuity models versus other models of care for childbearing women. *The Cochrane Library*, 2016(4). https://doi.org/10.1002/14651858.cd004667.pub5

Squires, N. (2018). Global health – What it means and why PHE works globally [blog]. UK Health Security Agency. https://ukhsa.blog.gov.uk/2018/09/04/global-health-what-it-means-and-why-phe-works-globally/

Taylor, S. (2018). 'Global health': Meaning what? *BMJ Global Health*, 3(2), e000843. https://doi.org/10.1136/bmjgh-2018-000843

Thaddeus, S., & Maine, D., (1994). Too far to walk: maternal mortality in context. *Social Science & Medicine*, 38(8), 1091–1110.

United Nations Population Fund (UNFPA). (2016). Stunning plunge in maternal deaths recorded in Maldives. *United Nations Population Fund.* https://www.unfpa.org/news/stunning-plunge-maternal-deaths-recorded-maldives

United Nations (UN). (2014). *Country Classification.* https://www.un.org/en/development/desa/policy/wesp/wesp_current/2014wesp_country_classification.pdf

United Nations (UN). (2015). *The Millennium Development Goals Report.* https://www.un.org/millenniumgoals/2015_MDG_Report/pdf/MDG%202015%20rev%20(July%201).pdf

United Nations (UN). (2023). *Sustainable Development Goals.* https://www.un.org/sustainabledevelopment/

World Health Organization (WHO). (n.d). *Maternal Deaths.* https://www.who.int/data/gho/indicator-metadata-registry/imr-details/4622

World Health Organisation (WHO). (2021a). *Spotlight: The Impact of COVID-19 on Global Health Goals.* https://www.who.int/news-room/spotlight/the-impact-of-covid-19-on-global-health-goals

World Health Organization (WHO). (2021b). *Ending Preventable Maternal Mortality (EPMM): A Renewed Focus for Improving Maternal and Newborn Health and Well-being.* https://www.who.int/publications/i/item/9789240040519

World Health Organization (WHO). (2023a). About WHO. https://www.who.int/about/

World Health Organization (WHO). (2023b). *Trends in Maternal Mortality 2000 to 2020: Estimates by WHO, UNICEF, UNFPA, World Bank Group and UNDESA/Population Division.* Geneva: World Health Organization. Retrieved from https://www.who.int/publications/i/item/9789240068759

World Health Organization (WHO). (2023c). *Global Progress in Tackling Maternal and Newborn Deaths Stalls Since 2015.* UN. https://www.who.int/news/item/09-05-2023-global-progress-in-tackling-maternal-and-newborn-deaths-stalls-since-2015--un

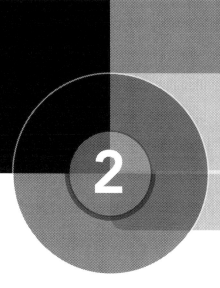

Public Health Policy and Midwifery

2

REBECCA WHYBROW

INTRODUCTION

Public health can be defined as the science and art of preventing disease, prolonging life and promoting health through the organised efforts and informed choices of society, organisations, public and private, communities, and individuals (Her Majesty's [HM] Treasury 2004). A life course approach to public health goes further acknowledging that a

> person's physical and mental health and wellbeing are influenced throughout life by the wider determinants of health. Consisting of a diverse range of social, economic, and environmental factors, alongside behavioural risk factors which often cluster in the population, reflecting real lives.

> (Public Health England [PHE] 2019a)

Implementing a life course approach to public health facilitates delivering evidence-based interventions that minimise risk factors and enhance protective factors at

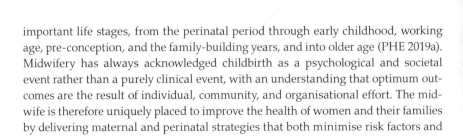

important life stages, from the perinatal period through early childhood, working age, pre-conception, and the family-building years, and into older age (PHE 2019a). Midwifery has always acknowledged childbirth as a psychological and societal event rather than a purely clinical event, with an understanding that optimum outcomes are the result of individual, community, and organisational effort. The midwife is therefore uniquely placed to improve the health of women and their families by delivering maternal and perinatal strategies that both minimise risk factors and enhance protective factors.

This chapter will explore how the midwifery model interacts with government policy on public health. To facilitate this, the chapter will start with a background to government policy on public health and midwifery, before considering the social and economic background to UK government policy. Current government policy will then be explored in more detail and linked to the factors influencing the ability of midwifery to fulfil its public health role.

BACKGROUND

With an increased recognition of the broader meaning of public health and an acceptance of the influence of disadvantage and inequality on health outcomes. The Independent Inquiry into Inequalities in Health (Acheson 1998) established a broad public health agenda that was followed through with 'Saving Lives: Our Healthier Nation' (Department of Health [DoH] 1999a) and 'Tackling Health Inequalities: A Cross Cutting Review' (HM Treasury 2002). 'Making a Difference: Midwifery Action Plan' (DoH 1999b) and the 'National Service Framework for Children, Young People and Maternity Services (NSF)' (DoH 2004) placed midwifery care and the public health role of the midwife at the centre of the public health agenda. Acknowledging that by placing maternity care in a community context, and actively engaging with disadvantaged communities, both short- and long-term improvements could be made, even before birth.

As a result, the Sure Start programme and subsequent Sure Start Children's Centres were created as part of the drive to improve outcomes for children and families, encouraging multi-agency working (Roberts 2000). Its evaluation by the Institute for Fiscal Studies (IFS) in 2018 found the programme had averted 5,500 hospitalisations of under 11-year-olds every year with effect greatest in poorer areas compared to the wealthiest (Cattan et al 2019).

With the 2008 recession and a new 'age of austerity' with the coalition government then in power, substantial cuts to public funding followed, including Sure Start funding by two-thirds and removing its ringed fenced funding, closing over 500 Sure Start centres across the country in the process (Cattan et al 2019). The subsequent conservative government launched their 'The Five Year Forward View' placing greater emphasis on patient choice and empowerment to improved health outcomes (National Health Service [NHS] England 2014). 'Personal Maternity Care Budgets' were adopted into this policy, the ambition being for services to become more personalised, with choice offered at every opportunity and across Clinical Commissioning Groups (NHS England 2014).

Brexit saw further policy shifts towards addressing regional inequalities, coined as 'levelling up'. The COVID-19 pandemic further reshaped public health policies, as it disproportionately affected those from racially diverse communities and those living in areas of social deprivation (PHE 2020). The UK and Ireland Confidential Enquiries into Maternal Deaths and Morbidity (MBRRACE-UK) 2022 report also showed widening maternal and perinatal inequalities in racially diverse communities in comparison to those identifying as white, especially within the most deprived areas (Knight et al 2022).

As a result, public health now focused on the life course approach, in which wider determinants of health are addressed through both risk reduction and enhancements strategies (PHE 2019a). Political, financial, and population health instability have undoubtably been a major feature of the last five years and as such implementation of policy has been challenging. What remains constant throughout is the importance of midwifery in improving public health and reducing health inequalities.

Public health is concerned with increasing life and healthy life expectancy and reducing differences between communities through developments in health improvements, wider determinants of health, health protection and healthcare provision (Office for Health Improvements and Disparities 2023). This next section will focus on obesity (health improvements), racial and economic inequalities (wider determinants) and COVID-19 (health protection).

OBESITY

Obesity limits life and healthy life expectancy and impacts pregnancy and birth. Data estimates that 25.3% of adults aged 18 and over were living with obesity in November 2020 to November 2021, an increase from 22.7% in 2015 to 2016 (Sport England 2022). This trend is also reflected in women and birthing people who are becoming pregnant, with the data illustrating that 18% of women were obese at the time of booking for their first pregnancy, rising further in a subsequent pregnancy to 23% (PHE 2019b) It's important to note that the increase in obesity is taking place alongside a decrease in physical exercise and poor adherence to dietary guidelines.

Obesity is more common in certain geographical areas and, more specifically, among some communities. For example, the number of people who are obese is higher in the North of England and Scotland than the South of England. With those under 25 also been found more likely to be obese and smoke compared to those in the older generation (Office for Health Improvement and Disparities 2022, Office of National Statistics 2022).

However, geography and age are not the key determinants of obesity, but rather the wider determinants of health, including economic and social inequalities; with those who are in the lowest income quintiles more likely to be obese. Between 2020 and 2021, 36.8% of people living in the most deprived decile were obese compared to 19.2% of people living in the least deprived decile (Office for Health Improvement and Disparities 2022).

These statistics demonstrate that when it comes to health and healthy behaviours, there is inequality in those making healthy choices and in health outcomes, with those who are poorest and most vulnerable in our society at most risk of poor outcomes, poor health in old age, and dying earlier (Marmot 2010).

RACIAL DIVERSITY AND MATERNITY INEQUALITIES

Health disparities can also be seen between racially diverse groups, although the picture here is more mixed. Before the COVID-19 pandemic peoples from the White Gypsy or Irish Traveller, Bangladeshi, and Pakistani communities having the poorest health outcomes across a range of indicators (Raleigh 2023). COVID-19 had a disproportionate impact on most racially diverse communities, causing overall mortality rates to exceed that of the white population until 2022, where pre-pandemic patterns returned. Unpicking the causes of racial inequalities in health is undoubtably complex. Available evidence suggests a complex interplay of many factors including deprivation, environment, health-related behaviours and the 'healthy migrant effect' (PHE 2020) – see Chapter 5.

Health inequalities are apparent during pregnancy, birth, and the postnatal period. MBRRACE-UK (2018–2020) found a 24% rise in maternal deaths over a two-year period (19% increase excluding deaths attributed to COVID-19) (Knight et al 2022). Black women were found to be 3.7 times more likely to die and Asian women 1.8 times more likely to die during or up to one year after the end of pregnancy (Knight et al 2022). It is important to note that 11% of the women who died during this timeframe were at severe and multiple disadvantages. The main elements of disadvantage were mental health diagnoses, substance use or domestic abuse (Knight et al 2022).

Prior to COVID-19 stillbirth rates were declining with a total of 3.8 stillbirths per 1,000 births in 2020. However, following COVID-19, these rates are back up to 4.1 per 1,000 births (Draper et al 2022). With black and black British babies over twice as likely to be stillborn (6.41 per 1,000 total births) with Asian and Asian British babies over 50% more likely to be stillborn (4.97 per 1,000 total births) indicating little change since 2010 (Harmer & Abrahams 2023). Data for 2016–2020 showed an increase in perinatal mortality with increasing deprivation, with stillbirth rates ranging from 2.67 per 1,000 total births in the least deprived quintile to 4.69 per 1,000 total births in the most deprived quintile; and neonatal mortality rates ranging from 1.21 per 1,000 live births in the least deprived quintile to 2.12 per 1,000 live births in the most deprived quintile (Draper et al 2022). Therefore, the data concludes that health inequality is a key determinant of maternal and perinatal mortality.

THE IMPACT OF COVID-19

A principal driver of public health policy is the prevention of transmission of communicable diseases determined by national vaccination programmes. Most high-income countries experience relatively low morbidity and mortality from communicable diseases. However, COVID-19 led to millions dying or left with severe morbidity worldwide. In the UK, COVID-19 disproportionately affected racially diverse communities, those with pre-existing health conditions and those living in the most deprived areas of the UK (Raleigh 2023). Women in the most deprived areas were 133% more likely to die from COVID-19 than those in the wealthiest areas – 114% in men (Stafford & Deeny 2020). Between March and December 2020, nine maternal deaths were attributable to COVID-19, equating to about 15% of all maternal deaths during this time (Knight et al 2022). COVID-19 has highlighted the stark inequalities that currently exist in the UK, and the urgent need to strengthen action to prevent and manage ill health in deprived and racially diverse communities (Raleigh 2023).

ORGANISATION OF PUBLIC HEALTH IN THE UK

The organisation and delivery of health services in UK has devolved since 1999, and whilst there are structural differences between England and the devolved nations in the organisation and delivery of care (including public health), there are similarities. This section will first look at England and outline the major changes that have taken place since 2019 (the start of COVID-19 and the election of the Conservative government under Johnson) and then outline the main differences and similarities between England's organisation of public health and that of the devolved nations.

ENGLAND

The organisation and delivery of public health has been through substantial change since 2012. PHE established in 2012 with distinct organisational and operational autonomy to provide leadership for health protection, including emergency preparedness, and health improvement and was controversially abolished in 2020 during the early stages of the COVID-19 pandemic. The Office for Health Improvement and Disparities (OHID) replaced it and is directly accountable to the Secretary of State for Health and Social Care and the Chief Medical Officer (CMO) for England. OHID aims to identify and address health disparities, focusing on communities and areas where health inequalities have greatest effect and act on the biggest preventable risk factors for ill health and premature death including tobacco, obesity, and harmful use of alcohol and drugs. Whilst under the leadership of the Chief Public Health Nurse, OHID leads international and national public health advice on nursing, midwifery, and allied health professionals.

There have also been significant changes to the organisation and delivery local health services since 2019 with the Health and Social Care Act 2012 replaced with the Health Care Act 2022, which provides a legislative framework supporting multi-agency and local collaboration rather than provider competition and working to address the wider determinants of health and the disconnect between health and social care at a local level. The Act formalised the adoption of integrated care systems (ICSs), partnerships of NHS bodies and local authorities, working with other relevant local organisations to plan and deliver joined up health and care services (DoH and Social Care 2022a). Each ICS is formed of an integrated care board (ICB) and an integrated care partnership (ICP). ICBs overseeing the commissioning of most NHS services, accountable to NHS England. With ICPs bringing together collaborators, not just the NHS, to develop a plan to address the wider determinants of health (DoH and Social Care 2022a).

SCOTLAND, WALES, AND NORTHERN IRELAND

Scotland, Wales, and Northern Ireland have chosen not to introduce competition, or a market, within their health systems (as brought in in England by the 2012 Health and Social Care Act). In Northern Ireland, this is due to structural reasons, but for Scotland and Wales, this has been an ideological choice.

Scotland has undergone structural changes to the organisation of public health in response to the COVID-19 pandemic. Public Health Scotland was founded in April 2020 with the creation of a new leadership body, development of shared national public health priorities and a whole-system approach to public health. Public Health Scotland reports to the Office of the Chief Medical Officer (CMO) via the Scottish Government Health Protection Team, Public Health Division, Population Health Improvement Directorate and no longer sits within National Health Scotland (Public Health Scotland 2022).

Public Health Wales National Health Service Trust is a statutory body that came into existence in 2009 under the Public Health Wales National Health Service Trust (Establishment) Order. It provides strategic and specialist support for local health boards with the aim of improving health and wellbeing and reducing health inequalities for the people of Wales (Public Health Wales 2009). The Public Health Agency, also established in 2009, fulfils a similar function in Northern Ireland. Both Northern Ireland and Wales are due to set out their new public health strategies in 2023 which it is anticipated will focus on the integration of services and the reduction of health inequalities (Public Health Agency 2009).

PREVENTION AND INTEGRATION: OVERARCHING AIMS OF THE CHANGES TO THE ORGANISATION AND DELIVERY OF PUBLIC HEALTH

The changes to the organisation and delivery of public health across the UK have several aims. The first being to ensure effective oversight of national public health department and to ensure future pandemic preparedness. The second being to reduce health inequalities and address the wider determinants of health through better integration of services. In England, ICS and their respective ICB and ICPs co-ordinate and commission services. The partnership and delivery arms of the ICS, ICB, and ICPs are sub-divided into system level collaborative, place level structures including Health and Wellbeing Boards and neighbourhood primary care networks. At every level, integration of services, including NHS Trusts, local authorities, mental health services, voluntary sector organisations, Healthwatch and primary care services such as GPs and dental services, is mandated to establish more joined up health services that address public health needs more holistically (DoH and Social Care 2022a.)

Following the publication of The Best Start for Life: A Vision for the 1,001 Critical Days' report, the Start for Life programme that includes the commissioning of Family Hubs was established (Leadsom 2022). Aiming to provide families with the integrated support they need to care for their children from conception, throughout the early years, and into the start of adulthood. The 'Family Hubs' will incorporate multi-agency professionals such as midwives, health visitors, special educational needs co-ordinators (SENCO) to provide integrated care to families living in areas of social deprivation who are most at risk (Leadsom 2022).

Similarly, following the publication of the Women's Health Strategy in 2022, the government has announced funding for new Women's Hubs, to address fragmentation in care provision, better access to care for menstrual problems, contraception, pelvic pain, and menopause care and could also offer cervical screening (DoH & Social Care 2022b). However, until these integrated health hubs have undergone economic and health outcome evaluations, their effectiveness in terms of reducing health inequalities remains uncertain.

THE ROLE OF MIDWIFERY IN PUBLIC HEALTH

Public health policy for maternity services and midwives in England and Wales is no longer set out in a single document but rather is integrated across several key policy documents that include:

- Better Births (and Saving Babies Lives Care Bundle).
- CORE20 plus5- an approach to reducing healthcare inequalities.
- The best start for life: a vision for the 1,001 critical days
- The Healthy Child Schedule of Interventions Guide' sets out Community, Universal, Targeted and Specialist Interventions for healthcare professionals in the pre-conceptual period, during pregnancy and birth and up to eight weeks following birth.
- The Office for Health Improvements and Disparities (OHID) Public Health Outcomes Framework for Child and Maternal Health – Pregnancy and birth records and reports on factors related to conception, pregnancy, and delivery.

BETTER BIRTHS AND CORE20 PLUS 5

The NHS England's Better Births Strategy led to the development and implementation of midwifery-led continuity of care, defined as a way of delivering maternity care so that women receive dedicated support from the same midwifery team throughout their pregnancy, as the preferred model to achieve the ambition of more personalised care and its potential effects on public health (Cumberlege 2016). The Cochrane Review into 'Midwifery-led continuity models versus other models of care' found midwifery continuity models reduced pre-term birth and fetal loss before 24 weeks and was particularly effective in women living in areas of deprivation (Sandall et al 2016). The NHS Long Term Plan committed to 35% of women being placed on a continuity of carer pathway by March 2020, with similar approaches being taken in the devolved Nations. (NHS England 2019a).

In 2021, The National Healthcare Inequalities Improvement Programme (HiQiP) was set up to deliver quality healthcare for all, ensuring equitable access, excellent experience, and optimal outcomes. The implementation arm of HiQiP 'Core20 PLUS 5' (formed from the most deprived 20% of the national population as identified by the national Index of Multiple Deprivation (IMD) and PLUS groups such as racially diverse communities; people with a learning disability and autism) has identified five areas for improvement, the first being Maternity Care (NHS England 2021).

The impact of COVID-19 has meant that in England there is now no set target date for maternity services to deliver Midwifery Continuity of Carer until maternity services in England can demonstrate sufficient staff levels to be able deliver it (May et al 2022) and where safe staffing is in place, NHS England continues to encourage the rollout of midwifery continuity of carer, prioritising those from racially diverse and the most deprived communities (NHS England 2021). A recent Care Quality Commission (CQC) statistical release reported those who have given birth using this model were still more likely to report not seeing the same midwife, with only 37% of respondents seeing the same midwife for their antenatal care in 2022 down from 41% 2021, and 27% seeing the same midwife postnatally down from 30% in 2021 (CQC 2023). From a public health perspective, this scaling back has the potential to impact on perinatal morbidity and mortality. As a midwife it is important to recognise the challenges facing the workforce post-COVID-19 and it remains to be seen whether the momentum on implementing continuity of carer can be regained over the coming years.

SAVING BABIES LIVES CARE BUNDLE

The Saving Babies Care Bundle (SBLCB) is a key midwifery public health document providing evidence-based best practice for providers and commissioners of maternity care across England to reduce perinatal mortality (NHS England 2016, 2019b) with the aim to halve rates of perinatal mortality from 2010 to 2025 and have achieved a 20% reduction by 2020 (Harmer & Abrahams 2023).

It is made up of six elements and associated clinical guidance, process, and outcome measures (NHS England 2016, 2019b). For example, element 1 focuses on reducing smoking in pregnancy by implementing NHS-funded tobacco dependence treatment services within maternity settings, in line with the NHS Long Term Plan and NICE guidance. Evidence suggests that the risk of several poor pregnancy outcomes can be reduced to that of a non-smoker if a successful quit is achieved early in pregnancy (NHS England 2016, 2019b). Smoking like many other public health issues is influenced by the wider determinants of health including economic and social inequalities; with those who are in the lowest income quantiles more likely to smoke. Therefore, efforts to reduce smoking in pregnancy require not only a focus on pregnancy advice and support and but also on underlying determinants of ill health, which are of course more challenging to address and go beyond the scope of maternity care — see Chapter 12 – Smoking Cessation in Pregnancy.

THE BEST START FOR LIFE: A VISION FOR THE 1,001 CRITICAL DAYS'

The best start in life: a vision for the 1,001 critical days report identified the need to improve the health and development outcomes for babies in England, stating "the first 1,001 days from pregnancy to the age of two set the foundations for an individual's cognitive, emotional and physical development" (Leadsom 2022, p. 13) Whilst interventions and support for children and their carers' in the first 1,001 are in place here in the UK, service provision and access is variable. The report sets out six action areas to improve cognitive, emotional and physical development of children in the first days of their life (Leadsom 2022) (Table 2.1).

The most notable and important action areas for midwives is arguably implementation of 'Family Hubs' and 'The Start for Life' programme, aiming to reduce inequalities in health and education outcomes for babies, children and families across England by ensuring that support provided is communicated to all parents and carers, including those who are hardest to reach and or most in need of it (Leadsom 2022). Midwives, it is intended, will be an important feature of the Family Hub provision, with ICSs and ICBs overseeing the integration of midwives into these Hubs, whether these will be successfully adopted and whether midwives will be successfully integrated into the Hubs remains to be seen. Similarly, it is too soon to report on the impact of this policy change although critics would argue that it is a reinvention of the Sure Start programme which provides a blueprint for success.

Table 2.1 Six action areas

Ensuring families have access to the services they need.
1. Seamless support for families: a coherent joined up Start for Life offer available to all families.
2. A welcoming hub for families: Family Hubs as a place for families to access Start for Life services.
3. The information families need when they need it: designing digital, virtual and telephone offers around the needs of the family.
Ensuring the start for life system is working together to give families the support they need
4. An empowered Start for Life workforce: developing a modern skilled workforce to meet the changing needs of families.
5. Continually improving the Start for Life offer: improving data, evaluation, outcomes and proportionate inspection.
6. Leadership for change: ensuring local and national accountability and building the economic case.

Source: Leadsom (2022, p. 34).

SCHEDULES OF INTERVENTIONS FOR MIDWIVES

Midwifery is situated within the idea of a life course framework, as envisaged in the Marmot review (Marmot 2010). Within a life course framework, disadvantages and related health inequalities start before birth and continue to accumulate throughout life. In practice, the public health role of the midwife across is that the public health interventions should take place at four levels:

- Universal
- Targeted
- Specialist
- Community

The Healthy Pregnancy Pathway located on the e-learning for health website – see resources – provides guidance to midwives at each level of intervention in relation to:

1. Pre-conceptual care
2. Pregnancy and birth
3. Postnatal Care (up to 6–8 weeks post birth).

Whilst the Healthy Child Programme Schedule of Interventions Guide – see resources – covers interventions at the four levels from birth to six months. There are multiple public health issues including healthy weight, place of birth, tobacco use, perinatal mental health, screening, immunisations, safeguarding, and breast-feeding to name a few.

PUBLIC HEALTH OUTCOMES FRAMEWORK FOR MIDWIVES

The Public Health Outcomes Framework, healthy lives, healthy people: Improving outcomes and supporting transparency sets out a vision for public health, including desired outcomes and the indicators that help government and providers understand how well public health is being improved and protected (PHE 2019c). It concentrates on two high-level outcomes – healthy life expectancy and differences in life expectancy and healthy life expectancy between communities – to be achieved across the public health system. The outcomes focus not only on how long people live, but on how well they live at all stages of life. Maternal and child health are of course extremely important to achieving healthy life course and therefore a significant quantity of data in these areas is collected (PHE 2019b). In practice, much of the data from England and Wales is collected by midwives and inputted into the Maternity Services Data Set (NHS Digital 2023b) with Scotland and Northern Ireland collecting similar data in the Maternity and Neonatal Care Data Hub and Northern Ireland Maternity System. The importance of accurate data collection by midwives cannot be stressed enough, as it is this data that informs national public health policy as well as regional and community-based interventions (Table 2.2).

The role of the midwife in delivery of public health is far reaching. Midwives may be involved in the set up and delivery of continuity of care models and 'Family

Table 2.2 Examples of data collected

Percentage of deliveries to women from racially diverse groups	General fertility rate
Under 18s conception rate	Under 18s conceptions leading to abortion
Folic acid supplements before pregnancy	Early access to maternity care
Obesity in early pregnancy	Drinking in early pregnancy
Drug misuse in early pregnancy	Smoking in early pregnancy
Under 18 mothers	Smoking status at time of delivery
Caesarean section rate	Multiple births
Low birth weight of term babies	Low birth weight of all babies
Very low birth weight of all babies	Premature births (less than 37 weeks gestation)
Stillbirth rate	Neonatal mortality rate
Admissions of babies under 14 days	Infectious diseases in pregnancy screening
Sickle cell and thalassaemia screening	Healthy life expectancy at birth (male & female)
Life expectancy at birth (female & male)	Baby's first feed breastmilk
Breastfeeding prevalence at 6–8 weeks after birth – current method	Baby's first feed breastmilk (previous method)

Hubs'. Whilst all midwives will work towards achieving the six elements set out in the saving babies lives care bundle. Midwives are expected to deliver care using the four levels of interventions set out by the OHID and are required to accurately collect and input public health data via the maternity services data set that will inform national, regional, and local public health policy.

BARRIERS TO IMPLEMENTATION OF PUBLIC HEALTH POLICIES

The last five years has seen significant change in relation to public health policy and the organisation of public health services brought about by political instability and the emergence of COVID-19 as identified above.

A longitudinal analysis of patient experience has found that overall patient experience of services has decreased since COVID-19 and is now lower than pre-pandemic levels with important unwanted regional variation (CQC 2022). To improve health services and public health the ICSs requires good leadership (which takes time to bed-in) and a sufficiently sized workforce to meet the needs of patients, arguably one of the biggest challenges currently facing healthcare services particularly in Midwifery (CQC 2022). Local partnership working is required with neighbouring NHS Trusts working with each other, with primary care and social care as well as charities to improve the experiences and outcomes of their local population (DoH and Social Care 2022a). How this works and what mitigating risks need to considered is still being understood examples of good practice exists such as moving staff where there is most need but is limited (CQC 2022).

To improve population health, ICSs need to be able to respond to local issues and not just implement wider health strategies. The CQC highlight Maternity Voices Partnerships (MVP) as potentially innovative solutions to delivering locally adapted health services. For example, some MVPs have recently focused on improving care for racially diverse communities in their area and appointing cultural diversity champions for their local area (CQC 2022).

Responsibility for the 'Family Hubs' which will involve significant transformation and systems change, requiring collaboration and commitment from across the children's early help system and the local community, lies with the ICSs (Leadsom 2022). ICSs are currently in the process of creating collaborative partnerships to harness commitment to a shared approach and outcomes, as well as co-produce a strategy to deliver 'Family Hubs'. There may be barriers to implementing this in terms of integrating midwives employed by NHS Foundation Trusts into 'Family Hubs' and the current midwifery workforce shortages (Royal College of Midwives 2022).

The success of ICSs and ICBs will undoubtably impact maternal public health as issues such as improvements in smoking in pregnancy, diabetes, infant feeding, and perinatal mental health require strategies and integrated care pathways at all levels of service provision encompassing a range of healthcare care needs. As such the barriers to successful implementation of ICSs are relevant to midwifery.

SUMMARY

- A life course approach to public health acknowledges a person's physical and mental health and wellbeing are influenced throughout life by the wider determinants of health.
- Midwives are uniquely placed to improve the health of women and their families by delivering strategies that both minimise risk factors and enhance protective factors.
- Family Hubs and Women's Hubs are an important strategic change to the delivery of integrated services with midwives playing an important role in their delivery.
- Implementing continuity of care models for pregnant women in the 'Core20 PLUS 5' group is a national midwifery priority.
- Implementing Saving Babies Lives Care Bundle and the Healthy Pregnancy and Health Child policies are also a maternity priority.

REFERENCES

Acheson, D. (1998). *Independent Inquiry into Inequalities in Health*. London: The Stationary Office.

Cattan, S., Conti, G., Farquharson, C., & Ginja, R. (2019). *The Health Effects of Sure Start*. London: IFS.

CQC. (2022). Systems: challenges and opportunities. Systems: challenges and opportunities – Care Quality Commission. State of Care 2021/22 - Care Quality Commission (cqc.org.uk)

CQC. (2023). *Maternity Survey 2022*. London: Care Quality Commission. Retrieved from https://www.cqc.org.uk/publication/surveys/maternity-survey-2022

Cumberlege, J. (2016). *Better Births: Improving Outcomes of Maternity Services in England. A Five Year Forward View for Maternity Care.* Retrieved from https://www.england.nhs.uk/publication/better-births-improving-outcomes-of-maternity-services-in-england-a-five-year-forward-view-for-maternity-care/

DoH. (1999a). *Saving Lives: Our Healthier Nation.* London: The Stationary Office.

DoH. (1999b). *Making a Difference: Strengthening the Nursing, Midwifery and Health Visiting Contribution to Health and Healthcare.* London: The Stationary Office.

DoH. (2004). *National Service Framework: Children, Young People, and Maternity Services.* London: The London Stationary Office.

DoH and Social Care. (2022a). Health and Care Act. https://www.legislation.gov.uk/ukpga/2022/31/contents/enacted

DoH and Social Care. (2022b). *Women's Health Strategy for England.* https://www.gov.uk/government/publications/womens-health-strategy-for-england/womens-health-strategy-for-england#ministerial-foreword

Draper, E., Gallimore, I.D., Smith, L.K., Matthews, R.J., Fenton, A.C., Kurinczuk, J.J., Smith, P.W., & Manktelow, B.N. (Eds.). (2022). *MBRRACE-UK Perinatal Mortality Surveillance Report. UK Perinatal Deaths for Births from January to December 2020.* Leicester: The Infant Mortality and Morbidity Studies, Department of Health Sciences, University of Leicester. Retrieved from https://www.npeu.ox.ac.uk/assets/downloads/mbrrace-uk/reports/perinatal-surveillance-report-2020/MBRRACE-UK_Perinatal_Surveillance_Report_2020.pdf

Harmer, C., & Abrahams, K. (2023). Saving babies lives 2023 a report on progress. JPU_Saving_Babies_Lives_Report_2023.pdf (sands.org.uk)

HM Treasury. (2002). *Tackling Health Inequalities: Summary of 2002 Cross-Cutting Review.* London: Department of Health.

HM Treasury. (2004). *Securing Good Health for the Whole Population.* London: Treasury Office.

Knight, M., Bunch, K., Patel, R., Shakespeare, J., Kotnis, R., Kenyon, S., & Kurinczuk, J. (Eds.). (2022). *Saving Lives, Improving Mothers' Care Core report: Lessons Learned to Inform Maternity Care from the UK and Ireland Confidential Enquiries into Maternal Deaths and Morbidity 2018–20.* Oxford National Perinatal Epidemiology Unit. MBRRACE-UK. MBRRACE-UK_Maternal_MAIN_Report_2022_UPDATE.pdf (ox.ac.uk)

Leadsom, A. (2022). *Family Hubs and The Best Start for Life Programme Guide.* London: HM Government.

Marmot, M. (2010). *Fair Society, Healthy Lives: The Marmot Review.* A Strategic Review of Health Inequalities in England. London. GOV.UK (www.gov.uk)

May, R., Dunkley-Bent, J., & Jolly, M. (2022). *B2011-Midwifery-Continuity-of-Carer-letter-210922.* London: National Health Service England. Retrieved from https://www.england.nhs.uk/publication/midwifery-continuity-of-carer/

National Health Service Digital. (2023a). Saving Babies' Lives: Version 3. A Care Bundle for Reducing Perinatal Mortality. PRN00614-Saving-babies-lives-version-three-a-care-bundle-for-reducing-perinatal-mortality.pdf (england.nhs.uk)

National Health Service Digital. (2023b). About the Maternity Services Data Set. https://digital.nhs.uk/data-and-information/data-collections-and-data-sets/data-sets/maternity-services-data-set/about-the-maternity-services-data-set

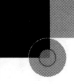
National Health Service England. (2014). *Five Year Forward View*. London: NHS (england.nhs.uk)

National Health Service England. (2016). *Saving Babies' Lives. A Care Bundle for Reducing Stillbirth*. London: NHS. saving-babies-lives-car-bundl.pdf (england.nhs.uk)

National Health Service England. (2019a). *NHS Long Term Plan*. London: NHS.

National Health Service England. (2019b). *Saving Babies' Lives Version Two. A Care Bundle for Reducing Perinatal Mortality*. London: National Health Service England. Saving-Babies-Lives-Care-Bundle-Version-Two-Updated-Final-Version.pdf (england.nhs.uk)

National Health Service England. (2021). *Core20PLUS5 (adults) – An Approach to Reducing Healthcare Inequalities*. London: NHS England

Office for Health Improvement and Disparities. (2022). *Obesity Profile: Short Statistical Commentary July 2022*. London: Department of Health and Social Care. Retrieved from https://www.gov.uk/government/statistics/obesity-profile-update-july-2022/obesity-profile-short-statistical-commentary-july-2022

Office for Health Improvement and Disparities. (2023). The Public Health Outcomes Framework. https://fingertips.phe.org.uk/profile/public-health-outcomes-framework

Office of National Statistics. (2022). *Adult Smoking Habits in the UK: 2021 Data and Analysis from the Census 2021*. London: Office for National Statistics. Retrieved from https://www.ons.gov.uk/peoplepopulationandcommunity/healthand socialcare/healthandlifeexpectancies/bulletins/adultsmokinghabitsingreatbritain/2021#:~:text=1.-,Main%20points,Annual%20Population%20Survey%20(APS)

Public Health Agency. (2009). The Regional Agency for Public Health and Social Well-being (Membership) Regulations (Northern Ireland) 2009 (legislation. gov.uk) The Regional Agency for Public Health and Social Well-being (Membership) Regulations (Northern Ireland) 2009 (legislation.gov.uk)

Public Health England. (2019a). *Health Matters: Prevention – Life Course Approach*. Retrieved from https://www.gov.uk/government/publications/health-matters-life-course-approach-to-prevention/health-matters-prevention-a-life-course-approach

Public Health England. (2019b). *Health of Women Before and During Pregnancy: Health Behaviours, Risk Factors and Inequalities*. An updated analysis of the maternity services dataset antenatal booking data. London: PHS (Crown Copyright). Retrieved from https://assets.publishing.service.gov.uk/government/uploads/system/uploads/attachment_data/file/844210/Health_of_women_before_and_during_pregnancy_2019.pdf

Public Health England. (2019c). *Public Health Outcomes Framework 2019/2020: A Consultation*. London: Public Health England (publishing.service.gov.uk).

Public Health England. (2020). *Disparities in the Risk and Outcomes of COVID-19*. London: PHE.

Public Health Scotland. (2022). *A Scotland Where Everybody Thrives: Public Health Scotland's Strategic Plan 2022 to 2025*. A Scotland where everybody thrives: Public Health Scotland's strategic plan 2022 to 2025- Our Organisation – Public Health Scotland.

Public Health Wales. (2009). *Public Health Wales Standing Orders and Reservation and Delegation of Powers*. Wales: NHS.

Raleigh, V. (2023). *The Health of People from Ethnic Minority Groups in England.* https://www.kingsfund.org.uk/publications/health-people-ethnic-minority-groups-england#footnote2_o6228ad

Roberts, H. (2000). What is sure start? *Archives of Disease in Childhood*, 82(6), 435–437. https://doi.org/10.1136/adc.82.6.435

Royal College of Midwives. (2022). NHS Staff Survey 2022. 2022-nhs-staff-survey. pdf (rcm.org.uk)

Sandall, J., Soltani, H., Gates, S., Shennan, A., & Devane, D. (2016). Midwife-led continuity models versus other models of care for childbearing women. *Cochrane Database of Systematic Reviews*, 2016(4), CD004667. https://doi.org/10.1002/14651858.CD004667.pub5

Sport England. (2022). Active lives survey November 2020–21 report. https://www.sportengland.org/research-and-data/data/active-lives

Stafford, M., & Deeny, S. (2020). *Inequalities and Deaths Involving COVID-19. What the Links Between Inequalities Tell Us.* https://www.health.org.uk/news-and-comment/blogs/inequalities-and-deaths-involving-covid-19

RESOURCES FOR BOOK WEBSITE

The Healthy Pregnancy Pathway located on the e-learning for health website. https://e-lfh.org.uk/healthy-pregnancy-pathway/index.html, provides guidance to midwives at each level of intervention in relation to:

The Healthy Child Programme Schedule of Interventions Guide. https://www.e-lfh.org.uk/pathways-healthy-child/birth-to-6-months/community.html

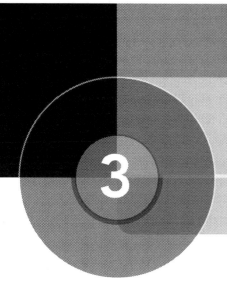

Health Promotion: The Core Role of the Midwife

SAM BASSETT

INTRODUCTION

Midwives are by the very nature of their profession promoters of health and clearly identified as a central part of the International Confederation of Midwives (ICM) definition of the midwife.

> Midwifery is an approach to care of women and their newborn infants whereby midwives promote women's personal capabilities to care for themselves and their families.

(ICM, 2017, p. 1)

As well as featuring strongly in the Nursing & Midwifery Council (NMC) Standards of proficiency for midwives.

> They (Midwives) provide health education, health promotion and health protection to promote psychological and physical health and well-being and prevent complications. Evidence shows the positive contribution midwives make to the short- and long-term health and well-being of women, newborn infants, and families.

(NMC, 2019, p. 4)

Whilst individuals are likely to see a nurse only whilst unwell for a short period of time, midwives have the potential for a much more holistic role. Midwives have regular contact with women, and their families often for an extended period of time. Offering a unique opportunity to promote the health and wellbeing of women,

DOI: 10.4324/9781003350071-3

birthing people, and their families with the potential to make noticeable sustained positive changes (Chief Nursing Officer (CNO), 2010). One that can be enhanced even further when relationships are allowed to flourish through continuity of carer (Clayton et al., 2022).

Therefore, health promotion is not just an extended role of the midwife but considered a core skill. Using relevant evidence, this chapter will now look at the concepts and influences of health, health needs assessment (HNA) of health promotion and the role the midwife plays in the delivery of health promotion.

BACKGROUND

Throughout history, the concept of health has been valued, attributed in many cases to wealth. Mahatma Ghandhi validated this in 1948 when he was quoted as saying, "It is health that is the real worth and not pieces of gold and silver" (Gandhi, 1948). Alluding to the fact that Society cannot prosper unless its people are healthy. Historically, though the determinants of health were poorly understood with the main public health tool available for many years being the use of quarantine to prevent the spread of disease. Great advances in public health were not really seen until the 19th century when Edwin Chadwick and Thomas Southwood Smith, pioneers of modern public health, acknowledged that public health was more than just preventing the spread of disease, but rather a way to make life better for all. Alongside other innovators of the time, they advocated that for the poor to be able to thrive they needed better living conditions (Moorhead, 2002).

As a result, public health became more recognised as a way of improving health with many parliamentary acts following. For example, in the UK, the goal of the Clean Air Act published originally by the UK government in 1956 and amended in 1968 and 1993 was to reduce the number of pollutants in the air that we breathe and improve health. Today, COVID-19 pandemic excluded, it is recognised that most major health problems come less from infectious diseases and more from chronic diseases or what are known as noncommunicable diseases (NCDs). Often a result of a combination of genetic, physiological, environmental, and behavioural factors, the main types of NCDs are cardiovascular disease (such as heart attacks or stroke), cancers, chronic respiratory diseases (such as asthma) and diabetes. In total they are responsible for around 74% (41 million) of all deaths globally with 77% (31.4 million) of these occurring in low- and middle-income countries (WHO, 2023a).

WHAT IS HEALTH?

The word *health* is derived from an old English word *hale* meaning 'wholeness, being whole or sound' (Oleribe et al., 2018). As a result, many definitions have focused on health being the body's ability to carry out its biological functions with any disruption viewed as a disease.

Historically in the Western world, we have been most familiar with the 'medical model', with health defined as the absence of pathology. This embraces the Cartesian view attributed to the philosopher Descartes in the 17th century, with the belief that mind and body are essentially separate entities. Viewing the body as a lifeless machine with the assumption that ill health has a pathology, in which the 'machine' needs to be repaired or fixed by the healthcare professional (Keller, 2020).

However, today our understanding has changed significantly, reflected by Merleau-Ponty a 20th century phenomenological philosopher, who first presented the notion of the 'lived body'. With the belief that the body is not an object, but "a multiphasic, experiential being of finite freedom" (Gold, 1985, p. 664). This approach places the emotional and psychosocial needs of an individual as just as important as their pathology, diagnosis, assessment and treatment. With healthcare professionals needing to acknowledge patients as unique individuals with their own inherent needs (Keller, 2020).

This so-called lay concept perspective of health is characterised by three main qualities: wholeness, pragmatism and individualism (Svalastog et al., 2017). With wholeness viewing health as a holistic phenomenon, being woven with all other aspects of an individual's life – everyday, working, family, and community. Pragmatism reflecting health as a relative phenomenon. Where health is experienced and evaluated according to what individuals find reasonable to accept given their age, medical conditions, and social situation. For example, older people may see health and social networks as more important than economic resources (Hill et al., 2007). Whereas, young people may see health as being fit and strong with a subsequent reluctance to access health care for fear of potentially being unable to work as a result (Hagell, 2015). Finally, individualism relates to health being a highly personal phenomenon, with health being highly influenced by perception. Whilst being part of a society and feeling close to other people appears important to all, values are very individualised with every human being unique with the strategies for improving their health needing to fully reflecting this.

The WHO definition of health, "health is a complete state of physical, mental and social well-being and not merely the absence of disease or infirmity" (WHO, 1946, p. 2), may be seen to incorporate all the concepts above, but there are many arguments against this definition, mainly around the ambiguity of the terms used, for example, what is meant by 'wellbeing' or how do you measure 'complete' physical, mental and social well-being?

REFLECTION

- Consider your own concept(s) of health by thinking about someone you consider 'healthy' and someone else you consider not healthy.
- Why do you put them in the category you have put them in?
- How do your thoughts fit into the concepts above?

PRACTICE POINTS

- Health can mean different things to different people and these views can change over a lifetime.
- When discussing health issues with women and their families, listen to how they perceive their health and use this to present a health message they may comprehend and accept.

PREGNANCY AND HEALTH

The definition of health given to us by the WHO can also be seen as a challenge for women during the childbirth continuum as they go through a period of physical, sexual, emotional, mental, spiritual, and social change. For example, the pregnant woman enduring nausea and vomiting, or a newly delivered woman experiencing perineal stitches, might view their health as anything but 'healthy' or ever class themselves in a 'complete state of well-being'! It also challenges the health professional versus lay person's views of health with midwives perhaps viewing all the above as a physiological process commonplace in pregnancy and childbirth. Conversely, if a midwife adopts a traditionally medicalised viewpoint where nothing is viewed as 'normal except in retrospect', this could also be at odds to a mother that embraces pregnancy and motherhood as healthy (Crafter, 1997). To combat this, the WHO adapts its definition, stating maternal health applies to the health of women during pregnancy, childbirth, and the postnatal period with each stage being a positive experience, ensuring women and their babies reach their 'potential' for health and wellbeing (WHO, 2023b).

In 2010, Midwifery 2020 was published recommending that midwives be the lead professional for all healthy women with straightforward pregnancies (for women with more complex needs the midwife will be the key coordinator of care within the multidisciplinary team) (CNO, 2010) reiterated further in 'Better Births' in 2016 (NHS England, 2016). However, this recognition comes with challenges as the demographics of childbearing women has changed dramatically over the last few decades in the UK with increasing age of mothers, medical and social complexities, mental health issues, and ethnicity to name but a few. Complicating matters these disadvantages have been highlighted to often be multiple for women increasing their overall risk of both morbidity and mortality even further (Knight et al., 2020; 2023). As a result, uncertainty is now a core aspect of the Midwife's role as they provide care across the spectrum of women no matter the context. The only constant being providing supportive, facultative care, including health promotion, seeking medical support as and when appropriate (Bowden, 2006).

Evidence has shown that optimal health no matter the context before a woman conceives and whilst she is pregnant improves outcomes for both mother and baby, with the benefits continuing well beyond birth (Korenbrot et al., 2002). However, we know inequalities in maternal and infant outcomes exist, with poorer outcomes experienced in certain groups. Therefore, understanding any potential patterns in health before and during pregnancy could be vital if we are to narrow the health gap for those most vulnerable. As such, since 2017, the Maternity Services Datasets (MSDS) in England has been collecting national data on adaptable healthy behaviours such as smoking, Folic acid, maternal body mass index (dietary), alcohol, and substance misuse. In addition, due to the importance of an early opportunity to discuss the best way to ensure a healthy pregnancy – antenatal booking within ten weeks of pregnancy (PHE, 2019). The dataset has evolved over the years adapting to collect prevalent data to maternity services. However, constant to this has been the aim to improve clinical care and health promotion with specific monthly datasets specific to relevant NHS Trusts being freely accessible to all via the intranet.

- Midwives care for women with no health issues to women with severe health issues.
- Providing holistic health promotion is an essential part of the role of the midwife whatever the circumstances.

WHAT IS HEALTH PROMOTION?

- What does the term health promotion mean to you?
- Write your own definition before you look at the WHO and other definitions given below.

The term 'health promotion' was first coined in 1945 by Henry E Sigerist, a renowned medical historian, who defined medicine as having four main remits: promotion of health, prevention of illness, restoration of the sick and rehabilitation (Kumar & Preetha, 2012). The WHO further define it as the process of enabling people to increase control over, and to improve, their health (WHO, 1986).

Fundamentals for health include peace, shelter, education, food, income, a stable ecosystem, sustainable resources, social justice, and equity (see Figure 3.1). Therefore, health promotion is not just the responsibility of a health service but has a far wider reach including international organisations, national governments, and local communities. All of which need to enable individuals to exert control over these determinants of health to achieve not only healthy lifestyles but also wellbeing.

Due to growing worldwide expectation that health could and should be improved for everyone the first international conference on Health Promotion was held in Ottawa in 1986. Comprising a variety of stakeholders including international

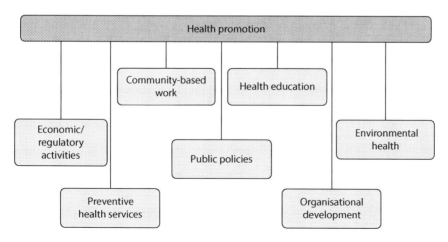

Figure 3.1 Activities encompassed within health promotion.

Source: Adapted from Manning (2017, p. 22).

organisations, national government, and local communities, the aim of 'Health for all' by the year 2000 was developed. To achieve this, the Ottawa charter was established comprising of three health promotion strategies: advocate (to boost the factors which encourage health), enable (allowing all people to achieve health equity) and mediate (through collaboration across all stakeholders). With five key actions: build healthy public policy, create supportive environments for health, strengthen community action for health, develop personal skills and re-orient health services (WHO, 1986).

This commitment to health promotion has continued with the development of the eight Millennium Development Goals (MDGs), a project inaugurated by the United Nations (UN) at the 2000 Millennium summit and endorsed by member states. Arguably representing the largest and most cohesive global collaboration to tackle poverty, education, gender equality, child survival, maternal health, combating disease and environmental sustainability ever launched. However, despite ambitious scale the MDGs soon faced criticism in their failure to reach the intended outcomes and unintended consequences such as the diversion of funds away from locally determined goals and initiatives (Fehling et al., 2013). As a result, in September 2015, the UN adopted the Sustainable Development Goals (SDGs) which lay the foundation for supporting global health and international development work for the next 15 years. Goal 3 explicitly stating, "Ensure healthy lives and promote wellbeing for all at all ages" (UN, 2015). Importantly, the SDGs also challenges health promoters to consider how they can work towards, and advocate for, approaches that are empowering, participatory, and salutogenic in orientation (Spencer et al., 2019).

ACTIVITY

- List some of the health promotion activities you do in your practice.

INFLUENCES OF HEALTH

When considering health, it is imperative to explore and understand what influences health, as there are both positive and negative factors often interwoven as illustrated in Figure 3.2.

In 2005, the WHO set up a commission to explore the causes and consequences of social and economic disadvantages on health. The final report was 'Closing the Gap in a Generation: health equality through action on the social determinants of Health' (WHO, 2008). The report clearly identified that the social condition into which people are born, live, and work is the single most important determinants of good or ill health. For example, children around the world face vastly different chances of survival depending on where they are born with the African region being the highest at 72 deaths per 1,000 live births compared to the European region of 7–8 deaths per 1,000 (WHO, 2023c).

Whilst it may be easy to assume then that health inequalities don't apply in a country such as England, the Marmot report in 2010 'Fair Society Healthy Lives' reported "that health inequalities causing people to die prematurely equated to

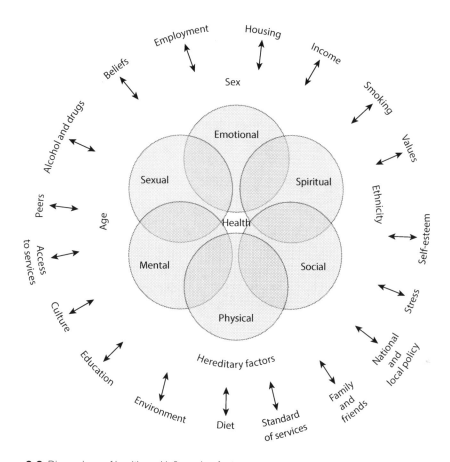

Figure 3.2 Dimensions of health and influencing factors.

Source: Adapted from Manning (2017, p. 23).

between 1.3 and 2.5 million extra years of life lost" (SRHIE, 2010, p. 9). In conclusion, recommending action across all the social determinants of health including:

- Good employment
- Higher educational attainment
- Safe, supported, and connected communities
- Poor housing and homelessness
- Living on a low income
- Social isolation, exclusion, and loneliness
- Stigma and discrimination

However, social and environmental elements are not the only determinants of health; age, sex, new and re-emerging diseases, mental health issues, and NCDs all require urgent responses as well (Kumar & Preetha, 2012). "The truth is that healthcare has a relatively limited impact on our health. The environment around us, our genetic inheritance, how we live our lives and the opportunities we have together largely determine our health" (PHE, 2014, p. 6). Whilst you may feel that midwives have little impact on the determinants of health, the fact remains that they can, and they do (McNeill et al., 2012). Pregnancy can motivate women to improve their health and as result they can be highly receptive to healthy lifestyle choices. Midwives are key in providing such information, and as such through meaningful conversation it is important that every contact counts. The role women play in the early years of their child's life from conception to the age of two is pivotal as illustrated in the report 'The Best Start for Health: A Vision for the 1,001 Critical Days' (DHSC, 2021). It is also important to note that the midwife's role in promoting the health and wellbeing can be far reaching as not only does this encompass women and their babies but it has the potential to influence partners, families, and friends and therefore Society as a whole.

PRACTICE POINT

- Although midwives cannot influence a person's genes or age, they can influence the beginning of a person's life by supporting the mother to be as healthy as she can be during pregnancy and beyond.

MIDWIVES AND HEALTH PROMOTION

Midwives constantly undertake health promotion but do not always recognise it as such. Key public health themes are set out in the RCM report 'Stepping Up to Public Health' including infant feeding; smoking cessation; screening; mental health/psychological wellbeing; obesity prevention; contraception and sexual health; sudden infant death (SID) prevention/safe sleeping; immunisations; infection/sepsis protection; pelvic floor exercises; intrapartum public health (skin to skin contact and delayed cord clamping); and general healthy lifestyle (RCM, 2017). The report also explores the barriers and facilitators to midwives providing this information with recognition that topics such as female genital mutilation (FGM), bereavement, drug and substance misuse, domestic violence, homelessness, honour-based violence, and forced marriage being discussed less often.

The theory of salutogenesis offers midwives a potential approach for public health promotion. Developed by the medical sociologist Aaron Antonovsky (1996), the theory focuses on factors that can support women to move towards greater health and well-being regardless of the objective presence of illness or disease. Proposing that the health of an individual is forever on a continuum fluctuating from good to poor. Integral to this are what Antonovsky defines as internal (attitudes and beliefs) and external (finances, family) generalised resistance resources (GRRs), which act as buffering or mediating mechanisms. For example, when resources are available and utilised positively experiences that cause tension can in fact be health-promoting. Conversely if resources are not available and/or used effectively this tension could lead to stress and poor health (Mathias et al., 2021).

The ability of an individual to use their GRRs and move towards health is termed by Antonovsky as a sense of coherence (SOC) explaining how they view the associated stressors of their life as comprehensible, manageable, and meaningful (Antonovsky, 1996). Comprehensibility referring to the level to which an individual organises their world to bring understanding, order, and structure. Manageability relating to an individual's belief that the resources needed are effortlessly found and straightforwardly accessible. Meaningfulness reflecting an individual's motivation to cope with the stressor and see the challenge as worthy of overcoming (Becker et al., 2010). Hence, an individual with a strong SOC has the ability to draw on a wide range of successful coping mechanisms from the GRRs available to them to deal with stressors positively and move towards health.

Therefore, a more positive approach to health promotion is for midwives to ask the question, 'How can I facilitate this person in moving towards better health?'. For example, how can I support a vulnerable woman to identify the positive factors that help maintain her balance between health and poor health continuum, as suggested by Antonovsky (1996). The identification of these positive factors can then support women to build on these and regain balance. Using the key salutogenic concepts of comprehensibility, manageability, and meaningfulness, Mathias et al. (2021) explored the salutogenic qualities of midwifery care using a best-fit framework synthesis proposing the following: Comprehensibility (cognitive aspects of health): being ways that midwives help women increase preparation and predictability during the childbirth continuum in providing a predictable caregiver, a predictable system and preparation for an unpredictable experience. Manageability (behavioural aspects of health): ways that midwives can enhance and support a woman's internal resilience by adding extra support when needed, and strengthening external resources through connections to family, community, and specialist care. Meaningfulness (emotional/spiritual aspects of health): ways that midwives encourage the commitment and engagement of childbearing women by providing care through a personalised relationship, by cultivating a woman's autonomy (Mathias et al., 2021, p. 266).

The importance of the midwife's role in public health across the childbirth continuum is further clearly illustrated in McNeill et al. (2012) logic model framework developed from 36 systematic reviews of public health interventions in midwifery (Figure 3.3). This framework being read left to right clearly displays relationships between the core elements of context, inputs, outputs and outcomes.

However, there are ever-changing and ever-growing demands on midwives as the evidence of their vital role in providing high-quality maternal and newborn care grows only further (Renfrew et al., 2014; Sandall et al., 2016; Renfrew, 2020). Perhaps then the more pressing hour of the moment is that midwives are provided with the requisite training, skills, and time to undertake health promotion in a way that is both meaningful and sustainable.

PRACTICE POINT

- Midwives have a window of opportunity to influence pregnant women about positive health choices.
- Make every contact count by giving bite sized pieces of information.
- Keep thinking about how to move women towards optimal health.

NEEDS IN HEALTH PROMOTION

The first element of any health promotion intervention is to establish what the needs actually are. Bradshaw taxonomy of need (1972) defines four types of needs:

1. Normative need: a desirable/expected standard specified by the professional, often in the form of a policy or recommendation.

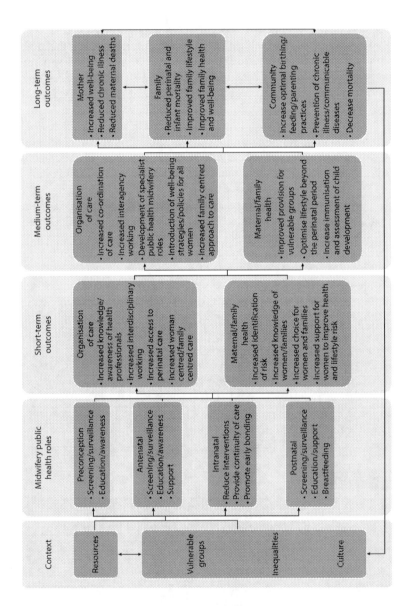

Figure 3.3 The logic model.

Source: From McNeill et al. (2012).

2. Felt need: what people actually want. This may eventually become an expressed need.
3. Expressed need: that is, the service requested/demanded by an individual, group or community.
4. Comparative need: occurs where the recipients of a service are compared with assess gaps and inequality in service provision. The need is to bring about equality and fairness.

An HNA is a systematic approach to understanding the needs of a community. A recommended public health tool it can provide health care professionals and other organisations evidence to address health issues and social inequalities (PHE, 2021). Using available epidemiology and demographic data, it considers social, economic, cultural, and behavioural factors that influence health, often then influencing local commissioning decisions (Mooney et al., 2011; Cross & Woodall, 2023).

However, HNA can be considered a top-down approach – meaning it is in the control of the professional providing the service, the managers, or commissioners of the local services (normative needs), or that of national organisations governments (corporate needs). As such, they may interpret a health need very differently to the profiled population of that area (felt or expressed needs). As a result, a bottom-up approach with service use involvement in HNA from the outset using a shared language is undoubtably key to ensuring maximum benefits which include:

- Strengthening community involvement in decision making
- Improved public patient participation.
- Improved team and partnership working
- Professional development of skills and experience
- Improved patient care
- Improved communication with other agencies and the public
- Better use of resources.

(Cavanagh & Chadwick, 2005)

PRACTICE POINT

- There are tensions to HNA. Who is doing the assessment?
- Their view of health such as biomedical or social models all play a part in the assessment.
- Being aware of these issues can support better evaluation of the health needs of an individual or group or area.

ACTIVITY

Think of a health need you have seen implemented in your practice area.

- Who identified the need for this intervention?
- How was the HNA undertaken?
- Do you think different needs might have been identified if another agency had been involved in the HNA?

Public health England (PHE) was established in 2012 with the aim of providing leadership for health protection, including emergency preparedness and health improvement. However, following criticism of the handling of the early stages of the COVID-19 pandemic, it was suddenly and unexpectantly abolished in August 2020 (Calvert & Arbuthnott, 2021). Eventually being replaced by two new bodies the UK Health Security Agency [UKHSA]) and the Office for Health Improvement and Disparities [OHID]) (Hunter et al., 2022). UKHSA taking on the role of health security regarding pandemic preparedness and external threats across the UK and OHID the role of wider public health, including health improvement and population health. Building on the work of PHE, OHID's priorities include tackling obesity, improving mental health, promoting physical activity, and addressing other population health issues (e.g. inequalities arising from obesity, smoking, mental health, and alcohol misuse).

To provide Local Maternity Services (LMS's) with the latest evidence, guidance, resources, and local practice examples in regard to six high priorities known to affect maternal and child outcomes in England, six maternity high-impact area documents were developed by PHE between 2019 and 2020.

- Improving planning and preparation for pregnancy
- Supporting parental mental health
- Supporting healthy weight before and between pregnancy
- Reducing the incidence of harms caused by alcohol in pregnancy
- Supporting parents to have a smokefree pregnancy
- Reducing the inequality of outcomes for women from Black, Asian, and Minority Ethnic (BAME) communities and their babies

Contributing to the strategic ambitions of NHS Universal Personalised Care Model (NHS England, 2019) and the modernisation of the Healthy Child Programme, these high impact areas also align with 'The Marmot Review ten years on' need for approaches to tackle health inequalities (Marmot et al., 2020). These documents now sit within the broader 'All our Health: personalised care and population health' framework (OHID, 2023) that brings together resources and evidence to help support evidence-based practice and service delivery building on the skills that healthcare professionals and other have to support women and 'Making Every Contact Count' (MECC) (NHS England, 2024).

Nonetheless needs are like health, as in the whole is more than the sum of their parts. There is an element of subjectivity with what the needs might be and what the goals are. A formula to present needs might be:

'A' needs 'X' in order to 'G', for example, 'A' = a woman who wants to breastfeed, needs 'X' = breastfeeding support, in order to 'G' = breastfeed successfully.

(Cross & Woodall, 2023)

Whilst this formula may appear too simplistic, whenever a health promotion activity is developed, it starts with a HNA NOT and HNA and identification of the need. However, identification of a need can be challenging. Where is the need coming from, a pressure group or your manager? If several needs are identified, whose need should be met first? There are many pitfalls with needs identification and seeking support, and clarification is an essential part of beginning the road to creating an intervention. The success and longevity of health promotion interventions depend on the identification of a genuine health need. On the contrary, it may fail if the identified health need is not deemed important by those it is intended for.

PRACTICE POINT

- The identification of health needs is an essential part of setting up a health promotion intervention.
- One must seek support and clarification at every step to ensure that the need identified is one that is considered equally important by the service users as well as the service providers.

SUMMARY OF KEY POINTS

- Health promotion is part of their role with midwives undertaking a lot of activities they do not always recognise as health promotion; vaccinations, screening programmes, breastfeeding support, discussing diet or alcohol use during pregnancy are just a few examples.
- Health has many different meanings and how someone defines health can change over their lifetime.
- Health is affected by different aspects such as where you live, what you eat, your genetic code, your gender, etc. Midwives can use this information to target health messages.
- The identification of needs is an essential part of a successful health promotion intervention. It can be affected by who is identifying the need and by the HNA which may not always acknowledge the social and environmental issues pertinent to that specific area.
- Midwives undertake a large amount of health promotion. Salutogenesis may provide a model to support midwives in this task.

REFERENCES

Antonovsky, A. (1996). The salutogenic model as a theory to guide health promotion. *Health Promotion International, 11(1),* 11–18. Available at https://www.salutogenesi.org/images/PDF/The_salutogenic_model_as_a_theory_to_guide_health_promotion.pdf

Becker, C.M., Glascoff, M.A., & Felts, W.M. (2010). Salutogenesis 30 years later: Where do we go from here? *Global Journal of Health Education and Promotion, 13,* 25–32. Available at https://www.proquest.com/openview/19a59611fd911e67f706f8 9a5e6fd689/1?pq-origsite=gscholar%26cbl=2037372

Bowden, J. (2006). Health promotion and the midwife. In *Health promotion in midwifery: Principles and practice,* edited by J. Bowden and V. Manning. London: Hodder Arnold, pp. 13–24.

Bradshaw, J. (1972). The concept of social need. *New Society, 19,* 640–643. Available at https://eprints.whiterose.ac.uk/118357/1/bradshaw_taxonomy.pdf

Calvert, J., & Arbuthnott, G. (2021). *Failures of state: The inside story of Britain's battle with coronavirus*. London: Harper Collins.

Cavanagh, S., & Chadwick, K. (2005). *Health needs assessment: A practical guide.* Health Development agency. Available at Health needs assessment: A practical guide (ihub.scot)

Chief Nursing Officers of England, Northern Ireland, Scotland and Wales (CNO). (2010). *Midwifery 2020: Delivering expectations*. Department of Health. https://www.gov.uk/government/uploads/system/uploads/attachment_data/file/216029/dh_119470.pdf and Midwifery 2020: Delivering expectations - GOV.UK (www.gov.uk)

Clayton, C.E., Hemingway, A., Hughes, M., & Rawson, S. (2022). The public health role of caseloading midwives in advancing health equity in childbearing women and babies living in socially deprived areas in England: The Mi-CARE Study protocol. *European Journal of Midwifery, 4*(6), 17. https://doi.org/10.18332/ejm/146012

Crafter, H. (1997). *Health promotion in midwifery: Principles and practice* (1st ed.). London: Hodder Arnold.

Cross, R., & Woodall, J. (2023). Information needs. In *Green & tones' health promotion, planning and strategies* (5th ed). London: Sage.

Department of Health and Social Care (DHSC). (2021). *The best start for life: A vision for the 1,001 critical days*. Available at https://www.gov.uk/government/publications/the-best-start-for-life-a-vision-for-the-1001-critical-days

Fehling, M., Nelson, B.D., & Venkatapuram, S. (2013). Limitations of the millennium development goals: A literature review. *Global Public Health, 8,* 1109–1122. Available at https://doi.org/10.1080/17441692.2013.845676

Gandhi, M.K. (1948). *Keys to health.* Ahmedabad: Navjivan Publishing House.

Gold, J. (1985). Cartesian dualism and the current crisis in medicine – A plea for a philosophical approach: Discussion paper. *Journal of the Royal Society of Medicine, 78,* 663–666. https://doi.org/10.1177/014107688507800813

Hagell, A. (2015). *Promoting young people's health literacy and understanding their help-seeking behaviour. AYPH Exploring Evidence series.* London: Association of Young People's Health, Public Health England. -

Hill, K., Kellard, K., Middleton, S., Cox, L., & Pound, E. (2007). *Understanding resources in later life views and experiences of older people.* York: Joseph Rowntree Foundation. Available at Understanding resources in later life (jrf.org.uk).

Hunter, D.J., Littlejohn, P., & Weale, P. (2022). Reforming the public health system in England. *The Lancet: Public Health, 7*(9), E797–E800. Available at https://doi.org/10.1016/S2468-2667(22)00199-2

International Confederation of Midwives (ICM). (2017). *ICM international definition of the midwife.* https://www.internationalmidwives.org/assets/files/definitions-files/2018/06/eng-definition_midwifery.pdf

Keller, K. (2020). The body as machine and the lived body in nursing. *Collegian, 27*(2), 238–244. https://doi.org/10.1016/j.colegn.2019.07.008

Knight, M., Bunch, K., et al. (eds.). (2020). *Saving lives, improving mothers' care. Lessons learned to inform maternity care from the UK and Ireland confidential enquiries into maternal deaths and morbidity 2016–18.* Available at https://www.npeu.ox.ac.uk/assets/downloads/mbrrace-uk/reports/maternal-report-2020/MBRRACE-UK_Maternal_Report_Dec_2020_v10_ONLINE_VERSION_1404.pdf

Knight, M., Nair, M., et al. (eds.). (2023). *Saving lives, improving mothers' care. Lessons learned to inform maternity care from the UK and Ireland confidential enquiries into maternal deaths and morbidity 2019–21* Available at https://www.npeu.ox.ac.uk/assets/downloads/mbrrace-uk/reports/maternal-report-2023/MBRRACE-UK_Maternal_Compiled_Report_2023.pdf

Korenbrot, C., Steinerg, A., Bender, C., & Newberry, S. (2002). Preconception care: A systematic review. *Maternal and Child Health Journal, 6,* 75–88. Available at https://doi.org/10.1023/A:1015460106832

Kumar, S., & Preetha, G. (2012). Health promotion: An effective tool for global health. *Indian Journal of Community Medicine, 37*(1), 2–12. http://dx.doi.org/10.4103/0970-0218.94009

Marmot, M., Allen, J., Boyce, T., Goldblatt, P., & Morrison, J. (2020). *Health equity in England: The marmot review 10 years on.* London: Institute of Health Equity. Available at https://www.health.org.uk/sites/default/files/upload/publications/2020/Health%20Equity%20in%20England_The%20Marmot%20Review%2010%20Years%20On_full%20report.pdf

Mathias, L.A., Davis, D., & Ferguson, S. (2021). Salutogenic qualities of midwifery care: A best-fit framework synthesis. *Women and Birth, 34*(3), 266–277. https://doi.org/10.1016/j.wombi.2020.03.006

McNeill, J., Lynn, F., & Alderdice, F. (2012). Public health interventions in midwifery: A systematic review of systematic reviews. *BMC Public Health, 12,* 955.

Mooney G, Wiseman S & Wiseman J (2011) Measuring needs IN Detels, R. (Editor). *Oxford textbook of public health* (5th ed.). Oxford University Press

Moorhead, R. (2002). William Budd and typhoid fever. *Journal of the Royal Society of Medicine, 95*(11), 561–564. https://doi.org/10.1177/014107680209501115

NHS England. (2016). *National maternity review: Better births improving outcomes of maternity services in England. A five year forward view for maternity care.* Available at https://www.england.nhs.uk/wp-content/uploads/2016/02/national-maternity-review-report.pdf

NHS England. (2019). *Universal personalised care: Implementing the comprehensive model.* Available at https://www.england.nhs.uk/wp-content/uploads/2019/01/universal-personalised-care.pdf

NHS England. (2024). Making Every Contact Count (MECC) programme. Available at https://www.e-lfh.org.uk/programmes/making-every-contact-count/

NMC. (2019). *Standards of proficiency for midwives.* standards-of-proficiency-for-midwives.pdf (nmc.org.uk)

OHID. (2023). *All our health: personalised care and population health.* Available at https://www.gov.uk/government/collections/all-our-health-personalised-care-and-population-health

Oleribe, O.O., Ukwedeh, O., Burstow, N.J., Gomaa, A.I., Sonderup, M.W., Cook, N., Waked, I., Spearman, W., & Taylor-Robinson, S.D. (2018). Health: Redefined. *The Pan African Medical Journal, 30,* 292. https://doi.org/10.11604/pamj.2018.30.292.15436

PHE. (2014). *From evidence into action: Opportunities to protect and improve the nation's health.* Available at https://www.gov.uk/government/publications/from-evidence-into-action-opportunities-to-protect-and-improve-the-nations-health

PHE. (2019). *Health of women before and during pregnancy: Health behaviours, risk factors and inequalities. An updated analysis of the maternity services dataset antenatal booking data.* Available at https://assets.publishing.service.gov.uk/media/5dc00b22e5274a4a9a465013/Health_of_women_before_and_during_pregnancy_2019.pdf

PHE. (2021). *Population health needs assessment: A guide for 0 to 19 health visiting and school nursing services.* Available at https://www.gov.uk/government/publications/commissioning-of-public-health-services-for-children/population-health-needs-assessment-a-guide-for-0-to-19-health-visiting-and-school-nursing-services

Renfrew, M.J. (2020). Scaling up care by midwives must now be a global priority. *The Lancet. Global Health, 9*(1), E2–E3. https://doi.org/10.1016/S2214-109X(20)30478-2

Renfrew, M.J., McFadden, A., & Bastos, M.H., et al. (2014). Midwifery and quality care: Findings from a new evidence-informed framework for maternal and newborn care. *Lancet, 384*(9948), 1129–1145. http://doi.org/10.1016/S0140-6736(14)60789-3

Royal College of Midwives (RCM). (2017). *Stepping up to public health.* Available at https://www.rcm.org.uk/media/3165/stepping-up-to-public-health.pdf

Sandall, J., Soltani, H., Gates, S., Shennan, A., & Devane D. (2016). Midwife-led continuity models versus other models of care for childbearing women. *Cochrane Database System Review, 4*(4), CD004667. https://doi.org/10.1002/14651858.CD004667

Spencer, G., Corbin, J.H., & Miedema, E. (2019). Sustainable development goals for health promotion: A critical frame analysis. *Health Promotion International, 3*(4), 847–858. https://doi.org/10.1093/heapro/day036

Strategic Review of Health Inequalities in England post-2010. (2010). *Fair society, healthy lives: The Marmot review.* https://www.instituteofhealthequity.org/resources-reports/fair-society-healthy-lives-the-marmot-review/fair-society-healthy-lives-full-report-pdf.pdf

Svalastog, A.L., Donev, D., Jahren Kristoffersen, N., & Gajović, S. (2017) Concepts and definitions of health and health-related values in the knowledge landscapes of the digital society. *Croatian Medical Journal, 58*(6), 431–435. https://doi.org/10.3325/cmj.2017.58.431

The Clean Air Act. (1956). Available at https://www.legislation.gov.uk/ukpga/Eliz2/4-5/52/enacted

The Clean Air Act. (1968). Available at https://www.legislation.gov.uk/ukpga/1968/62/contents

The Clean Air Act. (1993). Available at https://www.legislation.gov.uk/ukpga/1993/11/contents

United Nations. (2015). Sustainable Development Goals (SDG) Platform. Available at https://sdgs.un.org/partnerships

WHO. (1946). Preamble to the Constitution of the World Health Organisation as adopted by the International Health Conference, New York, 19 June–22 July 1946; signed on 22 July 1946 by representatives of 61 States (Official Records of the WHO, no 2, p. 100) and entered into force on 7 April 1948. Constitution of the World Health Organization (who.int)

WHO. (1986). *The Ottawa charter for health promotion.* Geneva: WHO. Available at https://intranet.euro.who.int/__data/assets/pdf_file/0004/129532/Ottawa_Charter.pdf

WHO. (2008). *Closing the gap in a generation: Health equality through action on the social determinates of health.* Available at https://www.who.int/publications/i/item/WHO-IER-CSDH-08.1

WHO. (2023a). *Noncommunicable diseases.* Available at https://www.who.int/news-room/fact-sheets/detail/noncommunicable-diseases

WHO. (2023b). *Maternal health.* Available at https://www.who.int/health-topics/maternal-health#tab=tab_1

WHO. (2023c). *World health statistics 2023 – Monitoring health for the SDGs.* Available at https://www.who.int/data/gho/publications/world-health-statistics

FURTHER READINGS – FOR BOOK WEB LINK

Bengt, L., & Eriksson, M. (2010). *The Hitchhiker's guide to salutogenesis: Salutogenic pathways to health promotion.* Helsinki: Fokhalsan Health Promotion Research.

Public Health England. (2014). *Public health contribution of nurses and midwives: Guidance.* https://www.gov.uk/government/collections/developing-the-public-health-contribution-of-nurses-and-midwives-tools-and-models

Royal College of Midwives. *Public health and health promotion online resources* Midwives and Public Health (rcm.org.uk)

Stockdale, J. (2011). *Achieving optimal birth using salutogenesis in routine antenatal education.* evidence-based-midwifery-september-2011.pdf (rcm.org.uk)

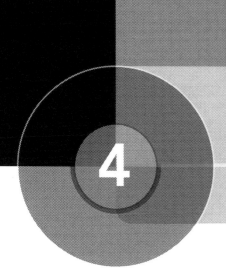

Factors Affecting Health Promotion: A Gendered Issue

CHARLOTTE DEWAR AND LUCY FLATLEY

INTRODUCTION

A large body of evidence has shown that in the UK, women frequently experience poorer health outcomes compared to men. The gender health gap relates to women's health in general, and also the specific health needs of the reproductive and childbirth continuum. In recent years, there has been UK policy and strategy response to this issue, including the Royal College of Obstetricians and Gynaecologists (RCOG, 2019) 'Better for Women' report which called for specific women's health strategy and recognised a number of key areas where women's health needs are unmet. The Women's Health Strategy for England was launched in 2022 (Department of Health and Social Care, 2022), recognising that greater focus is needed on women's health needs and that women are disproportionately affected by ill health and disability compared to men.

There are various factors which affect an individual's ability to respond to public health policy and health promotion interventions. This chapter explores the mediating factors that disproportionately influence a woman's capacity to make healthy choices in response to these interventions; her 'choice' pertaining to the product of her life chances and circumstances, rather than her actual free choices. The inability to engage with health promotion strategies not only affects the perinatal period but has lifelong and transgenerational implications. Therefore, it is imperative that maternity care is designed and delivered accordingly. Health behaviour theories and models help us understand individual choices and behaviours which impact health (this is explored in more detail in Chapters 7 and 9). This chapter broadly explores the following before considering the perinatal period and concluding with a discussion on midwifery practice:

- domestic responsibilities
- biological and social influences

DOI: 10.4324/9781003350071-4

- power and safety
- socioeconomic status

DOMESTIC RESPONSIBILITIES

The cultural acceptance of women being the more 'nurturing' sex designates them to form the core of the family unit and the gendered division of housework, childcare, and other caring responsibilities prohibit the prioritisation of their own health (Kashefi et al., 2018). Although views on gender roles are continuing to become more progressive (Phillips et al., 2018) and there has been a decline in the view that women should stay at home rather than take paid employment (Taylor & Scott, 2018); studies have shown that even when women work longer hours or earn more money, they still do more domestic labour than men (McMunn et al., 2020). In the literature exploring women's health behaviours, women frequently cite family commitments as a barrier to leading a healthy lifestyle (Lim et al., 2019). Time constraints; childcare needs; fatigue and subsequent low motivation; prioritising other family member's needs (Lim et al., 2019) and maternal guilt if they do prioritise themselves (Van der Pligt et al., 2018) are just some of the factors that influence women's health choices. Women also reported time constraints inhibiting their ability to source and cook healthy food (MacMillan Uribe & Olsen, 2019) and noted that fast-food restaurants were more child-friendly and affordable (Wright et al., 2017).

In addition to undertaking both paid employment and completing the biggest share of domestic chores, women are also disproportionately burdened with a greater 'mental load'. The 'mental load' depicts the project management of family life – including the thinking, scheduling and organising family members and the emotional impact of this work, including feelings of caring and being responsible for family members (Dean et al., 2021). The 'mental load' is invisible, boundaryless and relentless (Dean et al., 2021) and women are suffering physical and emotional health consequences as a result (Craig & Churchill, 2021). The 'mental load' causes greater bedtime worry and stress which results in less or poorer quality sleep (Hall et al., 2015), as well as reducing time for other things (Anxo et al., 2011) such as exercising and cooking healthy meals from scratch. The 'mental load' is exacerbated by social media pressure for the millennial woman to simultaneously be the perfect mother; career woman, homemaker, and friend whilst pursuing a healthy lifestyle. Whilst evidence suggests that health promotion delivered via social media can be successful in improving health behaviours for physical health (Petkovic et al., 2021), it is generally agreed that social media negatively impacts mental health and wellbeing, with a stronger association being noted for girls when compared to boys (Svensson et al., 2022). Health promotion, therefore, needs to sensitively consider these competing demands for a woman's time, whilst exercising caution not to add any undue pressure which could negatively impact health and wellbeing.

BIOLOGICAL AND SOCIAL INFLUENCES

There are biological and social influences that affect a woman's ability to lead a healthy lifestyle. Historically, women have been discouraged from exercising due to the belief that they were physiologically less able than men and that endurance activity may damage their reproductive health (Wallace, 2022). Despite a lot of positive change and women now equally representing men in the Olympic Games for example (International Olympic Committee, 2021), there is still a gendered difference towards exercise engagement. A higher proportion of men (70%) than women (59%) meet guidelines for aerobic exercise (NHS Digital, 2023), with men and women citing different reasons for exercising. Women report exercising for weight loss and toning, but men are much more likely to report exercising for enjoyment (Craft et al., 2014). Craft et al. (2014) also found that men were able to improve their quality of life with exercise, regardless of the reason reported. Conversely, for women, exercise to lose weight was associated with a lower quality of life whilst exercising to improve mood or health was associated with higher quality of life (Craft et al., 2014). Sport England's 'This Girl Can' is a UK nationwide campaign launched in 2015 which aims to readdress this narrative, making sport and exercise more inclusive, accessible, and enjoyable by removing barriers and celebrating active women (Sport England, n.d.).

A woman's menstrual cycle also impacts her lifestyle choices. Hormonal fluctuations can increase hunger and cravings for high-fat and high-carbohydrate foods, whilst depleting strength and energy levels (Wallace, 2022). Some women report the active avoidance of exercise during menstruation due to feelings of self-consciousness and menstrual symptoms (Kolić et al., 2021), despite research showing that exercise eases these symptoms (Kolić et al., 2021). Menstruation also puts women at a higher risk of iron deficiency anaemia, which can cause fatigue and a subsequent lack of motivation for exercise.

As previously discussed, fatigue is a commonly reported barrier to healthy lifestyle choices, and although research suggests that women get more sleep than men (Burgard & Ailshire, 2013), they are more likely to have poorer sleep quality caused by difficulty falling asleep, frequent night wakes and longer wakeful episodes (Meers et al., 2019). The reasons for this are both biological – with sleep disturbances reported to peak during periods, hormonal change such as puberty, pregnancy, and the menopause (Dorsey et al., 2021) – and social – with women experiencing greater sleep interruption due to her role as primary carer (Wallace, 2022).

ISSUES OF POWER AND SAFETY

Despite the feminist movements and progress with gender equality in the UK, many women still have choices and decisions affected by various factors. This can affect health behaviours at both an individual and community level.

Globally, one in three women will experience physical or sexual violence in their lifetime, with younger women being at the greatest risk (World Health Organization [WHO], 2021a). Domestic abuse is a significant issue for women in the UK with most recent figures suggesting that 6.9% of women in England and Wales experienced domestic abuse in 2022, with women being over twice as likely to experience abuse compared to men (Office for National Statistics [ONS], 2022a). Although the increase in prevalence has not increased in recent years, domestic abuse recorded crimes has increased, which reflects an increase in reporting of abuse (ONS, 2022a). Despite the rates of domestic abuse, the percentage of cases charged is 72%, meaning for a significant proportion of women their perpetrator is not prosecuted. In recent years both coercive control and economic abuse have been recognised as forms of domestic abuse. Both of these forms of abuse can impact on health behaviours.

Women's Aid defines coercive control as acts and patterns of controlling behaviour with the intent of frightening, harming, or punishing the victim (Women's Aid, 2022a). Financial abuse is a form of coercive control in which the perpetrator controls the victim's money and freedom with their money (Women's Aid, 2022b). This type of abuse can have severe impacts for women, depriving them of essentials and inhibiting their freedom (Women's Aid, 2022b). Research suggests that 25% of financial abuse victims do not have access to money for essentials (Women's Aid, 2019). Recommendations from research into financial abuse and the implications for Universal Credit by TUC and Women's Aid (Howard & Skipp, 2023) call for agencies to have training in coercive control to ensure women can be appropriately signposted to support and that some elements of Universal Credit, which relate to housing, should be paid to the landlord or bank to ensure housing security. The powerlessness that can result from a feeling of lack of control could have consequences for women's ability to make choices. (Chapter 17 discussed violence against women and girls in greater depth.)

Another pertinent issue is women's feeling of safety in the place where they live and its impacts on their health behaviours. This could affect their ability to walk rather than drive and impact on choices around exercise such as running or cycling. This area has received significant media attention and discussion in recent years following high-profile cases of women being attacked. A 2022 survey conducted in the UK found that in parks and open spaces, 82% of women reported feeling unsafe after dark, this is compared to 42% of men (ONS, 2022a).

The Safer Parks project has led to the initiation of new guidance for how parks should be designed and managed so that women and girls feel safe (The Safer Parks Consortium, 2023). The guidance is based on recent research (Barker et al., 2022) and has a focus on safety and wellbeing whilst ensuring the parks are an accessible and practical space to use. If implemented, this guidance has the potential to significantly impact women and girls' ability to spend time in parks which provide opportunities to be outside and exercise. This type of public health campaign is imperative in order to remove the barriers which women face in relation to power and control and enable them to make healthy choices to close the gender health gap.

SOCIOECONOMIC STATUS

Evidence suggests that socioeconomic status (SES) is associated with reduced life expectancy and that deprivation could have a similar impact to smoking and a sedentary lifestyle (Stringhini et al., 2017). A person's SES can affect their ability to make healthy choices, the reasons being multifaceted. There is a large body of literature which recognises the complex relationship between poverty, cognitive function, perception of self and behavioural patterns (Sheeny-Skeffington & Rea, 2017).

Poverty is an increasing issue in the UK and women are disproportionately affected. The most recent MBRRACE-UK report continued to find that women and birthing people living in the most deprived areas have the highest rates of maternal mortality and this is increasing (Knight et al., 2022). Women from racially diverse communities are also disproportionately more likely to die during the childbirth continuum compared to caucasian women (Knight et al., 2022). The effects are also cumulative, meaning those who are affected by more than one wider determinant of health are increasingly likely to have poorer outcomes.

BMC Medicine (2023) define food insecurity and food poverty as a household's inconsistent access to sufficient food to live a healthy life. There has been a large increase in food bank supply and demand since 2010 and the 'Born in Bradford' study reported that rates of food insecurity were higher than predicted and that food insecurity has a strong association with SES, particularly when receiving government benefits (Power et al., 2018). Other population groups that are also disproportionately affected by food security include: racial diversity communities; adults who receive Universal Credit; those who are unemployed and those who have disabilities (Department for Work and Pensions, 2021).

The UK has been experiencing a cost-of-living crisis since late 2021 (Crisis, 2023), this is likely to impact a range of factors such as issues around zero hours contracts, pay not matching inflation, Universal Credit, cost of childcare and maternity pay. Zero hours contracts are increasing in the UK and women from racially diverse communities are twice as likely to be on a zero hours contract compared to white men (TUC, 2022). The UK has ongoing issues with the gender pay gap; although slowly declining, a significant gap remains which was 8.3% for full-time employees in 2022 (ONS, 2022b). The cost of childcare in the UK is disproportionally high compared to wages (OECD, 2021), thus, investment in appropriately subsidised childcare would have a significant impact on women's choice around employment which affects socioeconomic and, ultimately, health status.

This section has outlined how socioeconomic status and inequity affects healthy lifestyles; however, health promotion may not be sufficient for addressing this (Zhang et al., 2021). Addressing the wider determinants of health by having a life course approach to health could have significant impact. Thus, making achieving optimum health in pregnancy pertinent, as this can have effects on the woman and baby's health across their life course. Just as income affects health, health impacts income; a lifelong condition or serious illness could impact employment and thus a person or household's financial circumstances (Joseph Rowntree Foundation, 2014).

A woman's socioeconomic status has been shown to have a complex relationship with choice ranging from nutrition to accessing services. Poverty can mean that engaging in health promotion is challenging. However, it is important to consider each person as an individual and not make generalisations based on SES which could lead to further marginalisation.

LEARNING ACTIVITY

Anita attends the children's centre for her 25-week routine midwife appointment and discloses to you that her partner has recently lost his job, she has financial concerns about when the baby will arrive.

Anita also discloses she is concerned about her flat which has some damp looking patches on some of the walls.

- What is the role of the midwife in this situation?
- Which other agencies could the midwife work with to support Anita and her partner?

THE PERINATAL PERIOD

So far, this chapter has considered barriers which affect health promotion for all women, however, the perinatal period presents an additional and specific set of challenges that affect women during pregnancy, postnatally and potentially for the rest of their lives.

Despite exercise being positively correlated with physical and mental health, the relief of pregnancy symptoms and favourable maternal and fetal outcomes (Budler & Budler, 2022), it can be challenging in the perinatal period. WHO recommends that pregnant women should do 150 minutes of physical activity every week (Bull et al., 2020), but research suggests that activity levels amongst pregnant women is incredibly low (Silva-Jose et al., 2022), with only 15% adhering to WHO's guideline. Nausea, vomiting, and fatigue are reported to be the biggest barriers to exercise in pregnancy (Sytsma et al., 2018), others include: lack of time, pain, swelling, obstetric complications, and concerns regarding safety (Sytsma et al., 2018). Midwives are also uncertain about the type and intensity of exercise that is safe during pregnancy (Marini et al., 2023), this lack of knowledge inhibits midwives from promoting exercise and women from taking it up during pregnancy. There is also poor provision of perinatal exercise services due to funding and inadequate interaction between policy makers and organisations – such as hospitals, community health providers, and local gyms (Saligheh et al., 2016). Additionally, private provisions are often too costly and inaccessible. There are also considerable inhibitors to exercise postnatally, and whilst fatigue and time are the most commonly reported (Saligheh et al., 2016); pelvic floor symptoms, including incontinence and pelvic organ prolapse, is a further significant barrier to exercise which is often overlooked (Dakic et al., 2022).

The barriers which inhibit exercise in pregnancy also inhibit healthy eating, particularly nausea and vomiting. Women reporting an increased severity of nausea also report a reduced range of foods consumed; with a decrease in the intake of vegetables and citrus fruits and an increase in the consumption of foods such as white bread (Crozier et al., 2017). Research suggests that nutrition knowledge is poor amongst pregnant women and both pregnant women and clinicians attribute this to being given/providing limited information (Lee et al., 2018). Pregnant women report getting their nutrition advice from a variety of sources including their midwife, GP, the internet and family and friends (Lee et al., 2018); thus, making it difficult to determine the official guidance from the myths such as; 'eating for two' or the need to drink full fat milk. Whilst most women do manage to make positive dietary changes in pregnancy (Lee et al., 2018); pregnancy symptoms, limited guidance from clinicians and conflicting advice make positive lifestyle choices difficult.

Excessive gestational weight gain is associated with adverse maternal and neonatal outcomes as well as postpartum weight retention (Champion & Harper, 2020) and can have a lifelong impact on women. Research suggests that approximately 75% of women weigh more one year postpartum than they were pre-pregnancy (Endres et al., 2015). Thus, the ramifications of excessive gestational weight gain are not limited to the perinatal period, making pregnancy a significant contributor to the obesity pandemic. There is a positive association between exclusive breastfeeding and postpartum weight loss (Tahir et al., 2019); however, only approximately 44% of infants aged 0–6 months worldwide are exclusively breastfed (WHO, 2021b). Weight management in pregnancy is therefore critically important, and whilst there is international guidance on weight gain in pregnancy (Centers for Disease Control and Prevention, 2022); there is no global consensus on maternal weight policies, including regular weighing in pregnancy (Scott et al., 2014). Midwives disclose a need for clearer guidelines for women and health professionals (Royal College of Midwives [RCM], 2018) and whilst women report being open to receiving healthy lifestyle messages in pregnancy, less than half discussed their weight with their midwife (RCM, 2018). Midwives report lack of time, training, and appropriate referral options, and many midwives are unsure about how to approach the subject in a sensitive and productive way, so they are inhibited by a fear of being judgmental (White & Davis, 2021).

It is paramount that the barriers to living a healthy lifestyle during the perinatal period are addressed, as the health implications – such as excessive gestational weight gain and pelvic floor damage – can have lifelong implications for women.

LEARNING ACTIVITY

You are conducting a booking appointment for Rachael whom you have never met before. She gives consent for you to take her height and weight and you calculate her BMI as 30.4 kg/m^2 which is in the obese range. Whilst you were taking Rachael's weight, she told you that she had put on 4 kg since finding out she was pregnant six weeks ago, that her morning sickness is making her crave salty foods and that she is too tired to even walk the dog in the evening.

- How would you sensitively discuss the implications of obesity in pregnancy and the importance of a healthy lifestyle?

RECOMMENDATIONS FOR MIDWIFERY PRACTICE

The sustained and regular interaction with maternity services throughout the perinatal period presents a unique and opportune time for women to engage with public health strategy. Thus, the role of the midwife in supporting health promotion is extensive and needs to be supported and underpinned by health policy which acknowledges the gender health gap, and the unique challenges women face in responding to health promotion; thereby prioritising women's health and focussing on prevention. The three-year delivery plan for maternity and neonatal services, published in 2023 (NHS England, 2023a), has committed to ensuring all women have access to pelvic health services as well as committing to improving equity for women and families and ensuring co-production of maternity services with service users. Improving prevention is one of the key aims of the Maternity Transformation Programme in England (NHS England, 2023b). To support maternity transformation on a local level, it is paramount that Local Maternity and Neonatal Systems and NHS trusts have specialist midwives to lead on this work. Having local experts is likely to increase awareness on the different aspects of prevention and support midwives to provide evidence-based care for women and families. Midwives also have a vital role of working with different agencies and referring and signposting women to support. The Family Hubs and Start for Life programme (Department of Health and Social Care and Department of Education, 2023) is a unique opportunity for health professionals to work together with a focus on a life-course approach to health.

PRACTICE ACTIVITY

You can read more about the Family Hubs and the Best Start for Life Programme on the following website: Family Hubs and Start for Life programme – GOV.UK

Which services could be developed to support women during this perinatal period at these hubs?

SUMMARY

- There is a gender health gap with women experiencing poorer health outcomes compared to men.
- There are various factors which disproportionately influence a woman's ability to engage with health promotion strategy, these include:
    - A greater responsibility for caring and household duties
    - Biological factors such as menstruation, pregnancy, and the menopause
    - Social attitudes to sport and exercise
    - Issues of power and safety
    - Socioeconomic factors
- These factors affect women's preconception health, impact, and are exacerbated by, the perinatal period, and if they are not addressed accordingly, can have lifelong and transgenerational ramifications.
- The perinatal period presents an opportune time for health promotion; thus, the public health role of the midwife is critical and must be supported by specific women's health strategy.

REFERENCES

Anxo, D., Mencarini, L., Pailhe, A., Solaz, A., Tanturri, M. L., & Flood, L. (2011). Gender difference in time use over the life course in France, Italy, Sweden, and the US. *Feminist Economist,* 17(3), 159–195.

Barker, A., Holmes, G., Alam, R., Cape-Davenhill, L., Osei-Appiah, S & Warrington Brown, S. (2022). What Makes a Park Feel Safe or Unsafe? The views of women, girls and professionals in West Yorkshire. University of Leeds. doi: 10.48785/100/108

BMC Medicine. (2023). Food insecurity: A neglected public health issue requiring multisectoral action. *BMC Medicine,* 21(130). https://doi.org/10.1186/s12916-023-02845-3

Brown, S. (2022). What makes a park feel safe or unsafe? The views of women, girls and professionals in West Yorkshire. BMC Sports Science, Medicine and Rehabilitation, 14(133). https://doi.org/10.1186/s13102-022-00524-z

Budler, L. C., & Budler, M. (2022). Physical activity during pregnancy: A systematic review for the assessment of current evidence with future recommendations. *BMC Sports Science, Medicine and Rehabilitation,* 14(133). https://doi.org/10.1186/s13102-022-00524-z

Bull, F., Al-Ansari, S. S., Biddle, S., Borodulin, K., Buman, M.P., Cardon, G., Carty, C., Chaput, J.-P., Chastin, S., Chou, R., Dempsey, P. C., DiPietro, L., Ekelund, U., Firth, J., Friedenreich, CM., Garcia, L., Gichu, M., Jago, R., Katzmarzyk, P. T., …

Willumsen., J. F. (2020). World Health Organization 2020 guidelines on physical activity and sedentary behaviour. *British Journal of Sports Medicine,* 54(24), 1451–1462. https://doi.org/10.1136/bjsports-2020-102955

Burgard, S. A., & Ailshire, J. A. (2013). Gender and time for sleep among U.S. adults. *American Sociological Review,* 78(1), 51–69. https://doi.org/10.1177/0003122412472048

Centers for Disease Control and Prevention. (2022). *Weight Gain During Pregnancy.* Retrieved from: https://www.cdc.gov/reproductivehealth/maternalinfanthealth/pregnancy-weight-gain.htm

Champion, M. L., & Harper, L. M. (2020). Gestational weight gain: Update on outcomes and interventions. *Current Diabetes Reports,* 20(3), 11.

Craft, B. B., Carroll, H. A., & Lustyk, M. K. (2014). Gender differences in exercise habits and quality of life reports: Assessing the moderating effects of reasons for exercise. *International Journal of Liberal Arts and Social Science,* 2(5), 65–76.

Craig, L., & Churchill, B. (2021). Unpaid work and care during COVID-19: Subjective experiences of same-sex couples and single mothers in Australia. *Gender & Society,* 35(2), 233–243.

Crisis. (2023). *The Cost-of-Living Crisis.* Retrieved from: https://www.crisis.org.uk/ending-homelessness/the-cost-of-living-crisis/#:~:text=The%20cost%20of%20living%20crisis%20refers%20to%20a%20period%20of,living%20crisis%20since%20late%202021

Crozier, S. R., Inskip, H. M., Godfrey, K. M., Cooper, C., & Robinson, S. M., SWS Study Group. (2017). Nausea and vomiting in early pregnancy: Effects on food intake and diet quality. *Maternal and Child Nutrition,* 13(4), e12389. https://doi.org/10.1111/mcn.12389.

Dakic, J. G., Cook, J., Hay-Smith, J., Lin, K., Ekegren, C., & Frawley, H. (2022). Pelvic floor symptoms are an overlooked barrier to exercise participation: A cross-sectional online survey of 4556 women who are symptomatic. *Physical Therapy,* 102(3), 1–10.

Dean, L., Churchill, B., & Ruppanner, L. (2021) The mental load: Building a deeper theoretical understanding of how cognitive and emotional labor overload women and mothers. *Community, Work & Family,* 25(1), 13–29.

Department of Health and Social Care. (2022). *Women's Health Strategy for England.* Retrieved from: https://www.gov.uk/government/publications/womens-health-strategy-for-england/womens-health-strategy-for-england

Department of Health and Social Care and Department of Education. (2023). *Family Hubs and Start for Life Programme.* Retrieved from: https://www.gov.uk/government/collections/family-hubs-and-start-for-life-programme

Department for Work and Pensions. (2021). *Family Resources Survey: Financial Year 2019–2020.* Retrieved from: https://www.gov.uk/government/statistics/family-resources-survey-financial-year-2019-to-2020

Dorsey, A., De Lecea, L., & Jennings, K. J. (2020). Neurobiological and hormonal mechanisms regulating women's sleep. *Frontiers in Neuroscience,* 14, 625397.

Endres, L. K., Straub, H., McKinney, C., Plunkett, B., Minkovitz, C. S., Schetter, C. D., Ramey, S., Wang, C., Hobel, C., Raju, T., & Shalowitz, M. U. (2015). Postpartum weight retention risk factors and relationship to obesity at 1 year. *Obstetrics and Gynecology,* 125(1), 144–152.

Hall, M. H., Casement, M. D., Troxel, W. M., Matthews, K. A., Bromberger, J. T., Kravitz, H. M., & Buysse, D. J. (2015). Chronic stress is prospectively associated with sleep in midlife women: The SWAN sleep study. *Sleep,* 38(10), 1645–1654.

Howard, M., & Skipp, A. (2023). *Unequal, Trapped and Controlled: Women's Experiences of Financial Abuse and Potential Implications for Universal Credit.* Retrieved from: https://www.womensaid.org.uk/wp-content/uploads/2015/11/Women_s_Aid_TUC_Financial_Abuse_Report_March_2015.pdf

International Olympic Committee. (2021). *The Women That Wowed: A Look at Some of the Best Female Performances at Tokyo 2020.* Retrieved from: https://olympics.com/en/news/the-women-that-wowed-at-tokyo-2020

Joseph Rowntree Foundation. (2014). *How Does Money Influence Health?* Retrieved from: How does money influence health? | Joseph Rowntree Foundation (jrf.org.uk)

Kashefi, M., Kermanshahi, S. M. K., & Fesharaki, M. G. (2018) The barriers to a healthy lifestyle in employed mothers of toddlers. *Journal of Holistic Nursing and Midwifery,* 28(4), 211–217.

Knight, M., Bunch, K., Patel, R., Shakespeare., J. Kotnis, R., Kenyon, S., & Kurinczuk, J. J. (Eds.) on behalf of MMBRRACE-UK. (2022). *Saving lives, improving mothers' care core report: Lessons learned to inform maternity care from the UK.* Oxford: National Perinatal Epidemiology Unit, University of Oxford.

Kolić, P. V., Sims, D. T., Hicks, K., Thomas, L., & Morse, C. I. (2021). Physical activity and the menstrual cycle: a mixed-methods study of women's experiences. *Women in Sport and Physical Activity Journal,* 29, 47–58.

Lee, A., Newton, M., Radcliffe., J., & Belski, R. (2018). Pregnancy nutrition knowledge and experiences of pregnant women and antenatal care clinicians: A mixed methods approach. *Women and Birth,* 31(4), 269–277.

Lim, S., Tan, A., Madden, S., & Hill, B. (2019). Health professionals' and postpartum women's perspectives on digital health interventions for lifestyle management in the postpartum period: A systematic review of qualitative studies. *Frontiers in Endocrinology (Lausanne),*10, 767.

MacMillan Uribe, A. L., & Olson, B. H. (2019). Exploring healthy eating and exercise behaviors among low-income breastfeeding mothers. *Journal of Human Lactation,* 35(1), 59–70.

Marini, S., Messina, R., Masini, A., Scognamiglio, F., Caravita, I., Leccese, V., Soldà, G., Parma, D., Bertini, V., Scheier, L. M., & Dallolio, L. (2023). Application of the COM–B framework to understand facilitators and barriers for practising physical activity among pregnant women and midwives participating in the WELL-DONE! Study. *Behavioral Sciences,* 13(2), 114. https://doi.org/10.3390/bs13020114

McMunn, A., Bird, L., Webb, E., & Sacker, A. (2020). Gender divisions of paid and unpaid work in contemporary UK couples. *Work, Employment and Society,* 34(2), 155–173.

Meers, J., Stout-Aguilar, J., & Nowakowski, S. (2019). Sex differences in sleep health. In M. A. Grandner (Ed.), *Sleep and Health,* 21–29. https://doi.org/10.1016/B978-0-12-815373-4.00003-4

NHS Digital. (2023). *Health Survey for England, 2021 part 2.* Retrieved from: https://digital.nhs.uk/data-and-information/publications/statistical/health-survey-for-england/2021-part-2#

NHS England. (2023a). *Three Year Delivery Plan for Maternity and Neonatal Services.* Retrieved from: https://www.england.nhs.uk/wp-content/uploads/2023/03/B1915-three-year-delivery-plan-for-maternity-and-neonatal-services-march-2023.pdf

NHS England. (2023b). *Maternity Transformation Programme.* Retrieved from: https://www.england.nhs.uk/mat-transformation/

OECD. (2021). *Net Childcare Costs.* Retrieved from: https://data.oecd.org/benwage/net-childcare-costs.htm

Office for National Statistics. (2022a). *Perceptions of Personal Safety and Experiences of Harassment, Great Britain: 16 February to 13 March 2022.* Retrieved from: https://www.ons.gov.uk/peoplepopulationandcommunity/crimeandjustice/bulletins/perceptionsofpersonalsafetyandexperiencesofharassmentgreatbritain/16februaryto13march2022

Office for National Statistics. (2022b). *Gender Pay Gap in the UK.* Retrieved from: https://www.ons.gov.uk/employmentandlabourmarket/peopleinwork/earningsandworkinghours/bulletins/genderpaygapintheuk/2022

Petkovic, J., Duench, S., Trawin, J., Dewidar, O., Pardo Pardo, J., Simeon, R., DesMeules, M., Gagnon, D., Hatcher Roberts, J., Hossain, A., Pottie, K., Rader, T., Tugwell, P., Yoganathan, M., Presseau, J. & Welch, V. (2021). Behavioural interventions delivered through interactive social media for health behaviour change, health outcomes, and health equity in the adult population. *Cochrane Database of Systematic Reviews,* (5). Art. No.: CD012932. DOI: 10.1002/14651858.CD012932.pub2. Accessed 27 August 2024.

Phillips, D., Curtice, J., Phillips, M., & Perry, J. (Eds.). (2018). *British Social Attitudes: The 35th Report.* London: The National Centre for Social Research.

Power, M., Uphoff, E. P., Stewart-Knox, B., Small, N., Doherty, B., & Pickett, K. (2018). Food insecurity and socio-demographic characteristics in two UK ethnic groups: An analysis of women in the Born in Bradford cohort. *Journal of Public Health,* 40(1), 32–40. https//doi.org/10.1093/pubmed/fdx029

Royal College of Midwives. (2018). *Call for Clear Guidance on Healthy Weight Management in Pregnancy from the Royal College of Midwives and Slimming World.* Retrieved from: https://www.rcm.org.uk/media-releases/2018/july/call-for-clear-guidance-on-healthy-weight-management-in-pregnancy/

Royal College of Obstetricians and Gynaecologists. (2019). *Better for Women.* Retrieved from: https://www.rcog.org.uk/about-us/campaigning-and-opinions/better-for-women/

Saligheh, M., McNamara, B., & Rooney, R. (2016). Perceived barriers and enablers of physical activity in postpartum women: a qualitative approach. *BMC Pregnancy Childbirth,* 16, 131.

Scott, C., Andersen, C. T., Valdez, N., Mardones, F., Nohr, E. A., Poston, L., Loestsche K. C. Q., & Abrams, B. (2014). No global consensus: A cross-sectional survey of maternal weight policies. *BMC Pregnancy Childbirth*, 14, 167.

Sheeny-Skeffington, J., & Rea, J. (2017). *How Poverty Affects People's Decision-Making Processes.* Joseph Rowntree Foundation. How poverty affects people's decision-making processes | Joseph Rowntree Foundation (jrf.org.uk)

Silva-Jose, C., Sánchez-Polán, M., Barakat, R., Gil-Ares, J., & Refoyo, I. (2022). Level of physical activity in pregnant populations from different geographic regions: A systematic review. *Journal of Clinical Medicine,* 11, 4638.

Sport England. (n.d.). *This Girl Can.* Sport England. Retrieved from: https://www. sportengland.org/funds-and-campaigns/this-girl-can

Stringhini, S., Carmeli, C., Jokela, M., Avendano, M., Muennig, P., Guida, F., Ricceri, F., d'Errico, A., Barros, H., Bochud, M., Chadeau-Hyam, M., Clavel-Chapelon, F., Costa, G., Delpierre, C., Fraga, S., Goldberg, M., Giles, G., Krogh, V., Kelly-Irving, M… Kivimaki, M. (2017). Socioeconomic status and the 25 × 25 risk factors as determiments of premature mortality: a multicohort study and meta-analysis of 1.7 million men and women. *The Lancet.* 389 (10075), 1229–1237. https://doi. org/10.1016/S0140-6736(16)32380-7.

Svensson, R., Johnson, B., & Olsson, A. (2022). Does gender matter? The association between different digital media activities and adolescent well-being. *BMC Public Health,* 22(273).

Sytsma, T. T., Zimmerman, K. P., Manning, J. B., Jenkins, S. M., Nelson, N. C., Clark, M. M., Boldt, K., & Borowski, K. S. (2018). Perceived barriers to exercise in the first trimester of pregnancy. *Journal of Perinatal Education,* 27(4), 198–206. https://doi. org/10.1891/1058–1243.27.4.198.

Tahir, M. J., Haapala, J. L., Foster, L. P., Duncan, K. M., Teague, A. M., Kharbanda, E. O., McGovern, P. M., Whitaker, K. M., Rasmussen, K. M., Fields, D. A., Harnack, L. J., Jacobs Jr, D. R., & Demerath, E. W. (2019). Association of full breastfeeding duration with postpartum weight retention in a cohort of predominantly breastfeeding women. *Nutrients,* 11(4), 938. https://doi.org/10.3390/nu11040938

Taylor, E. A., & Scott, J. (2018). Gender: New consensus or continuing battleground? In: D. Phillips, J. Curtice, M. Phillips & J. Perry (Eds.), *British Social Attitudes: The 35th Report* (pp. 56–85). London: NatCen Social Research,.

The Safer Parks Consortium. (2023). *Safer Parks. Improving Access for Women and Girls.* Retrieved from: https://www.westyorks-ca.gov.uk/media/10332/ safer-parks-final-050503-lr.pdf

TUC. (2022). *TUC: BME Women Twice as Likely to be on Zero-Hours Contracts as White Men.* Retrieved from: https://www.tuc.org.uk/news/tuc-bme-women- twice-likely-be-zero-hours-contracts-white-men

Van der Pligt, P., Ball., K., Hesketh, K. D., Crawford, D., Teychenne., M., & Campbell, K. (2018). The views of first time mothers completing an intervention to reduce postpartum weight retention: A qualitative evaluation of the mums OnLiNE study. *Midwifery,* 56, 23–28. https://doi.org/10.1016/j.midw.2017.09.013

Wallace, H. (2022). *The female factor: Making women's health count – and what it means for you.* London: Hodder & Stoughton.

White, C., & Davis, D. (2021). Barriers and enablers in maintaining healthy gesta-tional weight gain: A qualitative study. *Women and Birth,* 34(5), e461–e467.

Women's Aid. (2019). *The Domestic Abuse Report 2019: The Economics of Abuse.* Bristol: Women's Aid.

Women's Aid. (2022a). *What Is Coercive Control.* Retrieved from: https://www. womensaid.org.uk/information-support/what-is-domestic-abuse/coercive- control/

Women's Aid. (2022b). What Is Financial Abuse? Retrieved from: https://www.womensaid.org.uk/information-support/what-is-domestic-abuse/financial-abuse/

World Health Organization. (2021a). *Devastatingly Pervasive: 1 in 3 Women Globally Experience Violence.* Retrieved from: https://www.who.int/news/item/09-03-2021-devastatingly-pervasive-1-in-3-women-globally-experience-violence

World Health Organization. (2021b). *Infant and Young Child Feeding.* Retrieved from: https://www.who.int/news-room/fact-sheets/detail/infant-and-young-child-feeding

Wright, C., Mogul, M., Murray, R., Levinson, M., Momplaisir, F., & Shea, J. (2017) The development of a postpartum weight management intervention for low-income women: End-user perspectives as groundwork. *Progress in Community Health Partnerships,* 11(4), 409–416.

Zhang, Y., Chen, C., Pan, X., Guo, J., Li, Y., Franco, O. H., Liu, G., & Pan, A. (2021). Associations of healthy lifestyle and socioeconomic status with mortality and incident cardiovascular disease: Two prospective cohort studies. *BMJ,* 373. https://doi.org/10.1136/bmj.n604

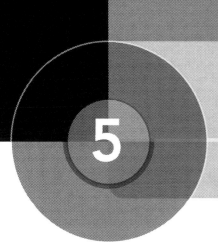

Health Promotion and Clients from Racially Diverse Communities

VERONA HALL

INTRODUCTION

The importance of addressing the issues surrounding racially diverse communities has grown exponentially in light of movements such as Black Lives Matter and Five X More, as well as recent reports which illustrate that these communities are at a noticeably higher risk of morbidity and mortality than white ethnic communities (Bharj & Salway, 2008; Haque et al., 2020; Kirkup, 2021). Although certainly there is more work to be done, this heightened awareness has led to changes, such as the identification of the need for culturally sensitive care (Benson et al., 2010; Cerdeña et al., 2020). It is important to note here though that this is not new information with Rocheron and Dickinson (1990) highlighting similar issues three decades earlier.

This issue is not isolated to the UK but is in fact a global issue. Affecting pregnant women and birthing people from racially diverse communities, not only in other high-income countries such as the USA, but around the world with non-white communities having poorer maternal health outcomes in general. With the UK's population becoming increasingly diverse, it is important to look at ways to address this imbalance, thus creating a more inclusive society. By understanding the factors that influence midwifery care, readers can evaluate whether they are upholding the fundamental rights of individuals, as well as embodying the International Confederation of Midwives (ICM) competencies for midwifery practice for inclusive midwifery care and practice (Barger et al., 2019).

The aim of this chapter is to examine the concepts of race, ethnicity and maternity outcomes. Whilst the author does not claim to have all the answers, the hope is to give the reader the opportunity to reflect on their own practice and the care provision provided by their hospitals and explore how we can find ways to work together to reduce this disparity improving maternity care for these women going forward.

DOI: 10.4324/9781003350071-5

TERMINOLOGY

There is currently little agreement in the UK about what language and terminology is acceptable when discussing how Black, Asian and minority ethnic (BAME) communities should be classified. This lack of agreement is viewed by many as perpetuating racial inequalities and 'white privilege' (Esegbona-Adeigbe, 2021).

Recently, the term 'BAME' has been heavily criticised. The UK Department of Ethnic Minority Advocates is currently investigating why the term is so problematic. The term 'BAME' is most often used when making comparisons between white and non-white populations, and appears effective in collecting and gathering statistics. However, the term 'BAME' often gives the false impression that all these individual communities share a singular or homogeneous ethnic identity. People assigned to a certain racial group do not necessarily share the same genetic ancestry with no underlying genetic or biological factors to unite them meaning that their health may not be accurately accessed leading to racial health disparities (Cerdeña at al., 2020).

The term 'people of colour' predominately used in the United States is becoming more commonly used now within the UK, viewed as a more positive term than BAME. Potentially, though it can be argued to be just as problematic, as it groups people who are racially diverse and share different experiences and identities without any regard for their differences.

Within the UK, the government have stopped using these terms in favour of the term racially diverse. This term seems to consider the diversity within ethnic groups, ensuring appropriate and correct terms are used and that ethnic diversity matters are not lost. It also allows practitioners to assess their biases and stereotypes to facilitate collaboration and cooperation, and to work in a culture-sensitive and people/family orientated manner (Barger et al., 2019).

By understanding the history and implications of the using certain words, the hope is that the practitioner will understand the complexity of the terminology used when talking about race and how it has changed over time. Furthermore, this understanding of language can reveal how prejudices and stereotypes influence the perception of racially diverse populations, and how this in turn can have negative consequences (Danso & Danso, 2021).

PRACTICE POINTS

- Think about what race or ethnic communities you are talking about, and by making sure the terms used accurately reflect the community.
- Refrain from using umbrella terms – no community is homogenous.
- Use current research to better identify, understand, and reflect on the experiences of different ethnic communities.
- Accept and acknowledge that ethnicity is an integral part of a person's identity, respect people's preferences, and be clear about how people describe their identities.
- Own your mistakes, and most importantly learn from them. It is not always possible to understand the terminology correctly. Apologise if you misunderstand terminology and cause offence.

UNCONSCIOUS BIAS AND RACISM

The meaning of race has changed over time to serve political objectives. It is a social power construct, not a scientific concept. For instance, race has historically been used to claim that racially diverse communities are biologically inferior (Roberts, 2011). However, race does not represent human variation well. The physical attributes distinguishing racial communities, which differ geographically and are not associated with underlying characteristics. Humans cannot be classified into biologically separate subgroups, according to genetic research (Mersha & Abebe, 2015; American Society of Human Genetics, 2018). However as different communities continue to mix and overlap, any existing genetic differences between them become less significant (Fuentes et al., 2019).

Race is often used as a shortcut in clinical medicine, even though there is no meaningful correlation between race and genetics. For example, when estimating renal function in Black patients, doctors adjust their calculations based on the assumption that Black people have more muscle mass than people in other races (Stevens & Levey, 2008). They may not be prescribed angiotensin-converting enzyme (ACE) inhibitors for hypertension, because they are thought to be less effective in them than in White patients (Stevens & Levey, 2008). Asian patients are thought to have higher visceral body fat than people of other races; they are more susceptible to developing diabetes at lower body mass indices (Hsu et al., 2015).

Research provides clear evidence of those from Black populations being used in medical trials and the outcome of which improved the care of those from white populations. For example, the Tuskegee Syphilis trial commenced in 1932 following the course of syphilis in black men and their families even after antibiotic treatment was available which continued till 1972. Dr J.M. Sim – considered to be the father of modern gynaecology – preformed many experimental surgeries on Black enslaved women, leading many modern authors to criticise his medical ethics and call for the re-naming of the instruments and procedures bearing his name to be changed to those who suffered these experimental procedures and recognise their suffering as most was carried out without pain relief (Wall, 2021).

Theories that stereotype about racially diverse communities impair the ability of doctors and health professionals to provide appropriate care is supported by evidence in the results of many reports (Lokugamage et al., 2019; Lokugamage & Meredith, 2020) and highlight how stereotypes and prejudice continue to silence racially diverse communities a sentiment that one might think has persisted 'since slavery'.

The perceptions and insights of racially diverse communities are key to exploring lived experiences, understanding social problems, and implementing action to eliminate inequalities and improve overall health for everyone. By understanding the unique perspectives of these communities, one can develop a more comprehensive understanding of social problems and work to create solutions that are more effective and inclusive (Fernandez Turienzo et al., 2021).

It is important to understand and recognise that colonialism has had a negative impact on health, both directly through aspects such as exploitation and disease and indirectly through aspects such as economic inequality (van Daalen et al., 2022). A way to dismantle racist structures globally is to identify, challenge and boycott those governments, organisations and persons that hold both overt and covert racists viewpoints. Additionally, we – both as individuals and as members of organisations that represent us – can support those who actively work to dismantle all forms of racism and bring about social change, as in the civil rights movement in the United States in the 1960s and the boycott of South Africa in the 1970s. The investigation and combating of these phenomena are crucial for health care provision and for midwives and other healthcare professionals globally, and in doing so will contribute to improved and sustainable health outcomes for those from these racially diverse communities (van Daalen et al., 2022).

Racism is multi-faceted and can be described on three important levels:

- Institutional (systemic) differentiates access to opportunities such as education, health care, employment, and housing.
- Personally mediated (interpersonal) prejudice or discrimination occurs when people are treated differently based on personal characteristics, which can be done implicitly or explicitly.
- Internalised is when the oppressed ethnically diverse community absorbs the negative views Society has of them and lowers their expectations of the care they will receive.

(Jones, 2000; Churchwell et al., 2020)

However not being 'racist' or 'biased' on a personal level is not enough. The goal is for all to be anti-racist and anti-bias at both a personal level and an institutional level. This distinction is important because it highlights how active participation

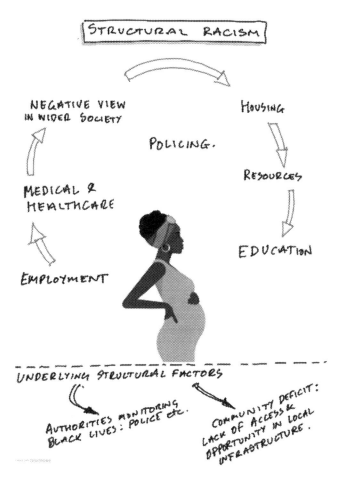

Figure 5.1 Conceptual framework of structural racism from the perspective of black African American women.

and understanding of structures, that systematically maintain and deprive individuals and communities of power, are necessary to create change (Douglass & Lokugamage, 2021) (Figure 5.1).

Racism is often so complex and multi-layered that it is not always conscious, obvious or easily visible to those perpetuating it. Systemic and structural racism are forms of racism that are widespread and deeply ingrained in systems, laws, written and unwritten policies, and ingrained practices and beliefs that create excuses, perpetuate widespread unfair treatment and oppression of racially diverse community, which in turn can and does lead to negative health consequences. Systemic racism is the structural and cultural racism that exists in institutions and society, while structural racism is the socioeconomic inequality that exists between different racially diverse communities (Chambers et al., 2021). It is therefore unsurprising that studies have found that racially diverse communities are less likely to take up health promotion initiatives.

You hear a colleague who is working with a student midwife say that she does not see colour. Her student asks if she is colour blind thinking that was what she is referring to. The midwife replies "No I mean treat everyone the same. I don't see a person's colour".

- What are your thoughts and feelings on hearing this?
- How could you deal with this situation?

WHAT WE KNOW

Maternity services data within the UK shows significant differences in care between women of racial diversity and those from white communities. With an almost four-fold difference in maternal mortality rates amongst women from Black ethnic backgrounds and an almost two-fold difference amongst women from Asian ethnic backgrounds compared to women from white ethnic backgrounds (Knight et al., 2016; Draper et al., 2021). Likewise, the highest infant mortality rate is also found among racially diverse communities in the UK (MacLellan et al., 2022; Matthews et al., 2022). Whilst the exact causes of the disparities are still to be fully determined, the history of racism and the growth of racist ideas and attitudes within the NHS, especially for women, has been well documented, with conscious and unconscious prejudice appearing to be a major contributing factor (Chambers et al., 2021; Peter & Wheeler, 2022; Ayorinde et al., 2023).

The UK government and Royal Colleges have released statements confirming that pregnant women from racially diverse communities face poorer health outcomes both in the short term and the long term (Douglass & Lokugamge, 2021). The NHS Long Term Plan has allocated funds to support the continuity of care for these women and those from the most deprived neighbourhoods (NHS England, 2019). This will help ensure that every woman has access to the care they need, regardless of their racial diversity or circumstances. This could create a significant difference, however without additional actions to get rid of inequalities and increase community engagement, it is doubtful that this will be enough (O'Mara-Eves et al., 2015).

Discussions about racism and unconscious bias are undoubtably uncomfortable and challenging. When one talks about racism, it is usually concerning white and non-white people. However, it is important to note that racism and unconscious bias can also be used between different racial and cultural communities. Although studies may use the terms 'white' and 'non-white' when discussing racism, it is important to remember that racism is not simply a black and white issue. With those with lighter skin often seen as more favoured or privileged (Herring, 2004).

Evidence indicates that midwives can have difficulty reconciling cultural and religious practices of women from racially diverse communities with hospital policies and guidelines and health advice. Clients felt they were judged harshly by the midwife (Aquino et al., 2015; Goodwin et al., 2018). Resulting in women and families feeling unsatisfied with their care and their relationship with their midwife. Goodwin et al. (2018) highlighted that midwives who failed to develop positive relationships with the women in their care were more likely to heavily condemn these women for their cultural practices for example fasting during Ramadan. While those midwives who established a positive relationship were more able to have a better understanding of these cultural practices and their impact on the client's care and the therapeutic relationship.

A literature review in 2021 exploring ethnic health inequalities in UK maternity services identified five clear themes:

- Communication
- The midwife-woman relationship
- Maternity services and systems
- Culture
- Social need

The review confirmed the issue of health inequalities and poorer maternity outcomes and questioned if any progress had happened in improving health inequalities among racially diverse communities within maternity services, in fact it was likely to have worsened (Marmot, 2020; Khan, 2021). As identified by Goodwin et al. in 2018, it is essential that current and future national policies consider the specific needs of women from racially diverse communities and support maternity care providers to modify their systems and services to meet these needs without judgement or bias (Goodwin et al., 2018).

The theme of culture (Khan, 2021) identified midwives and other maternity care health professionals as lacking in cultural awareness by the women. Impacting on attendance at antenatal appointments and parent education classes when female only staff could not be organised or guaranteed, and parent education classes could not be female only – both staff and attendees. Women from racially diverse communities also identified that requests for any cultural adjustments were not received positively, were time consuming and seen as a burden to an already busy workload for the staff. Disregard for the cultural needs will result in care that was not considered sensitive or responsive nor individualised (Aquino et al., 2015; Khan, 2021;).

To shift from a medical narrative that perpetuates disparity, change needs to happen. The current medical language and terminology used is based on white, Western ideology, which can be exclusionary to those from racially diverse communities (Churchwell et al., 2020). The use of the Apgar score tool is just one example, used to assess the adaptation of the baby to extra uterine life though colour, heart rate, respiration, muscle tone, and reflexes. It uses the phrase 'pink' to assess the level of oxygenated blood in the baby at birth. However, neonates with darker pigmentation may not appear pink and this may impact on the assessment and the care they receive. A pertinent factor given the higher mortality rate among babies of racially diverse populations (Mihoko et al., 2003).

Even in countries where maternal mortality rates are the lowest, there are still significant differences in outcomes between women from racially diverse communities (Khalil et al., 2023). These findings suggest there is a more complicated issue, both domestically and globally, which requires a greater understanding of this issue in order to develop interventions that lessen avoidable health consequences (Peterson et al., 2019).

Culturally sensitive interventions that engage with those from racially diverse communities with strong co-design interventions are necessary to address ethnicity-based health inequalities, while also acknowledging the implications of being racialised in the UK and it contributes to health disparities.

To fully understand the impact of maternity care on those from racially diverse communities, midwives and other health professionals need to identify opportunities for improvement. It is imperative to listen to the experiences of women, birthing people and their families from these communities. Their stories often go unheard or are only partially heard, leaving them with poor and suboptimal care as identified in the Black Maternity survey in 2022 (Peter & Wheeler, 2022) which highlighted some alarming experiences, some of which are illustrated in Figure 5.2.

HEALTH PROMOTION AND CLIENTS FROM RACIALLY DIVERSE COMMUNITIES

Health promotion is a comprehensive social and political process; not only encompassing action to strengthen individuals' skills and abilities but also action to change social, environmental and economic conditions to mitigate their impact on public and individual health. When midwives consider how women present and cope with health issues, they must always keep in mind the racial and cultural background of the women and their families.

The Western model of health and disease generally focuses on the idea that 'disease' is about the malfunctioning or decreased psychological and biological processes of a particular organ or body system. It may therefore be viewed differently in those clients from racially diverse communities. Patients may focus on the experience and psychocultural aspects of the illness and their respective society's response to it, rather than the 'illness' itself (O'Mahony & Donnelly, 2007). Understanding the body and how it functions, as well as the causes and treatments of disease, will be only part of the issue when looking at someone's health belief. Information exchange and health discussions by the midwife and the pregnant person will also vary greatly depending on their ethnicity, values, culture, worldview, and religion of both the midwife and the woman. It will also be impacted upon by their understanding of each other.

People's health beliefs are also shaped by their level of education. Some people may hold multiple belief systems, transitioning between them as their own education or that of the general population improves (Juckett, 2005; – see Chapter 9 for further information on health lifestyles and changing behaviours).

For women, childbirth is one of life's most significant events and it is culturally shaped and socially constructed (Ottani, 2002). For instance, while some African women may view childbirth as a natural event not requiring special medical care or attention this is in contrast to the Western model, which emphasises vigilant observation and prompt intervention when needed with nothing considered normal except in retrospect.

In a similar way, what people believe about the management of the illness may also be affected and determined by culture. For example, the use of herbs, foods and complimentary medicines plays a crucial role in many ethnically diverse cultures such as the balance of 'hot' and 'cold' foods and their role in maintaining the balance between health and illness, especially during pregnancy, birth, and the postnatal period. This may put the client and their family at odds with their midwife or

Women who do not speak English are an issue in our Asian culture and interpreting is an issue

I forgot to mention some Islamic practices. When I told the midwife, I wanted to add items to my birth plan, she looked annoyed and said we did this last week.

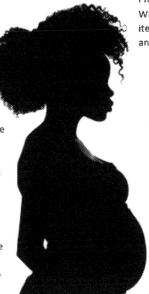

At my first visit with the midwife, she was surprised that I knew who the father was. As people like me usually don't know.

There was a sense that the midwives felt I could handle the pain. I was left alone to give birth to my baby in the toilet.

I didn't like taking the courses, because it was uncomfortable because there were a mix of women and men. Where is my privacy with these men?

The midwife said, moments after I gave birth, that we will see you next year anyway. Which I felt implying that because I'm Somali I'll just end up giving birth every year.

One midwife when doing the cervical sweep said the reason for slow dilation for me was due to an African pelvis – even though I was in pain I was mortified that she actually believed there was an African pelvis.

I had an episiotomy and, afterwards, the stitches fell out. I am high risk of infection due to my sickle cell. They kept refusing to have a look. By the time a doctor looked, the stitches had already fallen out and the wound was infected, causing a sickle cell crisis.

Figure 5.2 Black Women's experience of maternity services in the UK.

Source: Adapted from Peter and Wheeler (2022).

maternity health care professional potentially affecting health promotion activities (Lipson & Meleis, 1983).

In certain cases, some cultural accepted behaviours will not only put the client and their family at odds with the midwife and maternity health professional but also in conflict with Society as a whole, the government and its laws. As with female genital cutting (FGC) affecting over to 200 million girls and women worldwide including an estimated 170,000 in the UK. This culturally accepted behaviour has no proven health benefits and a long list of immediate and long-term health issues that will affect the person's physical, mental, sexual, and socio-economic domains of their health for the rest of their life (WHO, 2024). It is embedded in the social, religious and cultural ideals of femininity, modesty, and female sexual behaviour in some 30 countries in Africa, the Middle East and Asia (WHO, 2024). Although an illegal practice and identified by the WHO as a violation of the human rights of women and girls (WHO, 2024), many midwives and maternity health care professionals will care for women who have undergone FGC. The midwife needs to be careful to maintain a balance between cultural sensitivity, their own moral and ethical views, and the laws of the land in which they practice. This is vital in the care and support of clients who have undergone FGC, encouraging them to be open and not feel judged (WHO, 2022).

The underutilisation of public health and health promotion initiatives and services by those from racially diverse communities is an issue frequently reported in the media. It hit a peak during the COVID-19 pandemic, when within the UK, there was wide-scale suspicion and conspiracy talk and clear evidence of those from these communities dying at a higher rate than those from white populations (Meer et al., 2020). Uptake of the COVID-19 vaccine was affected leading to the public health agencies reaching out to prominent people from racially diverse communities to promote the importance of the COVID-19 vaccination in the media (Razai et al., 2021; see Chapter 18 on vaccinations and the impact of a global pandemic). However, it is also important to note the impact of a motivated, diverse, inclusive, and valued workforce, can never be underestimated. As documented by Ali et al. (2012), the diversity within the workforce makes a massive contribution in terms of quality patient care, higher patient satisfaction and engagement and improving uptake to public health and health promotion initiatives. By valuing the diversity of our workforce, we can improve the quality of care for all patients.

These patterns can also be seen in reproductive health outcomes. Women from Black communities have lower in vitro fertilisation (IVF) birth rates and tend to access and start IVF at a later age when compared to other racially diverse communities and those from white communities. Babies born to women from Black and Asian communities have an increased risk of premature births, low birth weight, and stillbirth than those from white communities. Access to public health screening programmes for cervical cancer and breast are similarly affected. With access likely to be lower in those from racially diverse communities. This may be in part due to the social construct of what it is to be a woman within these communities as well as poor and less frequent services and health service delivery. This then impacts on the diagnosis rates which is higher and poorer prognosis (Bolarinwa & Holt, 2023). Consider how to make healthcare system more inclusive and contemplate how to implement this

"I Don't See Colour"

Earlier you were asked to note your thoughts and feelings about a midwife who indicated to the student she was working with that she 'did not see colour and treated everyone the same'.

Some of your considerations may be indicated below:

- The midwife may feel this is a neutral stance – trying to show that they treat all pregnant clients the same irrespective of the colour of their skin.
- However, unless they have achromatopsia, a rare condition that causes a person to unable to see colours, we all see colours in some form.

- When meeting a person, the colour of their skin is a distinguishable feature that cannot be hidden or disguised.
- As midwives and maternity healthcare professionals, we should recognise those from racially diverse communities and work with them to be able to help us as midwives and maternity health professionals to better understand their needs and how to tailor care to those specific needs.
- To not see a person's colour may impact on their health outcome.

SUMMARY

This chapter has discussed health promotion and women and birthing people from racially diverse communities.

- The Western medical model is not always applicable in a Society with racial diversity.
- Racism is so deeply rooted that it counteracts colonisation.
- Unconscious bias and racism appeared to be the common thread throughout current research and are the key factor in the disparity that racially diverse communities have poorer maternity outcomes.
- It has highlighted the complexity of the terminology and the nervousness of not wanting to offend.
- There is a call for more education regarding the use of racially appropriate medical terminology.
- There is a call for more education and awareness about culturally sensitive care for all student and qualified midwives and other maternity care professionals.
- There are initiatives and campaigns that are trying to restore balance.
- Insights have been gained into how racially diverse communities in the UK population perceive the care they receive.
- The story leads us to understand why the racially diverse population that makes up the UK, there a lack of trust in the Western healthcare system by those from racially diverse communities.
- That midwives and other maternity health care professionals as both an individual and members of official organisations that represent them call out governments, policies, guidelines and individuals that hold both overt and covert racist views and beliefs.

Consider how to make healthcare system more inclusive and contemplate how to implement this

REFERENCES

Ali, S., Burns, C., & Grant, L. (2012). Equality and diversity in the health service: An evidence-led culture change. *Journal of Psychological Issues in Organizational Culture*, 3(1), 41–60.

American Society of Human Genetics. (2018). ASHG denounces attempts to link genetics and racial supremacy. *American Journal of Human Genetics*, 103(5), 636. https://doi.org/10.1016/j.ajhg.2018.10.011

Aquino, M. R., Edge, D., & Smith, D. M. (2015). Pregnancy as an ideal time for intervention to address the complex needs of black and minority ethnic women: Views of British midwives. *Midwifery, 31*, 373–379.

Ayorinde, A., Esan, O. B., Buabeng, R., Taylor, B., & Salway, S. (2023). Ethnic inequalities in maternal health. *British Medical Journal, 381*, 1–2. https://doi.org/10.1136/bmj.p1040

Barger, M. K., Hackley, B., Bharj, K. K., Luyben, A., & Thompson, J. B. (2019). Knowledge and use of the ICM global standards for midwifery education. *Midwifery, 79*, 102534.

Benson, J., Maldari, T., Williams, M. J., & Hanifi, M. H. (2010). The impact of culture and ethnicity on women's perceived role in society and their attendant health beliefs. *InnovAiT, 3*(6), 358–365. https://doi.org/10.1093/innovait/inp227

Bharj, K., & Salway, S. (2008). *Addressing ethnic inequalities in maternity service experiences and outcomes: responding to women's needs and preferences.* A race equality better health briefing paper. Race Equality Foundation. Addressing ethnic inequalities in maternity service experiences and outcomes: responding to women's needs and preferences. Briefing 11 (raceequalityfoundation.org.uk)

Bolarinwa, O. A., & Holt, N. (2023). Barriers to breast and cervical screening uptake among Black, Asian and minority ethnic women in the UK: Evidence from a mixed method systematic review. *BMC Health Services Research, 23*(390), 2–17. https://doi.org/10.1186/s12913-023-09410-x

Cerdeña, J., Plaisime, M., & Tsai, J. (2020). From race-based to race-conscious medicine: how anti-racist uprisings call us to act. *Lancet, 396*,1125–1128.

Chambers, B. D., Arega, H. A., Arabia, S. E., Taylor, B., Barron, R. G., Gates, B., … & McLemore, M. R. (2021). Black women's perspectives on structural racism across the reproductive lifespan: A conceptual framework for measurement development. *Maternal and Child Health Journal, 25*, 402–413.

Churchwell, K., Elkind, M. S., Benjamin, R. M., Carson, A. P., Chang, E. K., Lawrence, W., & American Heart Association. (2020). Call to action: structural racism as a fundamental driver of health disparities: A presidential advisory from the American Heart Association. *Circulation, 142*(24), e454–e468.

Danso, A., & Danso, Y. (2021). The complexities of race and health. *Future Healthcare Journal, 8*(1), 22–27.

Douglass, C., & Lokugamage, A. (2021). Racial profiling for induction of labour: Improving safety or perpetuating racism? *British Medical Journal, 375*, 1–2. https://doi.org/10.1136/bmj.n2562

Draper, E. S., Gallimore, I. D., Smith, L. K., Fenton, A. C., Kurinczuk. J. J., Smith, P. W., & Manktelow, B. N. (2021). *MBRRACE – UK Perinatal Mortality Surveillance report. UK perinatal deaths for births from January to December 2019.* MBRRACE-UK_Perinatal_Surveillance_Report_2019_-_Final_v2.pdf (ox.ac.uk)

Esegbona-Adeigbe, S. (2021). The impact of a eurocentric curriculum on racial disparities in maternal health. *European Journal of Midwifery, 5*, 36. https://doi.org/10.18332/ejm/140086

Fernandez Turienzo, C., Newburn, M., Agyepong, A., Buabeng, R., Dignam, A., Abe, C., … & NIHR ARC South London Maternity and Perinatal Mental Health Research and Advisory Teams Anna Horn. (2021). Addressing inequities in maternal health among women living in communities of social disadvantage and ethnic diversity. *BMC Public Health, 21*, 1–5.

Fuentes, A., Ackermann, R. R., Athreya, S., Bolnick, D., Lasisi, T., Lee, S. H., … & Nelson, R. (2019). AAPA statement on race and racism. *American Journal of Physical Anthropology*, *169*(3), 400–402.

Goodwin, L., Hunter, B., & Jones, A. (2018). The midwife–woman relationship in a South Wales community: Experiences of midwives and migrant Pakistani women in early pregnancy. *Health Expectations*, *21*(1), 347–357.

Haque, E. U., Choudry, B., & George, R. E. (2020). How can we improve health and healthcare experiences of Black, Asian and Minority Ethnic (BAME) communities?. In Matheson J, Patterson J and Neilson L (eds.), *Tackling causes and consequences of health inequalities: A practical guide* (pp. 233–244). CRC Press.

Hsu, W. C., Araneta, M. R. G., Kanaya, A. M., Chiang, J. L., & Fujimoto, W. (2015). BMI cut points to identify at-risk Asian Americans for type 2 diabetes screening. *Diabetes Care*, *38*(1), 150–158. https://doi.org/10.2337/dc14–2391

Jones, C. P. (2000). Levels of racism: A theoretic framework and a gardener's tale. *American Journal of Public Health*, *90*(8), 1212–1215.

Juckett, G. (2005). Cross-cultural medicine. *American Family Physician*, *72*(11), 2267–2274.

Khalil, A., Samara, A., O'Brien, P., Coutinho, C. M., Quintana, S. M., & Ladhani, S. N. (2023). A call to action: the global failure to effectively tackle maternal mortality rates. *The Lancet Global Health*, *11*(8), e1165–e1167.

Khan, Z. (2021). Ethnic health inequalities in the UK's maternity services: A systematic literature review. *British Journal of Midwifery*, *29*(2), 100–107.

Kirkup, B. (2021). The Health and Social Care Committee's Expert Panel: Evaluation of the Government's Commitments in the Area of Maternity Services in England. Written Evidence Health and Social Care Committee. House of Commons.

Knight, M., Nair, M., Tuffnell, D., Kenyon, S., Shakespeare, J., Brocklehurst, P., & Kurinczuk, J. (2016). *Saving lives, improving mothers' care: Surveillance of maternal deaths in the UK 2012–14 and lessons learned to inform maternity care from the UK and Ireland confidential enquiries into maternal deaths and morbidity 2009–14*. Oxuniprint. MBRRACE-UK: Mothers and Babies: Reducing Risk through Audits and Confidential Enquiries across the UK | MBRRACE-UK | NPEU (ox.ac.uk)

Lipson, J. G., & Meleis, A. I. (1983). Issues in health care of Middle Eastern patients. *Western Journal of Medicine*, *139*(6), 854–861.

Lokugamage, A. (2019). Maternal mortality—undoing systemic biases and privileges. *The BMJ Opinion blog*, 8.

Lokugamage, A., & Meredith, A. (2022). Women from ethnic minorities face endemic structural racism when seeking and accessing healthcare. *The BMJ Opinion* (online).

MacLellan, J., Collins, S., Myatt, M., Pope, C., Knighton, W., & Rai, T. (2022). Black, Asian and minority ethnic women's experiences of maternity services in the UK: A qualitative evidence synthesis. *Journal of advanced nursing*, *78*(7), 2175–2190.

Marmot, M. (2020). Society and the slow burn of inequality. *The Lancet*, *395*(10234), 1413–1414.

Matthews, R. J., Draper, E. S., Manktelow, B. N., Kurinczuk, J. J., Fenton, A. C., Dunkley-Bent, J., … & Smith, L. K. (2022). Understanding ethnic inequalities in stillbirth rates: A UK population-based cohort study. *BMJ open*, *12*(2), e057412.

Meer, N., Qureshi, K., Kasstan, B., & Hill, S. (2020). The social determinants of COVID 19 and BAME disproportionality. *Discover Society*, *30*.

Mersha, T. B., & Abebe, T. (2015). Self-reported race/ethnicity in the age of genomic research: its potential impact on understanding health disparities. *Human Genomics, 9*, 1–15.

Mihoko Doyle, J., Echevarria, S., & Parker Frisbie, W. (2003). Race/ethnicity, Apgar and infant mortality. *Population Research and Policy Review, 22*, 41–64.

NHS England. (2019). *The NHS Long Term Plan: NHS 2019.* Accessed 10 May 2023. NHS England » The NHS Long Term Plan

O'Mahony, J. M., & Donnelly, T. T. (2007). The influence of culture on immigrant women's mental health care experiences from the perspectives of health care providers. *Issues in Mental Health Nursing, 28*(5), 453–471.

O'Mara-Eves, A., Brunton, G., Oliver, S., Kavanagh, J., Jamal, F., & Thomas, J. (2015). The effectiveness of community engagement in public health interventions for disadvantaged groups: A meta-analysis. *BMC Public Health, 15*, 1–23.

Ottani, P. A. (2002). Embracing global similarities: A framework for cross-cultural obstetric care. *Journal of Obstetric, Gynecologic, & Neonatal Nursing, 31*(1), 33–38.

Peter, M., & Wheeler, R. (2022). *The Black maternity experiences survey a nationwide study of Black women's experiences of maternity services in the United Kingdom.* Black maternal experinces report — FIVEXMORE

Petersen, E. E., Davis, N. L., Goodman, D., Cox, S., Syverson, C., Seed, K., … & Barfield, W. (2019). Racial/ethnic disparities in pregnancy-related deaths-United States, 2007–2016. *Morbidity and Mortality Weekly Report, 68*(35), 762–765.

Razai, M. S., Osama, T., McKechnie, D. G. J., & Majeed, A. (2021). COVID-19 hesitancy among ethnic minority groups. *BMJ, 372*(513). https://doi.org/10.1136/bmj.n513

Roberts, D. (2011). *Fatal invention: How science, politics, and big business re-create race in the twenty-first century.* New Press/ORIM.

Rocheron, Y., & Dickinson, R. (1990). The Asian mother and baby campaign: A way forward in health promotion for Asian women? *Health Education Journal, 49*(3), 128–133.

Stevens, L., & Levey, A. (2008). National kidney foundation. Frequently asked questions about gfr estimates. 12-10-kidney.org/sites/default/files/441-8491_2202_faqs_aboutgfr_v5.pdf

van Daalen, K. R., Kaiser, J., Kebede, S., Cipriano, G., Maimouni, H., Olumese, E., … & Oliver-Williams, C. (2022). Racial discrimination and adverse pregnancy outcomes: A systematic review and meta-analysis. *BMJ Global Health, 7*(8), e009227.

Wall, L. L. (2021). The Sims position and the Sims vaginal speculum, re-examined. *International Urogynecology Journal, 32*(10), 2595–2601.

World Health Organisation. (2022). *Integrating female genital mutilation content in to nursing and midwifery curricula: A practical Guide.* Integrating female genital mutilation content into nursing and midwifery curricula: a practical guide (who.int)

World Health organisation. (2024). Female Genital Mutilation Female genital mutilation (who.int).

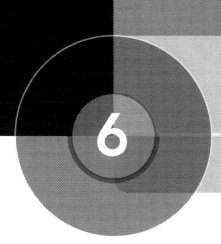

Health Promotion Considerations for Clients from the LGBTQ+ Community Embarking on Starting a Family

TERESA ARIAS, GRACE HOWARD, AND CLAIRE SINGH

INTRODUCTION

This chapter will introduce the reader to common life experiences of lesbian, gay, bisexual, trans, and queer+ (LGBTQ+) people during and around the perinatal period. For the purpose of this chapter, the term LGBTQ+ will be used throughout to describe this community of people (Greenfield & Darwin, 2021). It is hoped that by providing an insight into some of these experiences and challenges, midwives and health care professionals (HCPs) could be better informed and prepared to provide a safe clinical encounter for a member of this community. A glossary of terms used in this chapter is provided. The reader is encouraged to engage with the activities provided throughout the chapter. They have been set to support self-reflection and an appraisal of experiences of working within the health arena.

GLOSSARY OF TERMS

Definitions of terms used in this chapter have been provided to aid understanding but are not exhaustive. Though simplified for ease and chosen from a wide range of reliable sources (Silver, 2022; Stonewall, 2023). The experience of the LGBTQ+ community during conception, pregnancy, and birth remains largely invisible as pregnancy continues to be seen through a heteronormative lens (Charter et al., 2018; Darwin & Greenfield, 2019). In many countries, the numbers of people within the LGBTQ+ community are

DOI: 10.4324/9781003350071-6

undocumented and unknown as this data is rarely collected on sexual orientation of people who are pregnant or their partners. The UK Census for 2021 informs us that 3.2% population (1.5 million people) identify as lesbian, gay, and bisexual (Office of National Statistics [ONS], 2023a) and that 0.5% population (262,000) answered that they did not identify with the sex they were registered as at birth (ONS, 2023b). In the UK, this is the first time that enquiry has been made relating to gender identity. We also know that in the UK the live births registered to same sex couples is rising from 608 in 2011 to 2,533 in 2022 (ONS, 2023c), further emphasising that the 'one-size-fits-all' approach to maternity is not sufficient. These statistics are significant. The WHO (2022) reminds us that the right to health must be experienced without discrimination and that this extends to sexual orientation and gender identity. Midwives and HCPs therefore have a legal and moral duty to treat LGBTQ + people without discrimination.

Personalised care is, of course, the only way to give truly meaningful care as not every LGBTQ+ person is the same; however, research highlights that this group face some distinct challenges which may affect their access to healthcare, their experience of it and their ability to conceive (Greenfield & Darwin, 2021). It is hoped that by providing an insight into some of these experiences and challenges, midwives and HCPs can be better informed and prepared to provide a safe clinical encounter for a member of this community.

It is important to recognise that gender identity and sexual orientation is personal and complex. Some of these terms may not be favoured by every individual, therefore it is recommended that you ask the person to define the terms they feel comfortable with (Table 6.1).

Table 6.1 Glossary of terms

Bisexual	A person who is attracted to other people of the same or other genders/sexes.
Cis or cis-gendered	A person whose gender identity is the same as the sex assigned at birth.
Come out	Self disclosure of a person's sexual orientation, romantic orientation or gender identity
Dead-naming	Using an individual's previous name that no longer identifies with their gender.
Dysphoria	A disconnect between the person and their identity to the body they are in, often felt as discomfort or distress.
Gay	A person attracted to their own gender. This can also be used broader term for any sexual identity other than heterosexual.
Gender identity	An individual's psychological sense of self not linked to biological sex. Gender is a social construct which has been reinforced through cultural and societal norms.
Gender expression	An outward representation of gender through clothes, demeanour, actions
Gestational parent	The person who carried (gestated) the pregnancy.
Heteronormativity	The presumption of heterosexuality
Heterosexuality	A person attracted to the opposite gender.
Homosexuality	A person attracted to the same gender.

(Continued)

Table 6.1 (Continued) Glossary of terms

Lesbian	A woman who is attracted to other women.
Non-binary	A person who does not identify with the 'traditional' gender labels of male or female.
Pronouns	Can include (but not exhaustive): he/him, she/her, they/them, ze/zem. Please note that someone's choice of pronouns does not equal their gender or sex.
Queer	A person who is either not cis-gendered or heterosexual. Some members of the community still prefer not to use this term as it can be used as a slur.
Sexual orientation	Relates to who one is sexually attracted to. It is often, incorrectly, conflated with gender identity
Transgender	A person whose gender differs from their assigned sex at birth. In the UK, people who identify as transgender do not need to undergo surgery or take hormonal treatment.

Sources: Silver (2022); LGBT foundation (2023); and Stonewall (2023).

BACKGROUND

LGBTQ+ people face discrimination and exclusion worldwide (Hughes et al., 2016). There are still 70 countries across the globe where it is a criminal offence to be in a same-sex relationship; in 11 of these there is evidence of the death penalty being used as a punishment (Stonewall, 2020). This global concern has initiated responses from the United Nations (UN) acknowledging the direct impact of social discrimination on LGBTQ+ health and wellbeing (UN, 2015). More recently the WHO announced a guideline in development that will focus on evidence and guidance on implementation of interventions to increase access to and respectful care for trans and gender diverse people within health care sectors (WHO, 2023). This section will focus on the impact of social discrimination and isolation on the mental and physical health and wellbeing of LGBTQ+ people.

When compared to their heterosexual and cis counterparts, members of the LGBTQ+ community are at an increased risk of poor mental health (King et al., 2008; Stonewall, 2018). High numbers of LGBTQ+ people experience anxiety, depression, and suicidal thoughts which is highlighted in Stonewall's 2018 survey of over 5,000 LGBT people across the UK. In this report, over 52% of LGBT people stated they had experienced depression in the previous year, more than two in five (42%) saying they have felt, at some stage in the previous year, that life was not worth living. This troubling statistic increases to 70% if the LGBT person is aged between 18 and 24 (Stonewall, 2018). This same survey highlighted that 12% of trans people made an attempt on their own life in the previous year which is six times higher than their LGB counterparts.

It is important to consider the possible reasons and factors that contribute to higher mental illness in the LGBTQ+ community. Many people in this community experience forms of rejection or hostility that can lead to social isolation (Garcia et al., 2019). This can be from family members, friends, and colleagues potentially when they 'come-out', increasing the stress of daily life. As members of a minority group, there are fewer people to identify with and have true shared experiences. The separation and loneliness that can be experienced by LGBTQ+ people can be caused by feeling separate as Society deems them different (Elmer et al., 2022).

Members of the trans community are disproportionately affected by violence (Lombardi et al., 2002) and other trauma (Mizock & Lewis, 2008). Transphobia, a hatred towards or fear of those who are trans, has seen a sharp increase in the UK and other countries in the last five years (Gov.UK, 2023). Poor mental health and suicidality link with the stigma and traumatic encounters stemming from transphobia encountered within a community (Bockting et al., 2013; McNeil et al., 2017). These sobering facts are important to be aware of to help inform the care you will be giving and provide a wider context for potential mental health concerns or trauma.

EXPERIENCE OF HEALTH SERVICES

LGBTQ+ people report experiencing many obstacles in trying to access culturally competent and affirming healthcare including financial, personal, and cultural barriers. The anxiety around these barriers may result in a delay in accessing screening or preventative health care (Moseson et al., 2020). One in eight LGBTQ+ people experience unequal treatment by midwives and other HCPs and one in four have observed derogatory remarks made by midwives and other HCPs about LGBTQ+ people (Somerville, 2015). Hesitancy and fear are common feelings when accessing health services as previous encounters may have been unsatisfactory and even harmful. This can lead to anticipation of bias from the midwife or HCP which can result in increased avoidance in engaging with these services, increasing their risk of health disparities (Broholm et al., 2023).

Insensitive care given by midwives and other HCPs, ranging from ignoring the person's sexual orientation to the giving of inappropriate health care (The National LGB&T partnership, 2017) highlighting a lack of competence amongst midwives and other HCPs (Yingling et al., 2017). The assumptions made of sexual orientation and gender identity by midwives and HCPs mean that LGBTQ+ people are faced with having to decide when or of to disclose their personal details in an environment that does not feel familiar or safe to them.

It is necessary that we challenge our assumptions as midwives. This often starts with the self-reflection of our own prejudices, expectations, and judgements and minding our own unconscious bias. Tackling the knowledge, beliefs, and attitudes of HCPs is a process that involves both individual reflection and reflexivity and cultural and societal shift.

REFLECTION

- What have you learnt about the LGBTQ+ community from reading the section above?
- Have you cared for anyone from the LGBTQ+ community in your capacity as a midwife or HCP?
- If the answer is Yes, reflect on how you felt and why you might have felt this?
- If the answer is No, how would you feel in caring for a person from this community and why do you think you would feel like this?

PRE-CONCEPTION CONVERSATIONS FOR THE LGBTQ+ COMMUNITY

The pursuit of biological parenthood for persons from the LGBTQ+ community is not a decision that is taken lightly. This pursuit can include the potential birthing person, a partner, and a wider team of healthcare professionals. The availability of assisted conception methods may vary according to the country, but it is important to note that whichever method is chosen, there are physical and emotional considerations that may impact on the prospective parents. The appointments, medication,n and financial costs may also impact on the health and wellbeing of that person and family.

People from the LGBTQ+ community are likely to face a series of challenges including the need to 'prove' themselves as fit to become parents as part of the registered fertility clinic process. The pathway to parenthood for LGBTQ+ people ranges from home insemination to sophisticated technologies offered by fertility clinics; whichever route taken involves emotional commitment and physical preparation.

ACCESSING FERTILITY TREATMENT FOR LGBTQ+ PEOPLE

We will be addressing fertility treatments for people wishing to have a genetic link to their child (either the gestational parent or their partner). As we have discussed, for people from the LGBTQ+ community, their previous health service interaction may not always have been a positive one, so embarking on an assisted conception journey can be daunting and overwhelming. The first step is usually seeking advice and guidance via their medical practitioner.

USING FERTILITY CLINIC SERVICES

There are several methods of assisted conception available (see Table 6.2). Ongoing costs associated with fertility clinics include the storage of any eggs/sperm or embryos as there may be rolling annual storage fee. A time limit for this storage may depend on the payment of these annual fees.

Whether funding for accessing fertility clinic services is state or insurance funded or privately paid for, this should not change the standards of care expected. Counselling for prospective parents may be provided by the clinic however legal documentation is likely to be integral to the process of assisted conception. This process is particular to the country where these services are offered. The Human Fertilisation and Embryology Authority (FHEA) is the regulatory body that governs the legal process in the UK.

In the UK, if fertility clinics services are utilised, the legal protection of both parents is considered and addressed through the paperwork that both parents would be required to in full if they wish to be registered as the legal parents of the child, this may be different in other Countries. Finally, fertility clinics may not be a viable option for many people due to the financial costs. Home insemination by a sperm donor may be chosen instead but this may mean that rigorous health checks may not be considered or performed.

Table 6.2 Assisted conception methods that might be available your region/country of practice

	Method
Donor insemination	Sperm is put inside the vagina of the intended birthing person. There are several ways they can access sperm for conception. Via a registered sperm bank or by private sperm donation which is unregulated. It is advisable that if a private sperm donor is chosen that the sperm donor gets tested for sexually transmitted diseases. It is also important to note that outside of licenced fertility clinics, the history of possible inherited conditions is not always known.
Intrauterine insemination (IUI)	Intrauterine insemination is often chosen by lesbian parents as it is suitable for people who need to utilise donated sperm. It is the least invasive form of assisted conception and involves having the sperm inserted into the uterus.
Assisted IUI	Assisted IUI follows the path of IUI, with the addition of fertility drugs which offers more control over the birthing parents' menstrual cycle
In Vitro fertilisation (IVF)	IVF is often used if IUI has not been successful or there may be underlying fertility issues for the birthing parent, such as low egg quality. IVF can have a more physical impact on the person that is having the egg collection, due to the required assisted conception medication
Reciprocal IVF	Works in the same way as IVF with the assisted conception outside of the body, however it is a method chose by some same sex female couples where one of the females is impregnated with the egg of their partner that will have undergone IVF.

ACCESSING ASSISTED CONCEPTION SERVICES OUTSIDE OF A CLINIC AND LEGAL CONSIDERATIONS

As mentioned earlier, for LGBTQ+ people embarking on a pregnancy via a fertility clinic (State or private), they may be required to complete a lot of legal paperwork which confirms their right to be documented as the child's parent on the birth certificate. This is an important consideration for any person who does not pursue pregnancy through a fertility clinic but accesses sperm donor through private sperm donation or indeed a surrogate who is sought privately.

For a same sex male couple, the options are more limited to surrogacy. In some countries, surrogacy is legal, and is often a service that is non-profitable, meaning that the surrogate may only be paid expenses and may not be paid a sum of money to carry the child. There are specific legal considerations regarding surrogacy, that should be discussed, as the surrogate remains the legal parent of the baby at birth, until a later time that a parental order may be put in place, for the surrogate to be able to legally hand the baby over, this would then be followed by adoption. For midwives and other HCPs, this is something to consider, as the baby would be discharged to the care of the surrogate parent. As the process of surrogacy comes with many legal considerations, it is highly likely that all parties involved would be fully aware of this.

PRACTICE POINTS

- In the UK, there is a legal requirement by the FHEA to hold information about all the donors and all donor conceived children.
- Therefore, it is possible for the child born from donor conception to connect with the donor once they have reached the age of 18.
- Parents must be married or have used a registered clinic for the non-gestational parent to be registered as a parent on the child's birth certificate.

ACTIVITY

- Identify the legal requirements for LGBTQ+ parents in your region/country of practice- what are the requirements for birth parents to be registered as parents in your area?
- Is surrogacy legally in your region/ country of practice?
- How are fertility clinics in your region/country of practice accessed?
- What do you know about these services? Are these services privately funded through insurance/the birthing person/or available free via the health system?
- Are these services accessible to all of the LGBTQ+ community?

ACCESSING MATERNITY CARE

We have learnt that LGBTQ+ people's experience of life, healthcare and assisted conception may result in different challenges compared to their cis gendered, heterosexual counterparts. Applying this knowledge of common experiences, we will now consider how you might adapt your clinical practice to provide safe, inclusive, and personalised care to a member of the LGBTQ+ community during the perinatal period.

LANGUAGE AND COMMUNICATION

Language and communication are key cornerstones in working with all service users on a pregnancy journey; as HCPs, to give personalised care we have learnt to make adjustments to our language to enhance understanding and comprehension. When we work with a family whose language is different to ours, it is incumbent on the HCP to adjust communication such as using simpler terms or avoiding medical jargon. Minor communication adjustments can make a major difference to the experience of members of the LGBTQ+ community whilst understanding that language and communication is nuanced and personal to the individual.

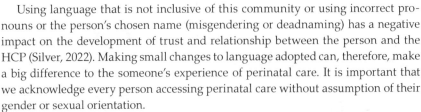

Using language that is not inclusive of this community or using incorrect pronouns or the person's chosen name (misgendering or deadnaming) has a negative impact on the development of trust and relationship between the person and the HCP (Silver, 2022). Making small changes to language adopted can, therefore, make a big difference to the someone's experience of perinatal care. It is important that we acknowledge every person accessing perinatal care without assumption of their gender or sexual orientation.

A simple act to communicate awareness of diversity in our population and avoid reinforcing heteronormative or gender normative values is to introduce one's name and pronouns. By asking how the person would like to be named and asking their pronouns, we communicate our intention to provide personalised and respectful care and avoid misgendering or deadnaming the person, which can cause distress. An example of an introduction is:

"Hello my name is Samantha, my pronouns are she/her. How would you prefer I address you and what are your pronouns?"

Midwives and HCPs may worry that cisgender patients may take offence or not understand this approach. A simple explanation could accompany this approach by signalling the intention to treat everyone respectfully without making assumptions based on appearance and name. The HCP should use the person's preferred name, and this should be documented and highlighted as such, along with any specific considerations for when/who the name and pronouns should be used. For example, some service users may have family members attend appointments with them and they may not be aware of their transition or sexual orientation. This must be respected.

Not acknowledging the chosen name or identified pronouns can cause psychological harm and jeopardise trust (Silver, 2022). It is also worth considering how best to apply this when addressing all patients in the waiting area, so as not to cause upset or harm, or risk of publicly 'outing' without the person's consent. Rather than calling out 'Mr or Miss', it may be prudent to say Patient Smith (Neira & Bowman, 2022).

To truly personalise the language that we use we need to ask the person. Talking about previous health care experiences, expectations and fears may be helpful in order for the HCP to tailor their care to those needs and enhance psychological and physical safety. It is important, however, to only ask questions that are relevant to the person's health care as this community have reported that they are often the asked questions that are not relevant to their health and demonstrates inappropriate curiosity (McEwing et al., 2022). Intrusive questioning of this sort, that seems unrelated to the provision of healthcare, has also been reported to contribute to feelings of discomfort in the clinical space (Stonewall, 2018; Malmquist et al., 2019).

A widely accepted approach when speaking to or about a group of parents is to use gender-additive language. For example, 'women and birthing people' or 'women and pregnant people' in order to both acknowledge the experiences of women using the services as well as those who identify differently (Green & Riddington, 2020).

Considering the needs of non-gestational parents, there can be feelings of exclusion from the pregnancy and birth process. The experience of some non-gestational mothers may feel that they are being 'othered' or isolated from the gestational mother in lesbian couples. Some non-gestational parents report being treated as though their role of parent is inferior to their partners, sometimes with the pregnancy carrier being referred to as the 'real parent' (Abelsohn et al., 2013). During the antenatal period, the opportunities for antenatal education can be negatively impacted if the HCP does not use terminology that is inclusive of LGBTQ+ families. Often the experience of attending antenatal classes may bring about another round of required explanation and 'outing', to other expectant parents and the expectant LGBTQ+ parent or parents having to address social awkwardness and questions.

LGBTQ+ parents may be especially anxious about the intrapartum period as the unpredictability of the unfolding events may limit the control over issues to do with maintaining their privacy and confidentiality. Assumptions should not be made regarding preferences of mode or place of birth as every person is different (Silver, 2022); however, the literature highlights a preference for continuity of midwife or HCP (Klittmark et al., 2019). Heteronormative language and presumptions cause further barriers during the postnatal period and the evidence emphasises the importance of providing care that is specific to the needs of the individuals (Klittmark et al., 2019; Malmquist et al., 2019).

Another topic that requires care tailored to the individual is infant feeding as without proper conversations about their infant feeding options, LGBTQ+ families are not being provided with informed choices. A topic that many midwives and HCPs still don't feel comfortable advising on is inducing lactation in the non-gestational parent. While inducing lactation is not a new phenomenon, it is under-researched, with much of existing evidence relating to adoptive mothers. A successful case of induced lactation with a transgender-woman who was able to successfully breastfeed her baby for six weeks was documented, proving inducing lactation is not just for those assigned female at birth (Reisman & Goldstein, 2018).

The assumption that trans-men or non-binary people will not want to breast or chest feed is a missed opportunity to explore wishes. It is true that some members of this community would prefer not to breast or chest feed for a variety of reasons, as in the cis, heterosexual community, but those who would like the opportunity feel ignored. This is especially true with people who have undergone top surgery, which can impact the amount of milk produced. This is different for every individual meaning there have been successful cases of breast/chest feeding with top surgery.

It has been demonstrated that HCPs provide inappropriate contraceptive advice to LGBTQ+ parents as the heteronormative lens influences the perception that all sexual activity may result in pregnancy. For lesbian couples, this is not the case. People using testosterone are still often (incorrectly) told this will make them infertile, meaning they are not given proper contraceptive advice of which they are entitled to. This lack of consideration and personalisation contributes to a lack of trust in the midwife or HCP (Silver, 2022).

ACTIVITY

Walk around your ward/clinical area and consider the following:

- Who is being 'welcomed' to the ward/clinical area and how is this communicated?
- Are all clients irrespective of their sexual diversity welcomed?
- If yes – how is this achieved?
- If no – what could you do to welcome all clients irrespective of their sexual diversity into your ward/ clinical area?
- What could be adapted in your unit guidelines/ policies to promote inclusion of the LGBTQ+ community?

SUMMARY

In this chapter, we have offered some opportunities for you to reflect on your practice and have highlighted aspects of the perinatal journey that have been evidenced as unsatisfactory for some LGBTQ+ people.

Educating oneself is essential when embarking on providing safe and sensitive care and the resources at the end of the chapter should assist you. The next section concludes this chapter and if you are just embarking on this intention to provide better care for LGBTQ+ people we would like to assist you on your journey by taking you back to the person's first encounter with perinatal services.

Creating a more inclusive welcome and environment for LGBTQ+ people can be the first step in working towards a more inclusive healthcare provision. It is acknowledged that every HCP, depending on where they are located, will need to consider how they do this within the framework of their practice and culture. Here are some suggestions:

- Advanced communication regarding what will happen during the first appointment may alleviate anxiety or LGBTQ+ people accessing the healthcare environment. This could include medical questions to be asked, physical and psychological examinations and screening tests.
- Service website or written literature could include links to LGBTQ+ organisations (Willenbrock & Santella, 2023).
- Explicit policy that relates to expected behaviours and care by staff members with clear escalation procedures when discriminatory practices observed (Menkin et al., 2022).
- Pronoun badges. Staff wearing pronoun badges as a way of signalling own gender identity. This serves to acknowledge gender identity as separate to gender expression and biological sex. It can also help LGBTQ+ people identify staff members who identify similarly, engendering a sense of comfort.
- Visual representations of different family compositions on display in the clinical setting.

One's own personal intentions are important for inclusive care provision; however, without senior leadership support and cultural safety education and integration throughout the service including front desk staff, efforts to sustain best practice may be lost (Menkin et al., 2022).

REFERENCES

Abelsohn, K.A., Epstein, R., & Ross, L.E. (2013) Celebrating the 'other' parent: Mental health and wellness of expecting lesbian, bisexual and queer non-birth parents. *Journal of Gay and Lesbian Mental Health,* 17:387–405. https://doi.org/10.1080/1935 9705.2013.771808.

Bockting, W.O., Miner, M.H., Swinburne Romine, R.E., Hamilton, A., & Coleman E. (2013) Stigma, mental health, and resilience in an online sample of the US transgender population. *American Journal of Public Health,* 103(5):943–951. https://doi. org/10.2105/AJPH.2013.301241.

Broholm, C., Lindell, D., Trossello, C., Lauren, J., Smith, B., Harris, A.B., Quinn Griffin, M.T., & Radix, A. (2023) "Ditch the white coats": What LGBTQ+ patients prefer in their primary care provider. *Journal of the American Association of Nurse Practitioners*, 35(1):41–52. https://doi.org/10.1097/JXX.0000000000000815.

Charter, R., Ussher, J.M., Perz, J., & Robinson, K. (2018) The transgender parent: Experiences and constructions of pregnancy and parenthood for transgender men in Australia. *International Journal of Transgenderism*, 19(1):64–77, https://doi.org/10.1080/15532739.2017.1399496.

Darwin, Z., & Greenfield, M. (2019) Mothers and others: The invisibility of LGBTQ people in reproductive and infant psychology. *Journal of Reproductive and Infant Psychology*, 37(4):341–343. https://doi.org/10.1080/02646838.2019.1649919.

Elmer, E.M., van Tilburg, T., & Fokkema, T. (2022) Minority stress and loneliness in a global sample of sexual minority adults: The roles of social anxiety, social inhibition, and community involvement. *Archives of Sexual Behaviour*, 51:2269–2298. https://doi.org/10.1007/s10508-021-02132-3.

Garcia, J., Vargas, N., Clark, J.L., Magaña Álvarez, M., Nelons, D.A., & Parker, R.G. (2019) Social isolation and connectedness as determinants of well-being: Global evidence mapping focused on LGBTQ youth, *Global Public Health*, 15(4):497–519, https://doi.org/10.1080/17441692.2019.1682028.

GOV.UK. (2023) Official Statistics Hate Crime England and Wales 2022–2023 Edition. Retrieved 13th November 2023 Hate crime, England and Wales, 2022 to 2023 second edition - Hate crime, England and Wales, 2022 to 2023 second edition - GOV.UK (www.gov.uk).

Green, H., & Riddington, A. (2020) *Gender inclusive language in perinatal services: Mission statement and rationale*. Retrieved January 13, 2023, from https://www.bsuh.nhs.uk/maternity/wp-content/uploads/sites/7/2021/01/Gender-inclusive-language-in-perinatal-services.pdf

Greenfield, M., & Darwin, Z. (2021) Trans and non-binary pregnancy, traumatic birth and perinatal mental health: A scoping review. *International Journal of Transgender Health*, 22(1–2):203–216. https://pubmed.ncbi.nlm.nih.gov/34806082/.

Hughes, T.L., Wilsnack, S.C., & Kantor, L.W. (2016) The Influence of gender and sexual oreintation on alcohol use and alcohol-related problems: Toward a global perspective. *Alcohol Research: Current Reviews*, 38(1):121–132.

King, M., Semlyen, J., Tai, S.S., Killaspy, H., Osborn, D., Popelyuk, D., & Nazareth I. (2008) A systematic review of mental disorder, suicide, and deliberate self harm in lesbian, gay and bisexual people. *BMC Psychiatry*, 8:70. https://doi.org/10.1186/1471-244X-8-70.

Klittmark, S., Garzón, M., Andersson, E., & Wells, M.B. (2019) LGBTQ competence wanted: LGBTQ parents' experiences of reproductive health care in Sweden. *Scandinavian Journal of Caring Sciences*, 33(2):417–426. https://doi.org/10.1111/scs.12639.

Lombardi, E. L., Wilchins, R. A., Priesing, D., & Malouf, D. (2002). Gender Violence: Transgender Experiences with Violence and Discrimination. *Journal of Homosexuality*, 42(1), 89–101. https://doi.org/10.1300/J082v42n01_05

Malmquist, A., Jonsson, L., Wikström, J., & Nieminen, K. (2019) Minority stress adds an additional layer to fear of childbirth in lesbian and bisexual women, and transgender people. *Midwifery*, 79:102551. https://doi.org/10.1016/j.midw.2019.102551.

McEwing, E., Black, T., Zolobczuk, J., & Dursun, U. (2022). Moving beyond the LGBTQIA+ acronym: Toward patient-centered care. *Rehabilitation Nursing*, 47(5):162–167. https://doi.org/10.1097/RNJ.0000000000000378.

McNeil, J., Ellis, S.J., & Eccles, F.J.R. (2017) Suicide in trans populations: A systematic review of prevalence and correlates. *Psychology of Sexual Orientation and Gender Diversity*, 4(3):341–353. https://doi.org/10.1037/sgd0000235.

Menkin, D., Tice, D., & Flores, D. (2022) Implementing inclusive strategies to deliver high-quality LGBTQ+ care in health care systems. *Journal of Nursing Management*, 30:46–51. https://doi.org/10.1111/jonm.13142.

Mizock, L., & Lewis, T.K. (2008) Trauma in transgender populations: Risk, resilience and clinical care. *Journal of Emotional Abuse*, 8(3):335–354. https://psycnet.apa.org/record/2008-18645-005.

Moseson, H., Zazanis, N., Goldberg, E., Fix, L., Durden, M., Stoeffler, A., Hastings J., Cudlitz L., Lesser-Lee, B., Letcher, L., Reyes, A., & Obedin-Maliver, J. (2020). The imperative for transgender and gender nonbinary inclusion: Beyond women's health. *Obstetrics and Gynecology*, 135(5):1059.

Neira, P., & Bowman, R.C. (2022). Improving perioperative nursing care for transgender and gender diverse patients. *AORN Journal*, 116(5):404–415. https://doi.org/10.1002/aorn.13808.

Office for National Statistics. (2023a) *Sexual Orientation, England and Wales: Census 2021*. Retrieved September 7, 2023, from https://www.ons.gov.uk/people populationandcommunity/culturalidentity/sexuality/bulletins/sexualorientation englandandwales/census2021#:~:text=Around%2043.4%20million%20 people%20(89.4,did%20not%20answer%20the%20question.

Office for National Statustics. (2023b) *Gender Identity, England and Wales: Census 2021*. Retrieved September 7, 2023, from https://www.ons.gov.uk/people populationandcommunity/culturalidentity/genderidentity/bulletins/gender identityenglandandwales/census2021. Retrieved September 7, 2023, from https://www.ons.gov.uk/peoplepopulationandcommunity/culturalidentity/ genderidentity/bulletins/genderidentityenglandandwales/census2021.

Office for National Statistics. (2023c) *User Guide for Birth Statistics Census 2021*. Retrieved November 13, 2023, from https://www.ons.gov.uk/peoplepopulation andcommunity/birthsdeathsandmarriages/livebirths/methodologies/ userguidetobirthstatistics.

Reisman, T., & Goldstein, Z. (2018) Case report: Induced lactation in a transgender woman. *Transgender Health*, 3(1):24–26. https://doi.org/10.1089/trgh.2017.0044.

Silver, A.J. (2022) *Supporting Queer Birth: A Book for Birth Professionals and Parents* (1st ed.). London: Jessica Kingsley Publishers.

Somerville, C. (2015) *Unhealthy Attitudes. The Treatment of LGBT People Within Health and Social Care Services*. London: Stonewall.YouGov.

Stonewall. (2018) *LGBT in Britain – Health Report*. https://www.stonewall.org.uk/ system/files/lgbt_in_britain_health.pdf.

Stonewall. (2020) *LGBTQ+ Facts and Figures: International*. Retrieved on September 7, 2023, from https://www.stonewall.org.uk/cy/lgbtq-facts-and-figures.

Stonewall. (2023) *List of LGBTQ+ Terms*. Retrieved January 20, 2023, from https:// www.stonewall.org.uk/list-lgbtq-terms.

The National LGB&T Partnership. (2017) *Best Practice in Providing Healthcare to Lesbian, Bisexual and Other Women Who Have Sex with Women.* https://national lgbtpartnershipdotorg.files.wordpress.com/2016/11/lbwsw-report-final.pdf.

United Nations. (2015) *Discriminated and Made Vulnerable: Young LGBT and Intersex People Need Recognition and Protection of their Rights, International Day against Homophobia, Biphobia and Transphobia – Sunday 17th May 2015.* Retrieved August 8, 2023, from https://www.ohchr.org/en/statements/2015/05/ discriminated-and-made-vulnerable-young-lgbt-and-intersex-people-need.

Willenbrock, D., & Santella, A.J. (2023) Re-envisioning the role of student health centers in offering LGBTQIA+friendly and sex-positive services. *Journal of American College Health*, 71(1):1–4. https://doi.org/10.1080/07448481.2021.1878190

World Health Organisation. (2022) *Human Rights.* Retrieved October 16, 2023, from https://www.who.int/news-room/fact-sheets/detail/human-rights-and-health#:~: text=The%20right%20to%20health%20must,based%20approaches%20is%20 meaningful%20participation

World Health Organisation. (2023) *WHO Announces the Development of a Guideline on the Health of Trans and Gender Diverse People.* Retrieved November13, 2023.

Yingling, C.T., Cotler, K., & Hughes, T.L. (2017) Building nurses' capacity to address health inequities: incorporating lesbian, gay, bisexual and transgender health content in a family nurse practitioner programme. *Journal of Clinical Nursing*, 26(17–18):2807–2817. https://doi.org/10.1111/jocn.13707.

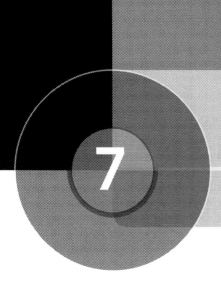

Models and Approaches in Health Promotion

JAN BOWDEN

Health promotion's focus can change and shift due to international sways. For example, the World Health Organization (WHO), national authority such as the Department of Health (DOH) and local power such as the public health unit, which now in many countries resides within local government. It can be impacted upon by health emergencies both at international, national or local levels such as the case with COVID-19 and the measles outbreak in the UK. Pair this with its broad field of action, incorporating many health-related professions e.g., midwifery, medicine, public health, education, primary care, the third sector, local councils to name but a few, and it soon becomes easy to see how it continues to be a contested field of study.

With its wide scope of practice and multitude of influences the approaches that underpin health promotion have also come from various disciplines, psychology, sociology, management, consumer behaviour and marketing (Nutbeam et al. 2022). Whilst health promotion approaches and models have been used in disciplines such as medicine and nursing for some time, their application to Midwifery has taken longer to develop. Perhaps, due in part to the unique and individual situations of pregnancy and childbirth, which do not lend themselves to categorisation of women, their families or their needs. Or because of our belief in our own autonomy as practitioners, facilitating a more holistic approach to care and the quest to find a model or an approach to meet these requirements.

DOI: 10.4324/9781003350071-7

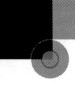

Historically, most models used within midwifery thus far have been adapted from nursing and medicine, which has illness as a starting point. However, the midwife must have a full understanding of the approaches and models used in health promotion to enhance the way that they deliver care.

Within this chapter, the approaches developed by Ewles and Simnett (2003) will be identified, then applied to models developed by Downie et al. (1996), Taylor (1990) and the midwifery specific model by Piper (2005), with their application to midwifery practice explored. These have been chosen as they are a foundation for most of the models used within health promotion.

BACKGROUND

The Lalonde Report (LaLonde 1974) provided the trigger for what is now termed 'health promotion'. Marc LaLonde, the then health minister for Canada, was the first to utilise the term identifying the activities that worked towards improving an individual's health. Within this, he recognised the complicated connections between biology, lifestyles, environment, and health care provision. Facilitating the exploration of the roles that government, societies, and the individual have in maintaining good health for all, providing the foundations that academics and researchers continue to use today. In turn, this has led to the development and design of theoretical frameworks and models, providing those engaged in health promotion with effective knowledge and guidance on which to practice. Though to note not all of these have been rigorously tested (Nutbeam et al. 2022).

WHY USE MODELS AND APPROACHES IN HEALTH PROMOTION?

Health promotion as identified earlier in Chapter 3 can be defined in many varied ways. There is no straightforward unity about the ideas that underpin health promotion or a single attempt to define what the principal goals of health promotion should be. Health promotion is neither neutral or value free, nor should it be. The main protagonists, including midwives, have differing views about the priorities and strategies which can be influenced by their personal views of the concept (McLellan et al. 2019). Views are based on values, beliefs, and experiences about health and health promotion that develop over time and experience. The importance of these differing views becomes apparent when working in a multidisciplinary team (MTD) where values are shared and made explicit. It is essential that health promoters listen and respect each other so they can work towards the same goals.

The development of unified models and approaches in health promotion and midwifery practice can be used as a tool to help us to communicate with each other more effectively, strengthening initiatives, which benefits everybody involved. The more sophisticated models and approaches will allow for individual holistic expression for both the midwife and the woman being cared for.

ACTIVITY

Before reading the next part of the chapter on approaches in health promotion. Think about the last client you undertook health promotion with for example one-to-one breastfeeding support in the postnatal period or discussion around the maternal vaccination in the antenatal period – e.g., flu and Pertussis.
  What health promotion approaches do you think you used in that conversation?

APPROACHES IN HEALTH PROMOTION

There is an abundance of approaches currently used within health promotion. Perhaps testimony to the speed with which health promotion philosophy has advanced. Some argue that due to the contested nature of health promotion, the relationship between the theory and the practice of health promotion should be explained, in as simple terms as possible to be understood (Nutbeam et al. 2022). In contrast, others argue that the rapid development of numerous approaches is a natural part of the topography of health promotion, which is large, loosely defined and under continuous development (Scriven et al. 2023). Some approaches are better known than others, often because they are more frequently used and quoted within health promotion practice. One such approach is that developed by Ewles and Simnett in 1985 (Scriven et al. 2023), which can easily be applied to midwifery health promotion.

EWLES AND SIMNETT'S APPROACHES IN HEALTH PROMOTION

Ewles and Simnett (1985) developed a framework of five approaches to health promotion, although originally designed for our colleagues in Nursing now considered as seminal in Midwifery Health Promotion literature (Table 7.1). They further elaborated on these in 1992 (Scriven et al. 2023) recognising that an intervention could be developed to improve health at a population, community and an individual level. From the outset being clear that there was no one single approach that was correct, with the ideal being a combination of them all:

> In our view there is no 'right' aim for health promotion, and no one right
> approach or set of activities. We need to work out for ourselves, which aim
> and which activities we use, in accordance with our own professional code

of conduct (if there is one), our own carefully considered needs and our own assessment of our clients' needs.

Ewles and Simnett (1992, p. 37)

However, these approaches are not without their denigration. Some highlighting their layout as simplistic and being on the edge in terms of idealism. With criticism that they fail to address the issue of values, attitudes, and beliefs held by both the health promoter and the woman and/or her family, which will have a significant impact on their use and success. The authors themselves also acknowledged this, whilst highlighting the enablement of further healthy debate on the health promotion theory and practice (Ewles and Simnett 2003). However, the delineation of the approaches is clearly very useful in developing health promotion theory knowledge, helping midwives through their use to understand how to clarify their aims and values.

Table 7.1 Approaches of health promotion

The Medical Approach

The concept here is based within the WHO definition of health. The aim to be free from medically defined diseases, illnesses, and disabilities. This approach involves active medical participation to prevent or improve ill-health and reduce morbidity and premature mortality. As seen globally during the COVID-19 pandemic and its following vaccination programme (James et al. 2021). The medical approach takes physical wellbeing as a marker on which to show success, with little or no reference to the psychological, social, or economic aspects of the cause and effect of disease. It values preventative medical procedures and the evidence showing its success using clinical trials and randomised control trials (Donaldson et al. 2018). Paternalism (one person deciding what is best for another) is a negative issue of this approach because full compliance is necessary on the part of the client/patient and can lend itself to blame when not.

Though used in midwifery practice, its suitability in low-risk pregnancy and childbirth continues to be debated (Mathias et al. 2021).

The Behaviour Change Approach

This approach is probably the most familiar to a midwife. The premise here is that an individual can be supported to change their health behaviours and attitudes to improve their health. Especially when faced with a behaviour that is impacting on their health, for example, poor diet or smoking. Most of the health service provision worldwide is investing time and effort on this approach (Nutbeam et al. 2022, Donaldson et al. 2018). It is cost-effective in terms of the outlay by governments and in terms of the savings made to the health service.

Elements of paternalism can be argued as being visible in this approach too as midwives will be convinced that changing a health behaviour is in the best interest of their clients-though this might not be a priority at that time for the woman or birthing person and compliance is necessary part of behaviour change to be successful.

(Continued)

Table 7.1 *(Continued)* Approaches of health promotion

The Educational Approach

Historically, this was the tradition approach in health promotion. With the midwife in the role of educationalist and the woman taking the role of the recipient of this trusted evidence. However, today this approach is seen very much as a two-directional between the midwife and the client. It needs to be well remembered that not all will seek information from the midwife but from other sources such as social media – see chapter on Health Promotion, Conversations, and Information.

Often seen as the first approach when engaging in health promotion (Upton & Thirlaway 2014, Thompson 2014). It has the capacity to reach many people and evidence seems to show that people are more informed and knowledgeable than ever before about health and the development of illness and disease (Donaldson et al. 2018). However, the midwife needs to be aware that health knowledge on its own will not change an unhealthy behaviour that would be far too simple. This approach should not be undertaken in isolation but in an environment where the woman's values and attitudes can be explored to help in their decision-making process.

The Client-Centred Approach

This approach – also known as the empowerment approach – lies as a key ethos for health promotion in the Lalonde report (Lalonde 1974). The aim is for the individual (or community) to take charge of their health and set their own goals to achieve that change, while working in collaboration with the health promoter, who assumes in this instance the role of a facilitator (Nutbeam et al. 2022, Piper 2005).

Women decide what the health issues are and sets the agenda. This is a 'bottom-up' approach – which is often more successful over a greater period of time rather than a 'top-down' approach in which those in power and authority set the agenda. The woman is seen as an equal and the knowledge and skills that she brings to the interaction are valued. The theme of self-empowerment is pivotal. Available data show this approach to be a successful one (Donaldson et al. 2018, Laverack 2017).

However, this approach does not provide 'quick wins', it requires a steady long-term approach to ensure success. This can be troublesome when looking at the finances and services required to support the individual or community to achieve change. The midwife may also find themself at the mercy of health targets, causing them to revert to approaches that are more easily achieved and measured.

The Societal Change Approach

This is Ewles and Simnett's only approach that does not directly concern the individual. Society is seen as central to health and the focus for changing health behaviours. It affects change physically, mentally, socially, and economically at a societal level. There by making the 'healthier option' easier to achieve for most of the population. This approach has had increasing credence within the UK and other countries across the world, especially in Canada.

It is not without its problems with some seeing it as an invasion of privacy and the development of a 'nanny' state, others question if the 'healthier option' is always the easiest (Donaldson et al. 2018) and has the potential to change depending on the political party in power at the time or the views of the majority of the population.

PRACTICE POINT

- Ewles and Simnett's five approaches provide clear examples of mapping in health promotion, and several approaches can be used in order to gain success.
- They might be considered too simplistic and fail to address issues such as values, attitude, and beliefs and their impact on health promotion.
- However, they provided foundations in the development of health promotion theory and continue to facilitate debate in this area.

REFLECTION ACTIVITY

Reflect on the activity you were asked to do prior to reading the section on approaches in health promotion.

Look at the list of approaches you were asked to identify and using the approaches of Ewles and Simnett identified above pinpoint what approach/approaches you used.

MODELS IN HEALTH PROMOTION

On scrutinising the available literature from various disciplines that use models, it is very apparent that many terms of reference are used loosely and interchangeably. Examples include models, theories, conceptual frameworks, approaches, paradigms, taxonomies and ideologies.

A model is a single physical representation of a set of ideas, often diagrammatic, that aids our understanding of the underlying philosophical issues of both theory and practice. A model aims to be objective and give shape to a theory and will conform to a pattern or reveal a pattern. Within disciplines such as health promotion, medicine, models are used equally in reference to theory and/or philosophy. However, in midwifery, the term model has, to a certain degree, been adopted to define the mode of care given to women for example continuity of carer.

Within this section, the term 'model' will be used unless an original author refers to their ideas by a different term.

The models by Downie et al. (1996) and Taylor (1990) and the midwifery specific model by Piper (2005) will be explored.

DOWNIE ET AL. MODEL OF HEALTH PROMOTION

Tannahill (1985, p. 167) described health promotion as 'a fashionable term that had acquired so many meanings as to become meaningless'. Proposing instead a model with three overlapping spheres of activity – health education, prevention, and health protection. Tannahill then worked in conjunction with a Professor of Moral Philosophy Downie identifying that although the original model had a broad base it was created from sound educational principles which stressed the importance of the sociopolitical factors involved in health and health behaviors (Downie et al. 1990,

p. 48). From this, they developed the three main overlapping areas further design-
ing a model which maps out seven possible domains of health promotion – positive
health, life skills, self-esteem, participation, and dimensions of health, choice, and
behavior with four aspects to health prevention (Downie et al. 1996) (Figure 7.1).

Health education – is defined as "all influences that collectively determine
knowledge, belief and behaviour related to the promotion, maintenance, and restoration of health in individuals and communities" (Smith 1979; cited in Downie et al.
1996, p. 27). This includes incidental as well as intentional education, and acknowledges the need for two-way education communication, in this case coming from
both the midwife and the woman.

Health prevention – encompasses avoiding, or reducing, the risk of different
forms of diseases, accidents and other forms of ill-health. Downie et al. (1996, p. 51)
defined the four aspects of prevention as:

1. Prevention of the onset or first manifestation of a disease process or some
   other first occurrence through risk reduction e.g., promotion of healthy eating
   and reducing the risk of Type 2 diabetes.
2. Prevention of the progression of a disease process or other unwanted state
   through early detection e.g. early detection of postnatal depression.
3. Prevention of avoidable complications of an irreversible, manifest disease, or
   some other unwanted state e.g. health promotion for Type 1 diabetes.
4. Prevention of the recurrence of an illness or other unwanted phenomenon e.g.
   an eating disorder such as anorexia nervosa.

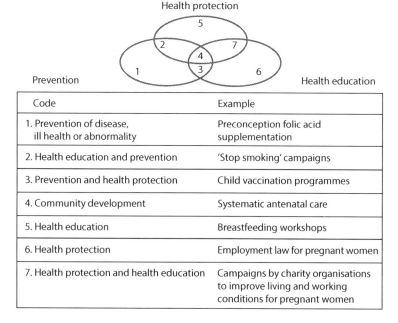

Code	Example
1. Prevention of disease, ill health or abnormality	Preconception folic acid supplementation
2. Health education and prevention	'Stop smoking' campaigns
3. Prevention and health protection	Child vaccination programmes
4. Community development	Systematic antenatal care
5. Health education	Breastfeeding workshops
6. Health protection	Employment law for pregnant women
7. Health protection and health education	Campaigns by charity organisations to improve living and working conditions for pregnant women

Figure 7.1 Model of health promotion.

Source: Reproduced from Downie et al. (1996), with kind permission of Oxford University Press.

Health protection – incorporates the environmental aspects safeguarding health by political, legislative, and social control, which using mechanisms to achieve positive health by attempting to make the environment hazard free, such as regulation, policy and voluntary codes of practice.

This model includes both individual and community action in health promotion but exclude curative medicine. It acknowledges the overlap in all the three areas of health promotion and offers community action as the ultimate in health promotion because it broadly incorporates health education, prevention of disease and health protection.

Rather than taking the perspective of the health promoter, favoured by the Ewles and Simnett approach, the Downie et al. model (1996) takes its perspective from health outcomes. Encouraging community-based health care with an educational approach that acknowledges all influences that lead to learning in clients and communities. As such, it does not include a medical approach in the curative sense (although they do acknowledge preventive medicine). Nor does the model include the client-centred and behaviour change approaches of Ewles and Simnett. A further limitation is that in attending to outcomes of health promotion, the process by which success is measured can be seen as a 'top-down' approach to health promotion, whereby the promotion is led by those in 'power' the government or the health care professional rather than the service user.

This model offers the midwife many permutations; however, it is not explicit in terms of the principal political or social values of each approach. It does not reveal the authors' preference as to the methods. By not doing so, perhaps it offers the midwife a greater autonomy than other models and approaches do, and this makes it more appealing to midwives who value their professional autonomy (Bowden 2017).

TAYLOR'S MODEL OF HEALTH PROMOTION

Taylor model (1990) is more of a sociological model to what the author refers to as health education. On examining their perspectives in today's terms, the model is actually referring to health promotion and takes the form of a paradigm map as shown in Figure 7.2.

Radical humanism – is that of self-development, particularly through personal growth, but with outreaching effects for community development. Removal from social regulation as far as possible is necessary, and in some cases, health professionals may be seen as social regulators, in that they are required to work strictly to rules and laws. An example could be a group of breastfeeding mothers running their own support group could be considered an example of the radical humanist approach.

Radical structuralism – though like radical humanism, radical structuralism is about moving towards change in the organisation of society, and more concerned with changing society to remove barriers to health than changing the individual. It may be exemplified by a nationwide campaign to encourage breastfeeding, including legislation to improve maternity leave, an advertising campaign to improve attitudes towards breastfeeding and the provision of widespread facilities for those choosing to breastfeed.

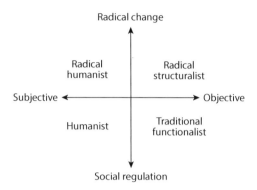

Figure 7.2 Perspectives of health education.

Source: Reproduced from Taylor (1990), with kind permission of the Health Education Journal.

Traditional functionalism – here it is the professional who possesses the expertise that is passed on to the layperson, who can then progress to healthier behaviours – a top-down approach. An example of traditional functionalism is the running of set antenatal education classes at defined times and places.

Humanism – here the focus is personal autonomy and empowering individuals through life skills development. A network of NHS breastfeeding counsellors illustrates the humanist quarter of the map.

This paradigm shows elements of Ewles and Simnett's medical and behaviour change approaches, with the radical structuralism having similarity with Downie et al.'s health protection approach, in that it is concerned with political and societal changes to improve the health of the public. However, the strong sociological background to Taylor's paradigm is very different from the more practical frameworks set by Ewles and Simnett and Downie et al making it difficult to make a direct comparison (Bowden 2017).

This model acknowledges both the 'top-down' where the control is from those in power for example the Department of Health or Midwife and the 'bottom-up' approaches placing health promotion within the control of the client/s and tends to have at its heart the client centred, empowerment perspective. It is the preferred approach as seen as having more success and longevity as the approach is client driven and more likely to meet the needs of the client (Donaldson et al. 2018).

THE PIPER MODEL OF HEALTH PROMOTION

Designed by Stuart Piper (2005) and based on earlier work by Beattie (1991), this model is unique in that it is specific for the midwife. Similarly, to Taylor' paradigm, it uses both the 'top-down' and 'bottom-up' approaches. It is split by an intersection, basically a power continuum between subjective knowledge and objective knowledge and an axis dividing individual and population. This then creates four distinct models of health promotion and clearly identifies the midwife's role in each quadrant (see Figure 7.3):

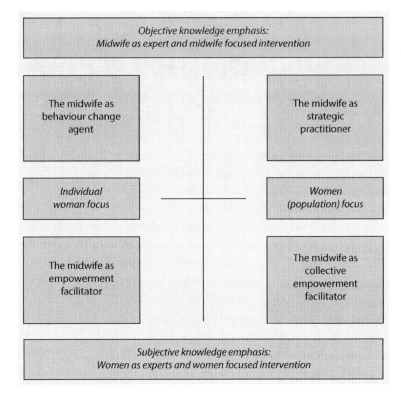

Figure 7.3 The Piper model of health promotion.

PIPER AND THE ROLE OF THE MIDWIFE

THE MIDWIFE AS A BEHAVIOUR CHANGE AGENT

This reflects a more traditional health promotion role of the midwife. Here the midwife is placed in a position of power and reflects a more medical and 'top-down' approach to health promotion which can be applied to all three levels of health promotion:

1. **Primary**: where health promotion is used to recognise or prevent the development of a health issue for example the mental health questions asked at the booking visit, they are asked of every woman and birthing person.
2. **Secondary:** where health promotion is used to prevent/limit complications from the health issue occurring or recognising a vulnerable woman for example the mental health questions identifying a woman with previous post-natal depression.
3. **Tertiary:** where health promotion is used to optimise outcomes and limit complications when they occur.

The intended outcomes are healthy women and babies with no complications. Taking as its premiss that women will make good decisions about their health when

Table 7.2 The midwife as a behaviour change agent

Aims	To encourage women to change unhealthy behaviours that may impact on their health either at the present time or sometime in the future
	Encourage compliance with treatments
	Attend the services they are referred to
Methods	Parent education classes, information giving
Impact	Increase the women's awareness, confirm the advice given and correct the unhealthy behaviour, increase uptake in the services offered
	Can been seen as paternalistic in its approach
	Issues around compliance, especially if unsuccessful
Outcome	A medically healthy mother and baby with no/minor complications
	Possible issues with guilt and stereotyping if outcome not achieved

Source: From Piper (2005).

Table 7.3 The midwife as an empowerment facilitator

Aims	To act as an advocate and support women as they become empowered
Methods	Advocacy, informed choice and informed consent. Client-centred engagement within a non-hierarchical framework
Impact	The woman leads her own health agenda with support from the midwife. A more bottom-up approach with, possibly, better success and longevity
Outcome	Increase in confidence and self-esteem. Women feel in control with improved decision-making skills
	Strengthen coping strategies and make childbirth a more positive experience
	An approach more favoured by the WHO and the RCM

Source: From Piper (2005).

given health promoting information. This is both simplistic nor acknowledges factors that act as barriers when changing health behaviours (see Chapter 9 on health, lifestyle, and behaviour change) (Table 7.2).

THE MIDWIFE AS AN EMPOWERMENT FACILITATOR

In complete contrast to that identified previously, here the midwife takes the empowerment facilitator role. With the aim of assisting an individual, or a group achieve their identified health promotion needs. This should be accomplished in a way that is non-hierarchical, non-coercive and empowering for the women maximising their opportunities for decision making as well as increasing self-esteem and confidence with regards to their health.

This quadrant of the model fits the current consumer culture within the NHS and the shift in the balance of power to the service user (Donaldson et al. 2018) (Table 7.3).

THE MIDWIFE AS THE STRATEGIC PRACTITIONER

Here the midwife, usually consultant midwives with public health as a specialism, as part of a MDT, promotes the wider issues involved in health and its promotion such as socioeconomic inequalities, environmental improvements and legislations such as welfare provision and maternity leave provision.

It is fair to say that not all midwives will engage with this part of the model on a regular basis unless their role indicates a strategic public health focus. However, every midwife can be involved in supporting/changing current public health policies and strategies, by lobbying the power holders via their professional organisations e.g., the Royal College of Midwives. Or by associating themselves with pressures groups that aim to address issues such as poverty and women, employment, baby loss e.g. the All-Party Parliamentary Group on Baby Loss (UK) (Table 7.4)

THE MIDWIFE AS COLLECTIVE EMPOWERMENT FACILITATOR

Appearing as a direct opposition to the previous role identified, here the midwife will work in a more 'bottom-up' approach, working with a collective group of women in response to their expressed health needs. The midwife is able in this role to encourage and support the development of social networks and improve social capital, especially those with social vulnerability such as young single mothers or those whose first language is not English (Thompson 2014) (Table 7.5)

This chapter has explored some of the available approaches and models used in midwifery practice. The examples given are known to midwives, who can use them to understand theoretical part of health promotion and work towards a minimum standard of high-quality health promotion practice.

Table 7.4 The midwife as the strategic practitioner

Aims	Influencing policy development and health care provision within Public Health within the job description of a consultant midwife with public health as a specialty
Methods	Lobbying, clinical audits and practice development Impact Organisational change, setting of professional/clinical standards at the national or local level
Outcome	Reduction in women and children's premature mortality and morbidity at national and local levels Reduction in the negative factors that impact on the health of a community or population Midwifery input at a strategic level and also at the development and pressure stage when supporting professional body and/or aligning with a pressure group

Source: From Piper (2005).

Table 7.5 The midwife as collective empowerment facilitator

Aims	Facilitating the building of social networks and social capital
	Supporting communal action by women with regard to 'their' expressed health needs
Methods	Public health consultation and intervention development led by women.
	A bottom-up approach with all its usual benefits of greater success and longevity
Impact	Developing and strengthening of social networks, especially for those women from the most vulnerable areas of society.
	Develop service user involvement and assist in 'opening doors' to power holders. Building self-confidence, self-esteem and empowerment
Outcome	Increased collective empowerment
	Social capital strengthened and developing the model to the linking stage
	A more fruitful project developed with a stronger chance of success and a longer time frame

Source: From Piper (2005).

SUMMARY OF KEY POINTS

- The numerous of models and approaches currently in use is often denounced for being perplexing and ineffectual, and not necessarily designed with midwives and their unique role in mind.
- Effective models and approaches serve to state the relationship between the theory and practice of health promotion. There is a moral requirement for the midwife to be clear about this relationship because, where an attempt is made to change people's behaviour, the ethical dimensions of such professional practice can be immense.
- Models and approaches in health promotion can help us to communicate more effectively by concentrating discussion on shared values and beliefs relevant to professional practice, and putting these into a framework that explicitly states acceptable standards of practice, to both the midwife and the women cared for.
- The application of health promotion models and approaches to some aspects of midwifery practice can offer a means by which agreed evidence-based frameworks standardise good practice as well as encourage further debate.
- The study and application of various health promotion models and approaches to midwifery practice can help us to understand different outlooks and develop innovative strategies suited to different communities.

REFERENCES

Beattie, A. (1991) Knowledge and control in health promotion: A test case for social policy and social theory. In Gabe Jonathon, Calnan Michael, & Bury Michael, Editors, *The Sociology of Health Service*. New York: Routledge.

Bowden, J. (2017) *Health Promotion Models and Approaches in Midwifery*. IN. CRC Press

Bowden, J., & Manning, V., Editors. *Health Promotion in Midwifery Principles and Practice* (3rd edition). Boca Raton, FL: CRC Press.

Donaldson, L., Rutter, P., & Scally, G. (2018) *Donaldson's Essential Public Health* (4th edition). Boca Raton: CRC Press.

Downie, R.S., Fyfe, C., & Tannahill, A. (1990) *Health Promotion Models and Values*. Oxford: Oxford Medical Publications.

Downie, R.S., Tannahill, C., & Tannahill, A. (1996) *Health Promotion. Models and Values* (2nd edition). Oxford: Oxford University Press.

Ewles, L., & Simnett, I. (1985) *Promoting Health: A Practical Guide*. London: Baillière Tindall.

Ewles, L., & Simnett, I. (1992) *Promoting Health: A Practical Guide* (2nd edition). London: Baillière Tindall.

Ewles, L., & Simnett, I. (2003) *Promoting Health: A Practical Guide* (5th edition). London: Scutari Press.

James, E.K., Bokemper, S.E., & Huber, G.E. (2021) Persuasive messaging to increase COVID-19 vaccine uptake intentions. *Vaccine*, 39: 7158–7165.

Lalonde, M. (1974). *A new perspective on the health of Canadians*. Ottawa, ON: Minister of Supply and Services Canada. Retrieved from Public Health Agency of Canada website: http://www.phac-aspc.gc.ca/ph-sp/pdf/perspect-eng.pdf

Laverack, G. (2017) The role of health promotion in diseases outbreak and health emergencies. *Societies*, 7(1): 2. https://doi.org/10.3390/soc7010002

Mathias, L.A., Davis, D., & Ferguson, S. (2021) Salutogenic qualities of midwifery care: A best fit framework synthesis. *Women & Birth*, 34(3): 266–277.

McLellan, J.M., O Carroll. R.E., Cheyne, H., & Dombrowski, S.U. (2019) Investigating midwives' barriers and facilitators to multiple health practice behaviour – A qualitative study using theoretical domains framework. *Implementation Sciences*. 14: 1–10. https://doi.org/10.1186/s13012-019-0913-3

Nutbeam, D., Harris, E., & Wise, M. (2022) *Theory in a Nutshell: A Practical Guide to Health Promotion Theories* (4th edition). Singapore: McGraw Hill Education.

Piper, S. (2005) Health promotion a practice framework for midwives. *British Journal of Midwifery*, 13(5): 284–288.

Scriven, A., Morgan, G., & Woodall, J. (2023) *Ewles & Simnett Promoting Health: A Practical Guide* (8th edition). India: Elsevier.

Tannahill, T. (1985) What is health promotion? *Health Education Journal*, 44(4): 167–168. https://doi.org/10.1177/001789698504400402

Taylor, V. (1990) Health education – A theoretical mapping. *Health Education Journal*, 49: 13–14.

Thompson, S.R. (2014) Approaches and models used in health promotion. In *The Essential Guide to Public Health and Health Promotion*. Croydon: Routledge.

Upton, D., & Thirlaway, K. (2014) *Promoting Health Behaviour: A Practical Guide* (2nd Edition). Oxford: Routledge.

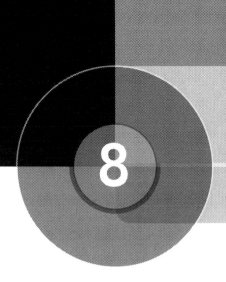

Evaluating Health Promotion: What Midwives Need to Consider

8

JAN BOWDEN

INTRODUCTION

As a relatively new field of health in comparison to others such as medicine and midwifery, evidence is vital for the planning and implementation of health promotion interventions. However, evaluation in health promotion is not as straightforward as it seems. The combination of factors such as: the long timescale of interventions, the numerous kinds of activities involved in an intervention and the number of stakeholders working in partnership, all of whom may have their own different objectives can muddy the waters in terms of the evaluation of health promotion interventions. Further difficulties may arise in the fact that health promotion can be an ambiguous affair with no assurances that specific effects will follow particular outcomes. In this chapter, the focus is on health promotion research, why evaluation is necessary, as well as the process and challenges of evaluating a health promotion intervention.

BACKGROUND: HEALTH PROMOTION AND VALUES

The responsibility of research is to try to cultivate new evidence that improves knowledge and understanding and moves health care forward for the betterment of the client and their families (Donaldson et al. 2018). It has been argued that health promotion research is quite distinct from other health disciplines. Woodall et al. (2018) go further identifying four attributes that makes health promotion research distinct when compared to other health disciplines.

DOI: 10.4324/9781003350071-8

THE FOUR ATTRIBUTES OF HEALTH PROMOTION RESEARCH

1. **Real-World Perspective:** Its application is to real-world issues that affect real-life clients. It does not focus on theoretical 'blue sky' research. Its focus is the development of evidence-based strategies that have direct action on health and its promotion. It is designed to explicitly inform practice.
2. **Research Values:** Like other health disciplines, health promotion is value-driven. However, its values are a little more difficult to agree upon and will subscribe to several sources such as the Ottawa Charter (WHO 1986), and the Galway Consensus (Barry et al. 2009). These values can overlap with those within Public Health, though health promotion will have a stronger focus on involvement, participation and developing empowerment of service users.
3. **The Professional Facilitation:** Health promotion highlights the importance of health promoter as a facilitator, promoting user/community involvement, reducing professional control, and working co-creatively with users/community to provide 'real-world' sustainable health promotion interventions.
4. **Methodologies:** The interdisciplinary nature of health promotion means the methodologies used are not unbendingly tied to a particular research paradigm. It is more diverse and flexible to explore the diverse health issues within a community. It will not meet the 'gold standard' of a randomised control trial (RCT), which can often see its results being deemed as not strong because of that.

Source: Adapted from Woodall et al. (2018).

LEARNING ACTIVITY

Before reading the next section, identify why you think evaluation is an essential element of health promotion

WHAT IS EVALUATION AND WHY DO IT?

Within health promotion, the simplest purpose of evaluation is to assess if the intervention achieves what it set out to. In today's health care climate of ensuring public monies are used sensibly and to good effect, this simple view is not good enough. Evaluation is not an afterthought and should be clearly visible at each stage of the planning cycle of the intervention as well as after the intervention has started and completed. Alongside identifying the economic efficiency and effectiveness of the intervention, it must also look at its longevity, sustainability, what worked and in what conditions and to what benefit to the population targeted within the intervention. This should cover both short and long terms (Green et al. 2015). Evaluation must consider the ethical issues of the intervention ensuring equity and the assessment of harm and not just physical harm (McFarlane 2014, Wills 2023).

Evaluation is guided by two essential principles: identifying and ranking the criteria and gathering data and information that will make it possible to measure to what degree these criteria are being or have been met. The following points can be used when a health promotion activity is being judged on its worth:

EFFECTIVENESS

This evaluation explores whether the activity has accomplished what it set out to do and to what extent the aims and objectives were met. It is essential to realise that, although in practice, the terms 'aims' and 'objectives' are used interchangeably. However, they are different. Aims tend to be general, while objectives contribute to the aims and are the 'nuts and bolts' of the planned intervention. Both are vital to the evaluation process. Poor identification of aims and objectives will make evaluation difficult and limited (Bauman & Nutbeam 2014, Wills 2023).

APPROPRIATENESS

This is assessing the relevance of the intervention to needs. The perception of needs will depend on who is defining them: the individual/group requiring the health intervention or the health promoter developing it. Both will have differing needs and therefore different expectations for the outcome of the intervention (Bradshaw 1972, Scriven et al. 2023).

ACCEPTABILITY

This assesses whether the intervention is being carried out sensitively. Sometimes overlooked, it may have an ethical or moral impact that affect its application either in the community for which it was intended or if rolled out to other communities. A 'one-size-fits-all' is not a guarantee. Also, the portrayal of those requiring the intervention may lead to typecasting that affects the impact of this current intervention and future ones within these communities. For example, the initial health promotion on HIV and AIDS in the 1980s in the UK portrayed the genesis of HIV firmly in Africa and the 'developing' world. This promoted racial typecasting, causing immense distress to many racially diverse communities, affecting uptake of testing and treatment and distrust in future interventions as well missing out other at-risk groups (Donaldson et al. 2018).

EFFICIENCY

This considers whether time, finances, and resources have been well spent given the benefits of the intervention. In recent years, the ratio of costs to benefits has increased in importance. Assessment needs to involve *cost-effectiveness analysis* (the comparison of the financial costs of similar projects) and *cost-benefits analysis* (the comparison of the cost of the project with the financial benefits resulting from achieving the goal) (Bauman & Nutbeam 2014, Will 2023).

EQUITY

This measures accessibility of the intervention. It goes beyond the identification of the numbers that an intervention reaches. Equity evaluates the social composition that the intervention has reached. Within health promotion, there is a call that the standard should be equity over equality, intentionally aiming health interventions at those in the most socially excluded and vulnerable groups and therefore those most at need (Trinh-Shevrin et al. 2015).

For evaluation to be successful, it must be built into the health promotion project from the planning stage and be always ongoing and explicit during the lifetime of that intervention. The complexity comes when this process of evaluation becomes formalised and with it the potential to become open to inspection and criticism from others (Bauman & Nutbeam 2014).

Despite the difficulties evaluation provides the best sort of feedback on which to develop health promotion interventions. The responses of the users of the intervention are essential allowing the health promoter – in this case, the midwife – to develop their health promotion knowledge and skills.

In recent years, there has been much debate about the reasons for the development of this evaluation culture within health. Some argue that it has a political and ideological function to legitimise the actions of governments – a tick box list to show they have done what they said they would, rather than focus on clients and patients and how they have benefitted (Bauman & Nutbeam 2014, Donaldson et al. 2018). Irrespective of this debate, there are many possible reasons about why evaluation is required and needed within health promotion and Figure 8.1 identifies possible reasons for evaluation. It is important to stress that Figure 8.1 offers only some suggestions and is not finite and you may well be able to add more.

WHO IS IT FOR AND WHO SHOULD DO IT?

Evaluation is undertaken for many reasons, as seen in Figure 8.1, and from this, it can be argued that there are several groups and individuals for whom evaluation is beneficial and necessary. Ideally, evaluation is best undertaken in a way that will allow each of the different stakeholders involved in the project to see if their aims and objectives have been met:

FINANCIAL BACKERS

Those providing the financial backing for the intervention will want the evaluation to show the efficiency of the project and its cost-effectiveness. This would allow them to see if their money had been well spent and to assess whether it requires continued longer-term funding or a possible reduction in funding.

HEALTH PROMOTERS

The health promoters may want the evaluation to show that their aims and objectives have been met and was an acceptable way of working with the clients/community. They may also use it to 'push' for the intervention to be rolled out to other

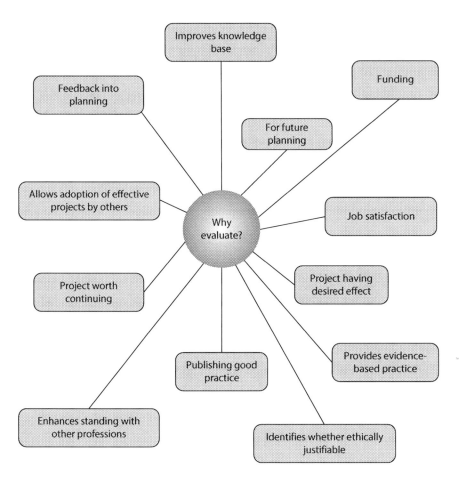

Figure 8.1 Why evaluate?

communities within their Trust areas or further afield. Health promotion managers may look upon the evaluation to assess performance and productivity of their team (Green et al. 2015).

USERS

The users may use the evaluation as a way of signifying some degree of control over health-related aspects of their lives and of gaining ownership of the intervention. A lack of user evaluation may show a lack of engagement with the target population on the part of the health promoters, which could have a potentially negative impact on the project in terms of success, longevity, and funding (Bauman & Nutbeam, Thompson et al. 2014).

POLICY MAKERS

Finally, the policy makers, e.g. local government, national government or international organisations such as the WHO, may use the evaluation to justify their

Types	Meaning
Eyewash	The evaluation focus is on the surface/outward appearance of the project only.
Whitewash	The aim of the evaluation here is to completely cover up an intervention's failure.
Submarine	The evaluation is used by the power holders, for example the government, to undermine the intervention.
Posture	This is a tick box exercise; evaluation is undertaken as it is expected but there is little to no intention to use the findings in any way.
Postponement	This is where the evaluation is sidestepped as a means of avoiding the outcomes to be identified and addressed.

Figure 8.2 Pseudo-evaluation.

Table 8.1 Advantages and disadvantages of internal and external evaluation

Internal evaluation	External evaluation
Knows background of project	Fresh viewpoint
Known and therefore accepted more readily	More objective
Easier to establish networks of communication	No allegiance to the project
Knowledge about the community for which the project is intended and therefore awareness of any issues	Unbiased attitude
Usually has some idea of weaknesses and strengths of the project	More likely to have research expertise
Financially beneficial as usually cheaper	More likely to have experience in evaluation
Too involved in the project	More likely to be made 'public'
Biased towards proving the success of the project	More likely to be thorough
Less likely to have research expertise	More likely to access the views of all the stakeholders including the users
Less likely to have experience in evaluation	More likely that all the stakeholders will receive the evaluation report
Time constraints prevent a thorough evaluation	Less accepted as seen as outsiders
Users may not be so honest with their evaluation because they know the evaluator	Networks of communication more difficult to establish
	More expensive than internal evaluation
	Lacks knowledge about the project and the community for whom it is intended
	Stakeholders may portray a 'united front' for the external evaluation

Source: Adapted from Naidoo, Jennie and Jane Wills. 2009. Health promotion foundations for practice (3rd ed.). London: Baillière Tindall; Katz, Jeanne and Alyson Perberdy. 2001. Promoting health knowledge and practice (2nd ed.). London: Palgrave Macmillan.

current health policies and strategies (Scriven et al. 2023). As well as provide drivers for future policies and strategies.

It is essential to examine who is going to evaluate the project and the impact they can have on the evaluation process. Most evaluation processes are undertaken internally, an accepted practice within health promotion. Internal evaluation allows for a more continuous process of evaluation to take place, because those evaluating are always available. It is seen as non-threatening, with stakeholders being more open about the project. However, there are challenges to this with evidence suggesting that it does not always fully evaluate the project because of issues such as lack of time and inexperience of the person undertaking the evaluation and are less likely to be made 'public', i.e., open for inspection (Bauman & Nutbeam 2014, Thompson et al. 2014, Wills 2023).

This means that poor projects are not always properly evaluated, which in turn means that a valuable learning experience is lost. Equally good interventions are not brought to the wider attention of others and their results not used to enhance the knowledge and practice base. Newburn (2001) explored this issue and developed a hypothesis of pseudo-evaluation and identified five types (Figure 8.2).

External evaluation is seen as more beneficial because it tends to be carried out by individuals who are well versed in the practice of evaluation. Though more expensive, it also tends to be more thorough with all stakeholders being asked their viewpoints. However, it is likely to suffer from issues associated with the evaluators being seen as outsiders and the stakeholders perhaps putting on a 'united front' (Bauman & Nutbeam 2014). Table 8.1 identifies the possible advantages and disadvantages of internal and external evaluation. Irrespective of whether evaluation is internal or external, 'a warts and all' approach to evaluation must be considered within health promotion to gain vital learning experience from both good and not so good interventions (Bauman & Nutbeam 2014, McQueen 2002).

USER EVALUATION

Health promotion is a complex process of intervention in an individual's or community's life at varying levels. Therefore, it must be justified and evaluated by the individual and community at whom it is aimed, allowing them to have their story heard. In recent years, the Department of Health (DoH), the NHS Executive and various research charities and funding bodies have emphasised the importance of user involvement (Donaldson et al. 2018). Questions regarding the use of service users need to be asked. Have they been included merely to satisfy regulations from the DoH and other funding bodies or is there a genuine conviction that their views are valuable to the evaluation process? By being used actively within the evaluation process, users will provide a fresh perspective on the health promotion intervention. It will provide user/community ownership of the intervention – a key value within health promotion – and allow the user to shape and guide the intervention and alter its organisational culture and structure (Farr 2012, Scriven 2017). Active user evaluation will add value and legitimacy to an intervention and potentially generate knowledge that could increase its significance and acceptance to other user groups (Scriven et al. 2023, Woodall & Cross 2022).

If users are given only a token involvement in evaluation, their role will be different and it is less likely that their story will be fully told, leaving them frustrated

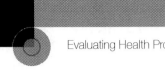

at not being heard or being allowed to be heard. Ownership will then be with the 'experts' and the organisational culture and structure will remain firmly within a professional remit. This, in turn, may affect the validity of the intervention and its sustainability within those at which it is aimed (Jones & Barry 2018).

To facilitate user involvement, consideration must be given to include users from the conception of the intervention and for them to undertake some training about their role within the project. Training for professionals must also be considered to allow them to understand lay perspectives and to work effectively with users in different situations (Smith et al. 2008, Staniszewska et al. 2012).

HOW BEST TO EVALUATE SUCCESS?

As identified earlier, evaluation in health promotion helps build a foundation of research and inquiry, demonstrating success. It allows effective health promotion practices to be identified and shared. It also allows these practices being further developed and enhanced. Evidence-based practice refers to the systematic process whereby decisions are made, and activities undertaken using the best evidence available (Sackett et al. 1996). This is often used in most other health fields informed by evidence from medical randomised control trials (RCTs). However, the RCT is not a tool that can be neatly fitted into health promotion. It is problematic for several reasons:

- It is impossible to isolate the effect of a health promotion project owing to the multiplicity of factors involved.
- An interventions success is in some part due to its spread to other groups beyond the target group.
- The length of time of interventions.
- The number of stakeholders within the intervention, each with their own aims, objectives, and viewpoints which they want to achieve.
- The awareness of health promoters of the social and cultural context in which they carry out their work.

Health promotion therefore suits a more social science approach to evaluation. It would allow for a much broader use of different methodologies from both the quantitative and the qualitative approaches. The different stakeholders and their individual viewpoints would also be considered, making the evaluation pluralistic (Green et al 2015). This of course may lead to the criticisms that there is a lack of methodological rigour and that the pluralistic approach is complex and lacks clarity (Bauman & Nutbeam 2014).

The difficulties in evaluating health promotion led Nutbeam and his colleagues to develop a six-stage model demonstrating an evaluation hierarchy which identifies how best to evaluate success in health promotion (Bauman & Nutbeam 2014). These stages are as follows:

PROBLEM DEFINITION

This draws upon the data used to identify the health issue which the intervention must improve. This information relies on epidemiological data and needs appraisal to define the problem, the factors influential to the problem and the scope for change.

SOLUTION GENERATION

This explores the behavioural and social research to expand the knowledge of the targeted population and the breadth of personal, social, environmental, and organisational features that may need to be adapted to form the basis for the intervention. It will also help to explain and predict change in those features as well as clarifying the potential content and approaches for the intervention. Stages 1 and 2 will help with the success and sustainability.

TESTING INNOVATION

This stage incorporates three areas that need to be considered and judged:

PROCESS EVALUATION

This is concerned with the assessment of the implementation and maintenance of the activity. Sometimes called formative or illuminative evaluation, it also focuses on the perception and responses of the participants to the health promotion intervention (Bauman & Nutbeam 2014). Moreover, it attempts to identify the factors that have hindered as well as ascertain those that have supported it. Process evaluation is a useful mechanism to gauge the acceptability as well as the appropriateness and equity of a health promotion project. Interviews, diaries, and observations are some of the 'soft' qualitative methods that process evaluation uses to gain details about a project. However, the use of qualitative evaluation methods is often dismissed because they lack the 'scientific' credibility of the 'hard' quantitative evaluation approaches and are often criticised for being unrepresentative (Bowden 2017).

IMPACT EVALUATION

The evaluation of an intervention must include identification of the effects of the intervention. The easiest and therefore the most popular way to undertake this is by assessing the immediate effect that the activity has on the recipients' knowledge, attitudes, behavior, and short-term health change (Scriven et al. 2023, Wills 2023). The midwife often collects this data at the time of finishing the activity or shortly after. Data collected tends to be of a quantitative nature, with all the usual criticisms.

Outcome Evaluation

This is considered the real test of whether the initial aims and objectives have been achieved. Outcome evaluation is more difficult and complex because it looks at evaluating the longer-term impact of the health promotion intervention. This may mean the midwife having to contact clients a year after the intervention has finished. However, despite these issues outcome evaluation tends to be much preferred. It attempts to evaluate changes that have stood the test of time. This evaluation often uses control groups and data that are expressed numerically, which increases its credibility because it is seen as more accurate and more like the quantitative approach (Bauman & Nutbeam 2014).

INTERVENTION DEMONSTRATION

This stage changes emphasis slightly from the assessment of process, impact, and outcome, and looks more closely at the conditions for success or lack of success. It will assess the achievement of the project under ideal circumstances and then look at whether the desired outcomes of the project can be achieved in a more 'real' environment. This is particularly relevant to the communities that are targeted, as well as the health promoters, because it looks at the achievability of the intervention in everyday life. It will also consider the unpredictable facets of health promotion practice and identify what basics need to be in place for it to be a success.

INTERVENTION DISSEMINATION

In this fifth stage, the emphasis is further moved to look at ways in which successfully evaluated interventions can be disseminated. This dissemination would advance evidence-based practice by investigating what others have done and, through use of their experiences, aid other health promotion projects (Wills 2023). Understanding how individuals and communities adopt and maintain a healthier lifestyle and what support is needed to assist this, determining what basics need to be in place to facilitate the success of an intervention as well as highlighting what needs to be done, by whom, to what criterion and to what cost, would be some of the benefits of intervention dissemination. However, it is rarely undertaken.

PROGRAMME MANAGEMENT

In the final stage, evaluation is tasked with assessing the maintenance of the intervention. Evaluation will incorporate the monitoring of the intervention's delivery in relation to its optimal conditions for success and, of course, value for money. Its sustainability and longevity will be continuously evaluated (Bauman & Nutbeam 2014).

LEARNING ACTIVITY

Before reading the next section, consider a health promotion intervention used in your practice e.g. breastfeeding or smoking cessation. What could impact on the results of that intervention?

CHALLENGES TO EVALUATION IN HEALTH PROMOTION

A midwife will face many issues when evaluating the midwife's role within health promotion or a midwifery-based/led health promotion intervention. Naidoo and Wills (2016) identified the following challenges that will be faced by the health professional when involved in health promotion evaluation:

- What needs to be measured?
- Are the effects entirely the result of the health promotion project?
- When to evaluate?
- What signifies success in a project?
- Is the effort worth it?
- What ethical issues are related to evaluation?

WHAT NEEDS TO BE MEASURED?

The essential tenet must be the measurement of the objectives decided on, which is undertaken in the planning stage of the intervention. This appears to be reasonably straightforward; however, the midwife may find numerous published studies that breach this simple golden rule. The biggest problem appears to be a lack of consensus between the stakeholders about the suitable measurements, e.g., trying to measure the involvement of a community in relation to breastfeeding or showing an increase in breastfeeding rates as a result of the development of breastfeeding workshops is not easy because of the other factors that may be involved, e.g., influence of peers, families, and media.

ARE THE EFFECTS ENTIRELY THE RESULT OF THE HEALTH PROMOTION PROJECT?

Health promotion does not provide a 'quick win' to improving health. The constantly changing situation makes it very difficult to be confident that the results of an intervention are solely the result of the input of that project (Naidoo & Wills 2016). Health promotion is a long-term process and, during that period, health-related knowledge, attitudes, and behaviours can change both for the health promoter and the targeted population. Society also continually reacts to varying factors, so the success of a health promotion project may be caused more by societal change than the actual intervention, e.g. the success of smoking cessation workshops for pregnant women who smoke may not be the result of the workshops themselves so much as society's changing views on smoking. An intervention's success is also in some part the result of its spread to other groups beyond the target population. It would be very difficult to prevent the health intervention 'seeping out' beyond its targeted population (Naidoo & Wills 2016).

WHEN TO EVALUATE?

As a result of the process of health promotion, an intervention will have different outcomes at different times during its lifetime. The timing of when to evaluate is vital to the success of a health promotion intervention, e.g. a breastfeeding promotion intervention may have several outcomes:

- Improvement in women's knowledge of breastfeeding.
- Increase in numbers of women attending breastfeeding workshops.
- Increase in local (and perhaps national) media coverage on breastfeeding.
- Persuasion of local restaurants, cafes, and shops to advertise that women may breastfeed within their environs.
- Encouragement of various organisations to adopt pro-breastfeeding measures, i.e., local employers.
- Reduction in the number of babies admitted to hospital with formula feed-related gastroenteritis.

(Adapted from Naidoo and Wills 2009)

Each of these outcomes will need to be evaluated at different times to be able to prove the success or indeed the failure of the intervention. However, there is no clear guidance to assist with the solution to this timing issue and health promoters tend to work on their own previous experience or the experience of others as to when to evaluate. For example, when working through the evaluation on the above-mentioned breastfeeding promotion intervention, the midwife may consider the following:

- An immediate evaluation of the project to ascertain the improvement in women's knowledge of breastfeeding.
- An interim evaluation at three to six months to identify the outcomes regarding the numbers of women attending the breastfeeding workshops and to assess there is an increase in media coverage local or national.
- A longer-term evaluation (maybe as long as five years) may be needed to assess if local businesses are adopting more pro-breastfeeding measures, café, and shops are advertising breastfeeding friendly status and if there is a reduction in the number of babies admitted to hospital with formula feed-related gastroenteritis.

This raises the issue of whether the success of the project is the result of the project alone or of changes within the community or society.

PRACTICE POINT

- There are many challenges that can affect the outcome of a health promotion intervention, such as when to plan evaluation to collect appropriate data, the impact of peers and family.
- Midwives need to be aware of these as many are outside the influence of a midwife, for example the media.

WHAT SIGNIFIES SUCCESS IN A PROJECT?

Investigation of what others have done and the use of their experiences to aid other health promotion interventions is one way of proving effectiveness. Effectiveness reviews assist health promotion in two ways: first by evaluating the quality of the research and second the quality of the intervention (Bauman & Nutbeam 2014). They also identify a means by which a foundation of knowledge is cultivated to pinpoint what the reasonable expectations of a successful intervention are. This is problematical for several reasons:

1. Health promotion's aim of changing health knowledge, behaviours, and attitudes on many different levels over a lengthy time period. It therefore requires a multi-pronged evaluation process that is fraught with difficulties.
2. The preferred 'gold standard' of an RCT does not fit well in health promotion where feelings, behaviours, attitudes, and changes to these are not easily expressed numerically.
3. Effectiveness reviews are the least common research found in the health promotion literature, partly due to a lack of interest in this area of research and partly due to the limited number of projects that have reached a stage of development that allows an effectiveness review to be undertaken.

IS IT WORTH THE EFFORT?

Appraising the value of one's work is an essential component of being a reflective practitioner. However, considering all the difficulties that evaluation in health promotion faces, a decision to undertake a more formal evaluation of that work and making it 'public' is not so easy. The dilemmas of what to measure, how to measure, when to measure and what constitutes success, are faced by all health promoters who undertake evaluation of their project. For a midwife measuring her own effectiveness in delivering a small-scale health-promoting intervention, reliability and validity are of little consequence. However, for larger project evaluation, these concepts must be addressed to make sure that the results obtained are genuine.

Ensuring that evaluation is built into the health promotion intervention from the planning stage and is always ongoing and explicit during the lifetime of that project is worth the effort. Providing the evaluation is explicated and fed back into the intervention, and to all those involved, it is worthwhile.

WHAT ETHICAL ISSUES ARE RELATED TO EVALUATION?

There are a few ethical issues that deserve consideration. The first is whose interests does the evaluation serve. The politics of vested interests in choosing an evaluation technique and the issue of who receives the findings, and what they do with them, are very pertinent when evaluating an intervention. Evaluation can be time-consuming for those involved and frustrating if they do not see any change resulting from the comments that they have made (Staniszewska 2012). This often happens if the evaluation highlights information that is difficult to interpret because of poor identification of the aims and objectives. It also occurs when the evaluation gives such a wide range of feedback that it is impossible to decide the effectiveness of the intervention or identify where improvements should be made.

Given that an evaluation has been reasonably well carried out and conclusions drawn, decisions must be made about who holds responsibility for incorporating the findings in future practice. If the conclusions recommend the investment of further resources, it may be impossible for the non-budget-holding evaluator to act. Aims and objectives almost always include an element of behaviour change, which may cause personal discomfort and influence the recipients' relationships with family and friends. The effect of education cannot be predicted and as seen in the film *Educating Rita*, where Rita's new knowledge leaves her abandoned by her husband and old friends and feeling misunderstood by her family, it can be a double-edged sword (Bowden 2017).

SUMMARY OF KEY POINTS

- Within the health care services, there is a drive to evaluate all aspects of health to ensure that all practices including health promotion are providing evidenced based care that does no harm to those being 'cared' for.
- As a relatively young field of health in comparison to others, there is added impetus for evaluation to take place to prove health promotion's worth, but often it is complex and undertaking poorly.

- Evaluation is formed of two essential parts: identifying and ranking the criteria and gathering data and information that will make it possible to measure to what degree these criteria are being or have been met.
- When judging the worth of a health promotion intervention, effectiveness, appropriateness, acceptability, efficiency, and equity must be considered.
- Health promotion is concerned with changing health knowledge, behaviours, and attitudes on many different levels sometimes over a lengthy time period. It therefore requires a multi-pronged evaluation process that is fraught with difficulties.
- The preferred 'gold standard' of RCT does not fit well in health promotion where feelings, behaviours, attitudes, and changes to these are not easily expressed numerically.
- Evaluation must include assessment of the ethical and moral issues of the interventions.

REFERENCES

Barry, M.M., Allegrante J.P., Lamarre, M.C., Auld, M.E., & Taub, A. (2009). The Galway Consensus Conference: International Collaboration on the development of core competencies for health promotion and health education. *Global Health Promotion* 16: 5–11.

Bauman, A., & Nutbeam, D. (2014). *Evaluation in a Nutshell: A Practical Guide to the Evaluation of Health Promotion Programmes* (2nd ed.). China: McGraw Hill Education.

Bowden, J. (2017). Evaluating health promotion activities. In Bowden, J., & Manning, V. (eds.). *Health Promotion in Midwifery Principles and Practice* (3rd ed.). Boca Raton: CRC Press.

Bradshaw, J. (1972). The concept of social need. *New Society,* 19: 640–643.

Donaldson, L., Rutter, P., & Scally, G. (2018). *Donaldson's Essential Public Health* (4th ed.). Boca Raton: CRC Press.

Farr, M. (2012). Collaboration in public services: Can service users and staff participate together. In Barnes, M., & Cotterell, P. (eds.). *Critical Perspectives on User Involvement*. Bristol: The Policy Press.

Green, J., Tone, K., Cross, R., & Woodall, J. (2015). Information needs. In: *Health Promotion, Planning and Strategies*. Sage: London.

Jones, J., & Barry, M.M. (2018). Factors influencing trust and mistrust in health promotion partnerships IUHPE. *Global Health Promotion,* 25(2): 16–24.

McFarlane, V. (2014). The same or different? Health promotion in ethically diverse communities. In Thompson, S.R. (ed.), *The Essential Guide to Public Health and Health Promotion*. Croydon: Routledge.

McQueen, D.V. (2002). The evidence debate: Evaluating evidence for public health interventions. *Journal of Epidemiology and Community Health,* 56: 83–84.

Naidoo, J., & Wills, J. (2009). *Health Promotion Foundations for Practice* (3rd ed.). London: Baillière Tindall.

Naidoo, J., & Wills, J. (2016). *Health Promotion Foundations for Practice* (4th ed.). London: Elsevier.

Newburn, T. (2001). What do we mean by evaluation. *Children and Society,* 15(1): 5–13.

Sackett, D.L., Rosenberg, W., Muir Gray, J.A., Haynes, B., & Scott Richardson, W. (1996). Evidence based medicine: What it is and what it isn't. *British Medical Journal,* 3: 71–72.

Scriven, A., Morgan, G., & Woodall, J. (2023). *Ewles and Simnett's Promoting Health: A Practical Guide* (8th ed.). India: Elsevier.

Scriven A (2017) *Ewles and Simnett's Promoting Health: A Practical Guide* (7th ed) India: Elsevier.

Smith, E., Ross F., Donovan, S., Mounthorpe, J., Brearley, S., Sitzia, P., & Beresford, P. (2008). Service user involvement in nursing, midwifery and health visiting research: The review of the evidence & practice. *International Journal of Nursing Studies,* 45(2): 298–315.

Staniszewska, S., Mockford, C., Gibson, A., Herron-Marx, S., & Putz, R. (2012). Moving forward: understanding the negative experiences and impact of patient and public involvement in health service planning, development and evaluation. In: Barnes, M., & Cotterell, P. (eds.). *Critical Perspectives on User Involvement.* Bristol: The Policy Press.

Thompson, S.R., Novak, C., & Thompson, K. (2014). Programme planning. In Thompson, R. (ed.). *The Essential Guide to Public Health and Health Promotion.* Croydon: Routledge.

Trinh-Shevrin, C., Nadkarni, N., Rebecca Park, R., & Kwan, S. (2015). Defining an integrative approach for health promotion and disease prevention: A population health equity framework. *Journal of Health Care for the Poor and Underserved,* 26(2): 146–163.

Wills, J. (2023). *Foundations of Health Promotion* (5th ed.). Scotland: Elsevier.

WHO. (1986). Ottawa charter for health promotion. *Health Promotion,* 1: iii–v.

Woodall, J., & Cross, R. (2022). *Essentials of Health Promotion.* Newcastle upon Tyne: Sage.

Woodall, J., Warwick-Booth, L., South, J., & Cross, R. (2018). What makes health promotion distinct? *Scandinavian Journal of Public Health,* 46: 118–122.

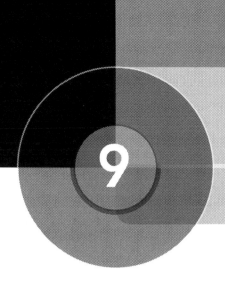

Healthy Lifestyles and Behaviour Change

9

JAN BOWDEN

INTRODUCTION

The impact of lifestyle and health behaviours on any individual is a complex one.

When poor lifestyle choices cause a negative impact on the health of a pregnant woman or birthing person, or directly on the fetus and neonate and some with the potential for intergenerational repercussions as with smoking and obesity, then lifestyle must be asked, support offered, and solutions suggested.

Health and the behaviours that assist in being healthy may not be considered important or relevant and may even be ignored until a person experiences ill-health themselves, or within their family and friends or brought to their attention by health publicity surrounding someone in the public eye. It may also be considered beyond the remit of the midwife and others within the multi-disciplinary team.

The United Nations' (UN) Sustainable Development Goals (SDGs) (2020) highlight the importance of promoting health in Goal 3: 'Ensuring Healthy Lives and Promote Health and Wellbeing at all Ages', with a primary focus on reducing the mortality rates for women, neonates, and children under five years old. The World Health Organization (WHO) are clear as to the midwife's crucial contribution to improving health outcomes and saving lives through a wide range of midwifery services including promoting health, screening, diagnosis, treatment, and follow up (WHO 2017).

Public Health and Health Promotion is undoubtedly central to the midwife's role and scope of practice as laid out within the International Confederation of Midwives (ICM) essential competencies of midwifery practice "assess the health status, screen for health risks and promote general health and wellbeing of women and infants" (ICM 2019, p. 1) and in the UK found within the Nursing & Midwifery Council's

Code: "Standard 3.1-pay special attention to prompting wellbeing, preventing ill health and meeting the changing health and care needs of people of all life stages" (Nursing and Midwifery Council [NMC] 2018, p. 7). The issues of lifestyles, health behaviours and the impact on health are a conundrum that can cause midwives frustration and annoyance both on a professional and personal level.

The aim of this chapter is to provide midwives with theoretical knowledge and understanding for promoting behaviour change including the determinants that influence it. It will provide a short background on health and lifestyles before examining useful health behaviour theories that midwives can use in their practice.

BACKGROUND

The link between lifestyle and health is not new. Hippocrates (460–370 BC) was amongst the first to recognise the interconnectedness between people, their lifestyles, and their health. Identifying that "those naturally fat are more liable to sudden death than those who are thin" (Donaldson & Rutter 2018, p. 312) and proposing that diet, exercise, water, and climate had a role in a person's health, a view that is now central to modern health and lifestyle thinking.

By the 19th century health had moved away from the concept that bodily fluids (the four humours) and smells (miasmas) were the cause of illness and disease, with the birth of a public health policy in the United Kingdom (UK). This policy centred on the new science of organism identification and their management by medicine. There is no doubt that this led to a decline in infectious diseases. However, data that recognised the progress made on health by social improvements to sanitation and housing, a better understanding of the role of nutrition, as well as the overall betterment to the lives of those living in poverty and therefore at greater health risk were overlooked (Upton & Thirlaway 2014, Donaldson & Rutter 2018).

Though dated the Department of Health (DoH) paper 'Our Health and Wellbeing Today' showed that within the UK life required less effort than ever before (DoH 2010). The living and working environments were safer with travel, household tasks, and even shopping requiring less effort than ever before (DoH 2010). Access to cheaper processed foods and alcohol, less physical activity in both men and women and more sedentary employment than ever before have seen a rise in illnesses and diseases that have poor lifestyle choice rather than infection or accident at its core (Donaldson & Rutter 2018, Public Health England [PHE] 2019).

HEALTH BEHAVIOURS

Behaviours which improve health are extremely advantageous to all and to Society as a whole. Bringing possible benefits that are health-positive, cost-effective, efficient, and low-risk with a reduction in health service expenditure (PHE 2022). This approach does not focus on just a cure, indeed there might not be one, but has roles in prevention and the reduction in complications where a health issue already exists, e.g., diabetes. These require a more psycho-social aspect to health and the need to work in collaboration with the client and other health-related services.

By changing behaviour, the focus moves away from a societal responsibility to an individual one. Many argue that this is as it should be – the Self Care Forum, a national charity in the UK promotes self-care as a nationally accepted point for health management, educating the populace with self-care skills to improve health and decrease pressure on the NHS (Webber et al. 2015). However, this can lead to a 'blame culture', when poor lifestyle choices lead to significant health issues, with the potential for the most vulnerable to be the most affected (Upton & Thirlaway 2014, Marmot et al. 2018).

LIFESTYLE BEHAVIOURS

Lifestyle behaviours are complex, altering depending on age, environment, social network, and personal beliefs as well as what is in the current landscape for that person, e.g., pregnancy. They are important in the development and continuation of social networks, coping with stress and the building and expansion of personal resilience (Upton & Thirlaway 2014).

TYPES OF BEHAVIOURS

ACTIVITY

Before reading the next section, list how many types of behaviours you know providing an example for each.

Then compare your list with those identified in Table 9.1

Table 9.1 Types of behaviours

Type of behaviour	Examples
One time/occasional behaviours: A behaviour that may be carriers out once of a few times in a life span	Breastfeeding, childhood vaccinations, Male circumcision, female genital mutilation (FGM).
Routine behaviours: A behaviour that is frequently undertaken with no or little conscious thought to it	Smoking, alcohol drinking, biting fingernails.
Traditional/custom based behaviours: A behaviour that is passed/shared within a family, a community or Society and is generational.	The eating of certain foods, FGM, Male circumcision, infant feeding- breast or formula.
Addictive/dependent behaviours: This behaviour gives a psychological or biological reinforcement, positively or negatively leading to repetition to gain further/ stronger reinforcement.	Taking drugs, binge eating, gambling, porn, plastic surgery, excessive exercise.

Source: Bowden (2017).

Behaviours may be undertaken in isolation of each other but are more than likely to cross in to more than one category, e.g., a routine behaviour such as smoking is also an addictive behaviour and may also be traditional/custom based if it is the norm for that family or social network (Upton & Thirlaway 2014).

Though positive and even pleasurable when started, the behaviour may have a negative outcome sometime in the future which was not considered or was ignored when started, e.g., smoking, and poor pregnancy outcomes, cardio-respiratory disease or cancer (Thompson & Almond 2014).

ACTIVITY

Before reading the next section, reflect on a time when you made a change to enhance your health, e.g., lose weight, exercise more, and stop smoking.

- Why did you want to make that change for a particular event like losing weight for a special event or a more long-term change?
- How did your friends, partner, and family view this change? What support did they offer?
- What were the pros and cons of the change?
- Were you successful? If so, what made you successful if not what affected your success?

LIFESTYLE BEHAVIOURS AND DETERMINANTS

Lifestyle behaviours and the complex determinants that influence them are considered to be under the control of the individual. Though the issue of control is a hotly debated area (Acheson 1998; Thompson & Almond 2014). Determinants such as sex, age, ethnicity and genetics are seen as unalterable. However, they can impact on the way health promoting messages are taken up. Research shows that the older a person gets the more likely they are to engage in positive health behaviours or modify negative ones. This is mainly due to life experiences and a better understanding of perceived risk (Edelman & Kudzma 2022). The midwife needs to consider this when caring for younger women, whose ability to assess risk – which is important in their development to adulthood – and alter behaviours might be affected by their lack of experience, knowledge, skills, and peer pressure (Zinn 2019) (Figure 9.1).

Studies show that women are more likely to adopt health promoting messages, access health services earlier and adopt healthier behaviours sooner than men (Kent et al. 2014, Rougan et al. 2014). However, women are more likely to prioritise their family's health over their own (Kent et al. 2014, Edelman & Kudzma 2022). Pregnancy appears to act as a catalyst for health behaviour change. The wellbeing of the unborn baby is said to increase women's responsiveness to health promoting messages and these alterations to her behaviour may continue beyond the birth, influencing the health of other family members (Bowden 2017).

However more recent studies indicate that women do not always change behaviour preconceptually, despite recommendations to be in optimal health for conception (Khekade et al. 2023). Also, evidence indicates that lifestyle and health behaviours decline in subsequent pregnancies in comparison to the first (Kandel

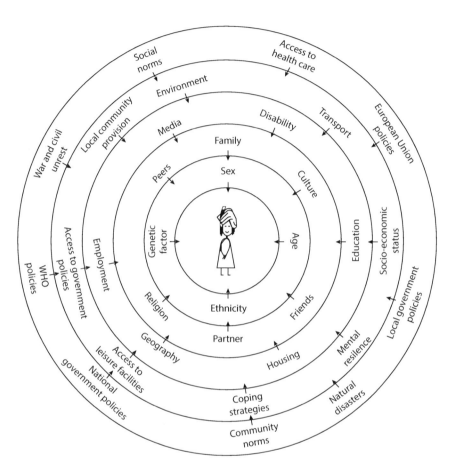

Figure 9.1 Factors and influences on health behaviour.

et al. 2021). The influence of the partner, family and friends on health behaviour and lifestyle change can be powerful. While encouraging healthier behaviours that are beneficial to the client and their baby, the midwife needs to recognise that this might put the woman or birthing person at odds with their social network (Rockliffe et al. 2021). Causing concern about 'fitting in' and worry about the level of support they will receive as well as having repercussions on their responsiveness to change behaviour (Zinsser et al. 2020).

PRACTICE POINTS

- Younger women may perceive risk differently to older women and impact on their receptiveness of health promotion messages and willingness to change.
- Healthy behaviours decrease with each pregnancy.
- Support networks might provide a positive or negative effect on the success and longevity of a health change.
- Women and birthing people might worry about 'fitting in' if they alter a behaviour that is viewed as a norm within their social network, leading to concern about the support they will receive and lessen their commitment to change.

HEALTH BEHAVIOUR THEORY AND MODELS

There are numerous theoretical models that attempt to explore health behaviours and with this how individuals can be supported to change less healthy lifestyles. These tend to take as their focus the key principles of biological drive, motivation, and cognitive dissonance (Table 9.2).

The oldest and most famous is the Health Belief Model (HBM) (Rosenstock 1966, Becker 1974). This model has been adapted to explore a variety of health behaviours including TB, sexual risk, and the transmission of HIV/ AIDS over its 57-year history (Linsley & Roll 2023, see Figure 9.2).

Behaviour change takes place as the individual recognises the health risk (perceived susceptibility), and its consequences to them both in the short and long terms (perceived severity), that they see benefits to changing the behaviour (perceived benefits) and that the cost outweighs the negatives (perceived barriers). The pregnant woman or birthing person would also need a degree of self-efficacy (Bandura 1997) to be confident in successful change as well as exposure to factors that provide "a cue to action", e.g., the booking appointment, or own health changes. Evidence suggests HBM is more efficient with preventative health promotion, e.g., screening and immunisation programmes and less effective with more complex longer-term behaviours that have additional social impact such as smoking and alcohol use (Corace et al. 2016).

LEARNING ACTIVITY

Tia, a 23-year-old woman, is pregnant for the first time. At her booking appointment, the midwife discussed the Pertussis and flu vaccines on offer to all pregnant people. Tia is unsure how to proceed with this offer.

- Using the HBM, explore how you could use this model to assist Tia in her decision making.

Table 9.2 Key principles of behaviour change models

Biological	Including the biological drives such as, hunger, thirst, sex, genetic factors, and physiological dependencies that may impact on a person's behaviour – these can de described as being out of a person's control
Motivational	This principle identifies the mediating effects of society and culture. However, it is hypothesised that the basic needs must be fulfilled first before attempting to address the impact of society and culture.
Cognitive dissonance	That a person has the awareness that certain lifestyles and behaviours can be harmful and will alter it accordingly. However, this is not always a given and the person may continue despite the harm or if there is an outcome they find beneficial such as smoking and appetite control.

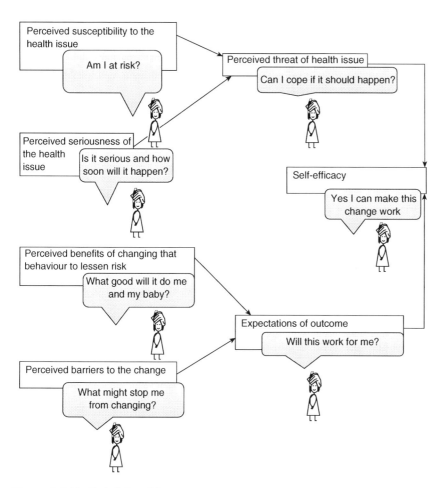

Figure 9.2 Health belief model.

REASONED ACTION AND PLANNED BEHAVIOUR

In their 'theory of reasoned action', Ajzen and Fishbein (1980) highlighted that change needed more than attitude and belief to be successful and inserted the word 'intention' between attitude and behaviour in their model. They believed by understanding the individual's intention alongside their attitude and beliefs that success could be more accurately identified (Ajzen & Fishbein 1980, Ajzen 1988). The main premise being that an individual will weigh up their beliefs, attitudes and felt social pressure in a logical process before arriving at their intention to change. Therefore, the individual's behaviour is one of 'reasoned action' and its application can be shown below on the predicted behaviour of a woman intending to formula feed (Figure 9.3).

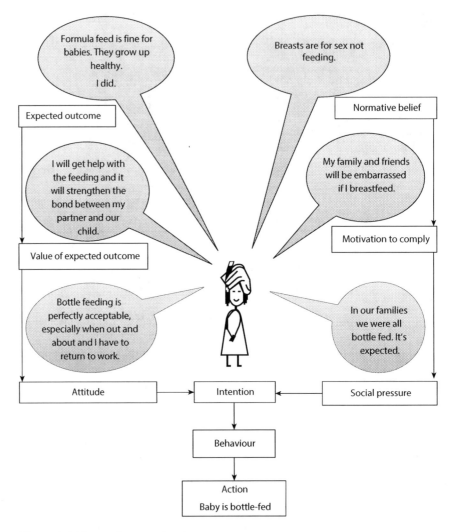

Figure 9.3 Theory of reasoned action.

Source: Modified from Ajzen and Fishbein (1980). Adapted by Crafter (1997).

THEORY OF PLANNED BEHAVIOUR

Ajzen (1991) introduced a further variable is his 'theory of planned behaviour' model by including the individual's perception of control over the situation. With the belief that the more favourable the individual's attitude, felt social pressure, and perceived control, the stronger the intention to change would be (Figure 9.4).

Although both models indicate success in behaviour change, they miss out the impact of the biological drives as seen in the HBM, the issue of the locus of control and the emotional input which is often variable and unpredictable (Ajzen & Fishbein 1980, Ajzen 1991). This is particularly so in pregnancy which, by its very nature, is a very emotional period for the woman or birthing person. Evidence suggests that this

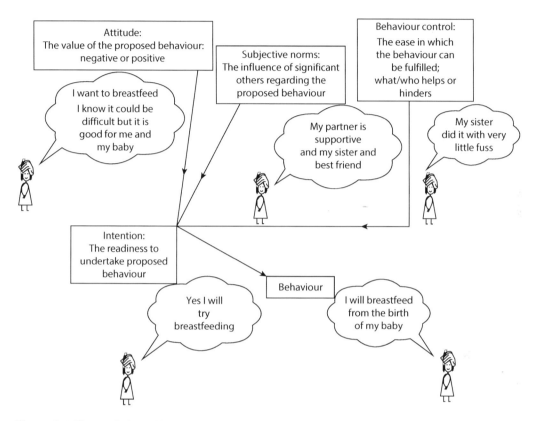

Figure 9.4 Theory of planned behaviour.

as a time where different ideas and values are formulated and attitudes and beliefs transition, though not necessarily influenced by the midwife or other health care professionals (Edvardsson et al. 2011; Grenier et al. 2021).

THE TRANSTHEORETICAL APPROACH TO HEALTH BEHAVIOUR CHANGE

The Transtheoretical Model of Behaviour Change theory (TTMBHCT) was designed by Prochaska and DiClemente in 1984, following a review of over 300 earlier psychotherapeutic interviews and the identification of 10 reoccurring processes (Green et al. 2015, Figure 9.5).

Originally designed to support smoking cessation, it describes the process undertaken by an individual to change their behaviour. It controversially indicated relapse as a given part of the process noting that this could occur in any stage even if the behaviour was considered 'cured'. Containing seven stages, if relapse occurs, and unfolding over many months it is dependent on support and the environment, by understanding this, the midwife will know how to support their client (Prochaska 2005) (Table 9.3).

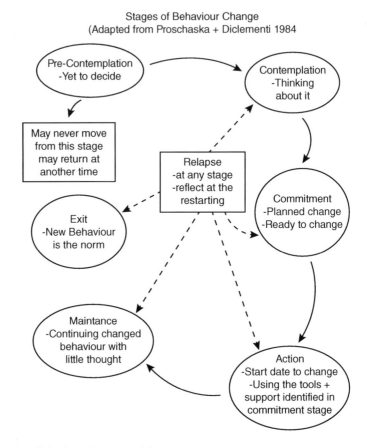

Figure 9.5 Behaviour change model.

Table 9.3 TTMBHCT and the role of the midwife

Precontemplation:

In this stage, the woman or birthing person is not anticipating change in the next six months; because they may feel that there is nothing at present to change or their current behaviour does not have the potential to harm.

Role of the midwife

The main roles here are:
- information giving which may provide that 'cue to action'.
- personalising information including risks and benefits and highlighting behaviours that may tip into unhealthy lifestyles as well as myth busting for example eating for two.
- recognising the 'elephant in the room' and actively discussing unhealthy behaviour. The midwife should not ignore this for fear of damaging the growing therapeutic relationship (Lee et al. 2012).
- realising that the client may be hostile to any attempt to discuss their unhealthy behaviour, suggesting that they have yet to reach the pre-contemplation stage (Prochaska 2005).

(Continued)

Table 9.3 (Continued) TTMBHCT and the role of the midwife

Precontemplation:

- equally the client may accept the health promotion advice and disclose concerns such as feeling powerless to stop or where to go for help. Giving the midwife the chance to further explore and look at referral, e.g., pregnancy smoking cessation services.

Contemplation stage

This is where there is engagement and a wish to change health behaviours (Prochaska 2005). The woman or birthing person will begin to address the health issue, the side effects, and its impact on themself and their child and how best to make the change and actively seek information.

Role of the midwife

The main roles here are:

- empowering the client and using their considerable skills to facilitate this process see below.
- using assessment skills such as using the 5A's assessment tool (see Figure 9.7)
- active listening and the using of client directed counselling techniques (see further resources)
- assisting the woman with finding best evidence (see Chapter 10 Health Promotion, Conversations and Information).
- referral as required.

Commitment stage

By entering this stage, the client is making a serious decision to change negative health behaviour. They may have a date by which they wish to start the change and have the beginning of a plan that will help them and show who they can turn to for support. The client may seek the help of the midwife to formalise this. Prochaska (2005) identified that this stage usually lasts no more than a month.

Role of the midwife:

The main roles here are:

- further development/formalisation of action plan.
- discussing coping strategies for when things get tough, including the development of a personal support group including identification of supporters and equally who to avoid.
- setting a date on which to commence the change.

Action stage

Here the woman or birthing person is making explicit modifications to improve their health behaviours. This may take up to six months (Prochaska 2005).

Role of the midwife

The main roles here are:

- support which is vital at this stage. This may include reminding them of their action plan and their personal support group.
- referral to additional services – if not already done.
- assessing ambivalence and promoting confidence and motivation.

(Continued)

Table 9.3 *(Continued)* TTMBHCT and the role of the midwife

<table>
<tr><th colspan="1" align="center">Precontemplation:</th></tr>
</table>

Maintenance stage

The behaviour is now at the point that is an accepted part of everyday life with little thought. The woman gains increasing satisfaction and confidence in themself and their coping strategies. They may also notice the benefits that the change has made.

Role of the midwife

The main roles here are:
- continued support.
- praising success especially if they begin to waver and if so prompt use of the action plan and coping strategies as per the commitment stage.

Exit stage

Here the health behaviour has been successfully changed and maintained with no temptation and 100% self-efficacy.

This stage is contentious as to its existence with less than 20% reaching this stage. Michie et al. (2011) identified that for the midwife and the woman it is important to recognise that for many the best they will achieve is the maintenance stage. This knowledge prevents a feeling of failure if the exit stage is not reached.

Role of the midwife

The main roles here are:
- discussing what the exit stage is.
- recognition of the success.

Relapse

It is important to realise that not all will be successful at the first attempt or indeed the second or third and to recognise that relapse is part of the changing health behaviour process and should not be deemed a failure on the part of the woman or birthing person (Prochaska & DiClemente 1984, Michie et al. 2011).

Role of the midwife

The main roles here are:
- supporting the client and reflecting with them to evaluate its cause. This will allow the midwife or others to offer support, particularly at the point where the relapse happened on the next attempt.
- reviewing the action plan and strengthen where necessary.
- developing additional coping strategies as the client starts the process again.
- discussing starting again from the beginning rather from where the relapse occurred which offers a better chance of success (Prochaska 2005).
- developing professional knowledge regarding the social – cognitive and behavioural strategies that can prevent or limit relapse episodes (Marlatt & Donovan 2005, Schuman-Oliver et al. 2020).

BEHAVIOUR CHANGE IN MIDWIFERY PRACTICE

Working with pregnant individuals to change harmful behaviours is challenging, especially when there has been relapse or there is resistance to change (Walker et al. 2020). It is also impacted upon by a lack of knowledge and confidence by midwives themselves, the current midwifery workload, and staffing issues (Khomami et al. 2021).

The behaviour models explored in this chapter give the impression that clients will make a rationale assessment as part of their decision making and change unhealthy behaviours. Midwives need to recognise this is often not always the case and that to alter harmful behaviours the following need to be considered:

- The change must be initiated by the individual.
- The behaviour is called in to question either by those close to the person or when it impacts on another part of the individual's life, e.g., obesity and difficulty in walking.
- The behaviour is not a coping mechanism.
- The new behaviour easily slots into everyday life.
- That the individual's life is not unduly difficult and there is a strong supportive social network.

(Pill & Stott 1990)

The COM-B model (West & Michie 2020) shows the midwife that the interconnected influences of Capability, Opportunity, and Motivation must be present for behaviour change to start and be successful. This very much fits with the salutogenic aspects of midwifery care, namely comprehensibility – the cognitive aspects of health, manageability – the behavioural aspect of health and meaningfulness – the emotional/spiritual aspects of health as identified by Mathias et al. (2021) and the RCM and looks at the strengths of a woman rather than their limitations with regards to health and behaviour change (Figure 9.6).

The key to these behaviour change conversations is that they are brief, and evidence based at the onset and may become longer in the future (Linsley & Roll 2023). Evidence shows that a health conversation lasting no more than three to five minutes can increase a person's chance of stopping smoking by up to 3% (Stead et al. 2013). This might not seem a lot but if as a midwife, you consider the number of clients you interact with on a daily and weekly basis that percentage grows and makes a large health impact (Thompson & Almond 2014). The time restraint also stops clients from feeling as though they are being lectured at and are less likely to put up barriers and fit in to the midwife's limited time.

Developing skills in motivational interviewing (MI), which is a collaborative client-centred interaction, will assist the midwife in her role as a behaviour change facilitator. MI is designed to explore the woman or birthing person's motivation, confidence and resolve to change. It allows the midwife to foster a respectful and collaborative environment in which to facilitate change while strengthening confidence and motivation and assessing for ambivalence (Miller & Rollnick 2013, 2023). This section will look briefly at some of these aspects.

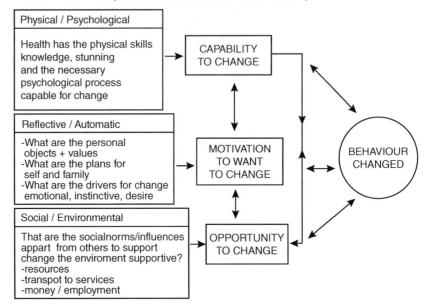

THE COMB MODEL OF BEHAVIOUR CHANGE
(ADAPTED FROM WEST + MICHIE 2020)

Physical / Psychological

Health has the physical skills
knowledge, stunning
and the necessary
psychological process
capable for change

Reflective / Automatic

-What are the personal
 objects + values
-What are the plans for
 self and family
-What are the drivers for change
 emotional, instinctive, desire

Social / Environmental

That are the socialnorms/influences
appart from others to support
change the enviroment supportive?
-resources
-transpot to services
-money / employment

CAPABILITY
TO CHANGE

MOTIVATION
TO WANT
TO CHANGE

OPPORTUNITY
TO CHANGE

BEHAVIOUR
CHANGED

Figure 9.6 COM-B model.

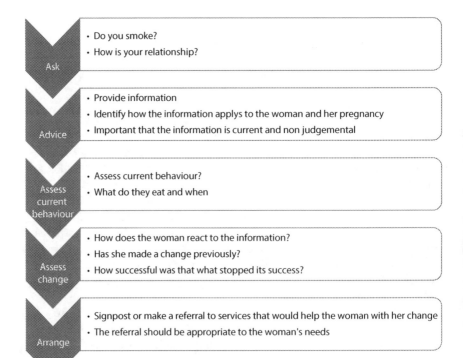

Ask
- Do you smoke?
- How is your relationship?

Advice
- Provide information
- Identify how the information applys to the woman and her pregnancy
- Important that the information is current and non judgemental

Assess current behaviour
- Assess current behaviour?
- What do they eat and when

Assess change
- How does the woman react to the information?
- Has she made a change previously?
- How successful was that what stopped its success?

Arrange
- Signpost or make a referral to services that would help the woman with her change
- The referral should be appropriate to the woman's needs

Figure 9.7 The 5As.

GETTING STARTED

Getting started is often the most difficult part, with those attending midwifery services usually aware of the health issues they have and the ones that a midwife wishes to discuss and explore.

The '5As' assessment tool is used in the UK Government's national intervention 'Make Every Contact Count' (MECC), where all health care professionals should make every contact count in terms of promoting and maintaining good health (NHS Future Forum 2011).

The '5 As' tool will help facilitate the midwife to open the discussion (Figure 9.7):

MOTIVATION AND CONFIDENCE

Assessing motivation and confidence in relation to change will allow the midwife to understand the level of support that the client might need. The use of a numbered range and supplement questions can facilitate this (Miller & Rollnick 2013, Wood 2020).

> **Example:**
> On a scale of 0 to 10 with 0 equal to no change and 10 indicating the most.
> How confident do you feel about eating more healthy foods/ exercising more/stopping smoking?
> If the birthing person indicates 5 or less a supplement question would be to ask as to why they have scored that low and what help they will need to make the number higher.
> Similarly, if the number is 6–8 then a supplement question of what they have in place to have scored well can be asked alongside is there anything else needed that could make that number higher.

AMBIVALENCE

Ambivalence is when there is a level of reluctance to change; the person appears to be in two minds as to what to do (Miller & Rollnick 2013, 2023). The reasons for this might be multifaceted, it might be due to lack of confidence in their ability to change, a lack of knowledge on which to base the change or there may be a 'block' to the change due to family or peer pressure for example. Evidence suggests that midwives when faced with an ambivalent client often provide information as to what they are not doing. Though this can be seen as being well intended it can lessen the positive effect of the intervention (Miller & Rollnick 2013, 2023, Upton & Thirlaway 2014). MI has been shown to be effective in dealing with ambivalence and encouraging a more effective and supportive dialogue to encourage behaviour change.

Ambivalence be helped with the following four steps which are a sequential and repetitive process (Miller & Rollnick 2013):

1. **Engagement**: the sooner the engagement the better the outcome.
2. **Focus**: a collaborative process that focuses on the health issue and the goals wishing to be achieved by the person.

3. **Evoke**: allowing the person to voice their ideas, concerns, and fears about the change and what it will achieve. This is crucial to MI.
4. **Plan**: the client reaches a 'tipping point'. This moves them from focusing on why they cannot change to how they can, with the development of a plan to continue and support the change.

SUMMARY OF KEY POINTS

- Changing behaviours is not easy to undertake and is affected by multiple factors, some of which the individual may have no control over.
- Health behaviour theories and models offer the midwife an understanding of the process of change, but they are not perfect exemplars.
- Pregnancy is often a time when a woman or birthing person is open to new ideas and may change their attitudes as they re-evaluate their lives, learn more about themselves and join a new social group of being parents. The midwife needs to bear in mind that vulnerable clients might find this difficult to achieve.
- Midwives need to be sensitive to the individual's values, the complex issues of health behaviour and the ethical dimensions of attempting to change an individual's values and attitudes.
- Midwives also need to be aware of their own values, beliefs, and attitudes, and how they may impact on the care that they give their clients.

REFERENCES

Acheson, D. (1998). *Independent Inquiry into Inequalities in Health*. London: Stationary Office.

Ajzen, I. (1988). *Attitudes, Personality and Behaviour*. London: Open University Press.

Ajzen, I. (1991). The theory of planned behaviour. *Organisational Behaviour and Human Decision Processes*, 50: 179–211. https://doi.org/10.1016/0749-5978(91)90020-T

Ajzen, I., & Fishbein, M. (eds.). (1980). *Understanding Attitudes and Predicting Social Behaviour*. Englewood Cliffs, NJ: Prentice Hall.

Bandura, A. (1997). *Self-Efficacy: The Exercise of Control*. New York: Freeman.

Becker, M. (ed.). (1974). *The Health Belief Model and Personal Health Behaviour*. Thorofare, NJ: Slack.

Bowden, J. (2017). Health, health lifestyles and behaviour change. In J. Bowden & V. Manning (Eds.). *Health Promotion in Midwifery Principles & Practice* (3rd ed., pp. 77–92). Boca Raton: CRC Press.

Corace, K., Srigley, J., Hargadon, D., Yu, D., MacDonald, T., Fabrigar, L., & Garber, G. (2016). Using behaviour chance frameworks to improve health care workers influenza vaccination rates: A systematic review. *Vaccine*, 34 (28): 3235–3242 https://doi.org/10.1016/j.vaccine.2016.04.071

Crafter, H. (1997). Attitudes, values and behaviour. In H. Crafter (ed.), *Health Promotion in Midwifery. Principles and Practice* (1st ed., pp. 54–64). Arnold London

Department of Health. (2010). *Our Health and Wellbeing Today*. Health and wellbeing of people in England: 2010- GOV.UK (www.gov.uk)

Donaldson, L., & Rutter, P. (2018). *Donaldson's Essential Public Health* (4th ed.). CRC Press. https://doi.org/10.1201/9781315154657

Edelman, C., & Kudzma, E. (2022). *Health Promotion Throughout the Lifespan* (10th ed.). United States Elsevier.

Edvardsson, K., Ivarsson, A., Eurenius, E., Garvare, R., Nystrom, M., Small, S., & Mogren, I. (2011). Giving offspring a health start: Parents experiences of health promotion and lifestyle change during pregnancy and early parenthood. *BMC Public Health*, 11: 936. https://doi.org/10.1186/1471-2458-11-936

Green, J., Tones, K., Cross, R., & Woodall, J. (2015). *Health Promotion planning & Strategies* (3rd ed.). London: Sage Publications Ltd.

Grenier, L., Atkinson, S., Mottola, M., Wahoush, O., Thabane, L., Xie, F., Vickers-Manzin, J., Moore, C., Hutton, E., & Murray-Davis, B. (2021). Be healthy in pregnancy: Exploring factors that impact pregnant women's nutrition and exercise behaviours. *Maternal & Child Nutrition*, 17: e13068. https://doi.org/10.1111/mcn.13068

International Confederation of Midwives. (2019). *Essential Competencies for Midwifery Practice*. Essential Competencies for Midwifery Practice | International Confederation of Midwives (internationalmidwives.org)

Kandel, P., Lim, S., Pirotta, S., Skouteris, H., Moran, L., & Hill, B. (2021). Enablers and barriers to women's lifestyle behaviour chance during the preconception period: A systematic review. *Obesity Review*, 22(7): e13235. http://doi.org/10.1111/obr.13235

Kent, L.M., Mortan, D.P., Rankin, P.M., Brett, G.M., Chang, E,. & Diehl, H. (2014). Gender differences in effectiveness of the complete involvement programme lifestyle intervention: An Australasian study *Health Promotion Journal of Australia*. 25: 222–229. https://doi.org/10.1071/HE14041.

Khekade, H., Potdukhe, A., Taksande, A., Wanjari, M., & Yelne, S. (2023). Preconception care: A strategic intervention for the prevention of neonatal and birth disorders. *Cureus*, 15(6): e41141. https://doi.org/10.7759/cureus.41141.

Khomami, M., Walter, R., Kilpatrick, M., de Jersey, S., Skouteris, H., & Moran, L. (2021). The role of midwives and obstetrical nurses in the promotion of health lifestyle during pregnancy. *Therapeutic Advances in Reproductive Health*. 15:1–12. https://doi.org/10.1177/26334941211031866

Lee, D.J., Haynes, C., & Garrod, D. (2012). Exploring the midwife's role in health promotion practice. *British Journal of Midwifery*, 20(3):178–186. https://doi.org/10.12968/bjom.2012.20.3.178.

Linsley, P., & Roll, C. (2023). *Health Promotion for Nursing Students UK*. London: Learning Matter.

Marlatt, G., & Donovan, D. (2005). *Prolapse Prevention: Maintenance Strategies in the Treatment of Addictive Behaviours* (2nd ed.). New York: The Guilford Press.

Marmot, M., Allen, J., Boyce, T,. Goldblatt, P., & Morrisons, J. (2018) *Health Equity in England the Marmot Review 10 Years On*. The Health Foundation. hHealth Equity in England: The Marmot Review 10 Years On - The Health Foundation

Mathias, L.A., Davis, D., & Ferguson, S. (2021). Salutogenic qualities of midwifery care: A best fit framework synthesis. *Women & Birth*, 34(3): 266–277.

Michie, S., van Stralen, M.M., & West, R.(2011). The behaviour change wheel: A new Method characterising behaviour change Intervention. *Implementation Science*, 6: 42. https://doi.org/10.1186/1748-5908-6-42

Miller, R.W., & Rollnick, S. (2023). *Motivational Interviewing Health People Change and Grow*. The Guildford Press.

Miller, R.W., & Rollnick, S. (2013). *Motivational Interviewing Helping People Change* (3rd ed.). Elsevier.

NHS Future Forum. (2011). *The NHS Role in Public Health. A Report from the NHS Future Forum.* https://www.gov.uk/government/uploads/system/uploads/attachment_data/file/216423/dh_132114.pdf

Nursing and Midwifery Council. (2018). *The Code: Professional Standards of Practice and Behaviour for Nurses, Midwives, And Nursing Associates.* NMC.

Pill, R., & Stott, N. (1990). *Making Changes: A Study of Working-Class Mothers and the Change Made in their Health-Related Behaviour Over 5 Years.* University of Wales College of Medicine.

Prochaska, J.O. (2005). Stages of change, readiness, and motivation. In J. Kerr, R. Weitkunat & M. Moretti (eds.), *ABC of Behavior Change. A Guide to Successful Disease Prevention and Health Promotion* (1st ed., pp. 111–127). Elsevier Churchill Livingstone.

Prochaska, J.O., & DiClemente, C.C. (1984). *The Transtheoretical Approach: Crossing Traditional Boundaries of Therapy.* Dow Jones-Irwin.

Public Health England. (2019). *Guidance: Prevention – A Life Course Approach.* London: Public Health England. Health matters: Prevention - a life course approach - GOV.UK (www.gov.uk)

Public Health England. (2022). *All Our Health: Personalised Care and Population Health. London: Public Health England.* https://www.gov.uk/government/collections/all-our-lives-personalised-care-and-population-health

Rockliffe, L., Peters, S., Heazell, A., & Smith, D. (2021). Factors influencing behaviour change during pregnancy: A systematic review and meta-synthesis. *Health Psychology Review,* 15(4): 613–632. https://doi.org/10.1080/17437199.2021.1938632

Rosenstock, I. (1966). Why people use health services. *Millbank Memorial Fund Quarterly,* 44: 94–121. https://doi.org/10.1111/j.1468–0009.2005.00425.

Rougan, A., Robroek, S.J.W., van Ginle, W., Lindeboom, D., Altink, B., & Burdorf, A. (2014). Barriers and facilitators for participation in health promotion programmes amongst employees – A 6 months follow up study. BMC Public Health, 14: 573. https://doi.org/10.1186/1471-2458-14-573

Schuman-Olivier, Z., Trombka, M., Lovas, D., Brewer, J., Vago, D., Gawande, R., Dunne, J., Lazar, S., Loucks, E., & Fulwiler, C. (2020). Mindfulness and behaviour change. *Harvard Review of Psychiatry,* 28: 371–394. https://doi.org/10.1097/HRP.000000000000027

Stead, L.F., Buitrago, D., Preciado N., Sanchez, G., Hartmann-Boyce J., & Lancaster, T. (2013). Physician advice for smoking cessation. *Cochrane Database of Systematic Reviews,* (5): CD000165. https://doi.org/10.1002/14651858.CD000165.pub4. Available: http://onlinelibrary.wiley.com/doi/10.1002/14651858.CD000165.pub4/abstract

Thompson, S.R., & Almond, M. (2014). Supporting people with behaviour change. In S.R. Thompson (ed.), *The Essential Guide to Public Health and Health Promotion* (1st ed.). Routledge.

United Nations. (2020). Sustainable Development Goals. http://www.ncbi.nlm.nih.gov/pubmed/26886241

Upton, D., & Thirlaway, K. (2014). *Promoting Health Behaviour: A Practical Guide* (2nd ed.). Routledge.

Walker, R., Choi, T., Quong, S., Hodges, R., Truby, H., & Kumar, A. (2020). "It's not easy" – A qualitative study of lifestyle change during pregnancy. *Women Birth,* 33(4):e363–370. https://doi.org/10.1016/j.wombi.2019.09.003

Webber, D.E., Gno, Z., & Mann, S. (2015). The responsibilities of the healthy: A manifesto for self-care. *Self Care,* 6(1): 2–9.

West, R., & Michie, S. (2020). A brief introduction to the COM-M model of behaviour and the PRIME theory of motivation. *Qeios,* 1–6. http://doi.org/10.32388/WW04E6

Wood, A. (2020). *The Motivational Interviewing Workbook.* Rockridge Press.

World Health Organization. (2017). *Optimizing the Contributions of the Nursing and Midwifery Workforce to Achieve Universal Health Coverage and the Sustainable Development Goals Through Education, Research and Practice.* Geneva: WHO. https://www.who.int/publications/i/item/9789241511971

Zinn, J. (2019). The meaning of risk taking – Concepts and dimensions. *Journal of Risk Research,* 22(1): 1–15. https://doi.org/10.1080/13669877.2017.1351465

Zinsser, L., Stoll, K., Wieber, F., & Pehlke-Milde, J. (2020). Changing behaviour in pregnant women: A scoping review. *Midwifery,* 85: 1–13. https://doi.org/10.1016/j.midw.2020.102680

FURTHER RESOURCES

Developed for NHS health trainers this handbook is a useful read as it talks through the behaviour change process with templates and exemplars that can be used in practice.

Making Every Contact Count Practical Resources: www.gov.uk/government/publications/making-every-contact-count-mecc-practical-resources

Michie, S., Rumsey, N., Fussell, A., Hardeman, W., Johnston, M., Newman, S., & Yardely, L. (2008) Improving Health: Changing Behaviour. NHS Trainer Handbook Manual. Depart of Health Publications (Best Practice Guidance Gateway Ref 9721) Improving health: changing behaviour. NHS health trainer handbook. (worktribe.com)

UK Government Package on using making every contact count within practice through the life stages.

Health Promotion: Conversations, Information, and 'Fake' News

RUTH SANDERS AND KENDA CROZIER

INTRODUCTION

In this chapter, we take a critical approach to the way that health promotion and information is viewed through a midwifery lens. We examine the multiple forms in which health promotion is discussed and shared between midwives and the women and families in their care, considered within the wider context of health information. The impact of the midwife on women's experiences will be explored, including the range of influences which may be present in women's lives, and how this information influences decision-making around birth and parenting. These considerations are underpinned by a shared decision-making approach.

Within in this chapter, the quality in health promotion literature, the rise and impact of 'fake' health news will be discussed. Difficult conversations with clients, facilitating individuals to take an active role in evaluating the information which is available to them will be explored and the influences on conversations about health information throughout the childbearing experience examined. Learning will be supported by a range of reflective and learning activities and practice points highlighted.

HEALTH PROMOTION LITERATURE

Health information is at the centre of health promotion and is disseminated via several strategies and resources (Lewis, 2019). The focus on health promotion in pregnancy is maximising healthy pregnancy through information on diet, exercise, and preparation for parenthood. There are messages aimed at lifestyle choices regarding weight (measured by Body Mass index), smoking (measured by carbon monoxide

DOI: 10.4324/9781003350071-10

monitoring) and substance and alcohol use (monitored by specific questions about quantity and frequency), and an increased emphasis recently on assessing mental health and wellbeing.

Historically health promotion information was directed towards midwives from sources such as government, professional organisations, hospital trust guidance, and research and professional journals (McCarthy et al, 2020; Song et al, 2012). These reputable sources were used by professionals to inform women and families, each individual practitioner making decisions about which information to share with the childbearing population. Information is delivered on this synchronous individual one to one basis as well as via asynchronous means at a population level from government agencies such as UK Health Security Agency Office for health improvement and disparities (formerly Public Health England), and each of the four countries in the UK has its own Department of Health which also uses mass media health campaigns (Foronda et al, 2016; NHS England, 2016). The World Health Organization (WHO) provides generic maternal and infant health information taken up by individual countries according to population need. The rise of information technologies and access to social media has fundamentally changed the relationship of information sharing in healthcare, with midwives no longer being the gatekeepers to childbearing information that they once were (Sanders & Crozier, 2018).

Healthcare improvement strategies including Better Births (National Maternity Review, 2016) and the Women's Health Strategy for England (Department of Health & Social Care, 2022) suggest best practice for communication and co-production, seeking to establish the information needs of service-users about maternity services. Guidance such as the NHS England's Accessible Information and Communication Policy discusses the need for staff to be flexible and creative in meeting individual needs, ensuring that information is 'accessible and inclusive' (NHS England, 2016, p. 5). The experiences of women and families requires continual monitoring due to the evolutionary nature of service changes and shifting perceptions as research changes current evidence (Redshaw et al, 2019).

Although midwives do still provide accessible information in the form of leaflets and booklets, they are no longer the sole provider of specialist information but one of multiple streams of information clients may engage with throughout pregnancy and postnatally. The emergence and proliferation of e-health has changed the way women and midwives interact, due to the range of free immediate information available in digital formats (Lagan et al, 2010, Sanders & Crozier, 2018; WHO, 2022), and midwifery practice must shift to ensure channels of effective communication between themselves and the communities they serve remain intact and fit for purpose (Sanders et al, 2016).

LEARNING ACTIVITY

Consider the public health information sources you utilise in your practice:

- Are they inclusive and appealing?
- Do they represent the public health messages relevant to the wide range of maternity population that you serve?
- Do you think these are valuable sources of information for service users?
- Are there elements you feel are missing from your local offering?

FUNDAMENTALS OF THE COMMUNICATION RELATIONSHIP

Fundamental to all health interactions and caring relationships is guaranteeing that patients are at the heart of all actions, decisions, and choices (Department of Health, 2013). Communication is essential for the delivery of high-quality, safe healthcare (Filby et al, 2016; Foronda et al, 2016; Marsh, 2019), with a plethora of evidence highlighting the connection between poor communication and negative patient experience, ineffective professional workflow, and poor outcomes (Independent Review Group, 2022).

Communication means to send, share and receive messages using verbal and non-verbal methods (Esegbona-Adeigbe, 2023), from the Latin "comunicare" – "to make common, share, participate, or impart" (Giger & Haddad, 2021, p. 19). Communication connects people, through written and oral language and behaviours such as gestures, facial expressions, body language and the use of personal space. It is contained within people's individual understanding and interpretation of the world, their communities and cultures, and because of this is rich with nuance, ideas, feelings, and sets of beliefs.

Communicating health information can be a complex process made up of numerous elements, including the raw information itself, the range of health messages and concepts within the information, the way in which this is imparted by the individual communicating the message and the perception or the way it is received by the individual it is aimed at, as well as the location in which this interaction occurs. The interaction between the information giver and information receiver is influenced by several factors (See Figure 10.1).

Communicating health messages is a core skill of midwifery practice, and effective communication is essential if people are to take an active role in their own health and wellbeing (Giger & Haddad, 2021). Midwives can take a flexible approach to communication, acknowledging that women and their family's modes

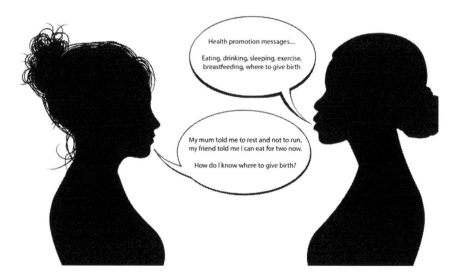

Figure 10.1 Giving and receiving messages.

of communication will depend on individual patterns and to some extent, social and cultural factors which impact their understanding and interpretation of information. Each pregnancy is a life changing and unique experience, navigating a series of complicated and dynamic decision-making processes in preparation for birth. Different psychosocial processes are involved, including exploration of choices for birth environment, labour support systems, discussions of mode of birth and strategies for birth and parenthood preparation. Decisions and options are influenced by societal and personal factors including socio-economic status, educational attainment, parity, previous birth experience, age and cultural, religious, spiritual backgrounds as well as identity, relationship status, and previous maternity experience (Sanders & Crozier, 2018; Yuill et al, 2020).

Information giving and the communication of health messages are the vehicles through which clients can make informed decisions about their choices for birth and the foundations for the health of their new family. Therefore, the models of shared decision-making which emphasise a partnership approach to care also suggest that individuals are not necessarily free to choose whatever they wish. Instead, they must make choices in a context of societal norms, both descriptive and injunctive relating to the ways people 'typically' do things and conforming or not to sets of anticipated behaviours (Brown, 2019). Information, therefore, will be filtered by people dependent on views, desires and feelings of uncertainty and caution acting to navigate their way through the terrain of birth and beyond (Madeley et al, 2023; Yuill et al, 2020).

Holistic communication is required in the midwifery context including verbal and non-verbal methods of communication, catered to each individual in a sensitive and person-centred way. This transcultural and flexible approach needs to be carried throughout the childbearing process from pre-conceptual care, antenatal discussion, labour facilitation and postnatal interactions to facilitate individualised and collaborative decision-making. Midwives therefore require an adept understanding

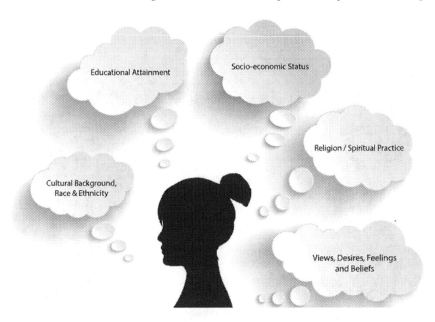

Figure 10.2 Factors to consider during communication.

to truly facilitate individuals' needs and preferences. This can be hampered by a lack of understanding on the part of the midwife, about the person they are supporting, as well as a limited time and training in health education (Creedy et al, 2021). There are many factors to be considered in communicating to meet the needs of the client in front of you as a midwife – see Figure 10.2.

REFLECTIVE ACTIVITY

Consider the influencing factors which might be present in your own communication with clients:

- Do you know where your maternity client's access and select information from?
- How do you have conversations with clients about the trustworthiness of information?
- What interactions make you feel that communication has been successful and why?
- How can you replicate this in future interactions?
- What beliefs and values inform your decision-making processes when providing care?
- How do you enable students to actively participate or lead positive communication when working with clients?

SOURCING INFORMATION: WHAT IS THE MIDWIFE'S ROLE?

The Department of Health's Women's Health Strategy for England (2022) aims to support health through the life course for women and girls, focusing on three main areas:

- Promoting good health
- Preventing negative health outcomes
- Restoring health and wellbeing

These are all aspects of midwifery care, understanding that women's health behaviours during pregnancy have life-long effects not only on women's own health but also upon the longer-term health of their children (Baron et al, 2017; Lippke et al, 2021).

Health information is in a constant state of evolution, responding to unforeseen circumstances and acknowledging the development of a changing evidence base as research continues. The COVID-19 pandemic, for example, required practitioners to seek new innovative modes of interaction due to limitations on physical distancing and social isolation (Atmuri et al, 2022). Midwives are expected to give specific advice about pregnancy and birth which will then impact longer term outcomes for women and children, making this a crucial opportunity for family health wellbeing (McCarthy et al, 2020).

Regan et al. (2013) found that nearly half of women in their study knew the kind of birth they wanted before they became pregnant, selecting information sources which confirmed their choices. People all carry a certain element of confirmation bias, seeking out information which matches their pre-pregnancy desires for birth, with information collected throughout the pregnancy journey adding and confirming those initial desires. This is supported in the above study with only 19%

of women reporting midwives as influential in their decision-making processes. Despite this, older studies, such as Larsson (2009), reported that 70% of the women in the study did not discuss information they had sourced from the Internet with their midwife, yet over half searched for information generated from midwives' discussion. Sanders and Crozier (2018) found that women often turned to informal information sources outside the healthcare professional's domain in response to conflicting advice from healthcare professionals as well as providing immediate relief from minor queries or concerns. Midwives need to continually update their knowledge base to remain current with emergent research but often this happens in an ad hoc and sporadic manner, due to a lack of protected time leaving professionals at risk of imparting out of date or inaccurate information (De Leo et al, 2019).

Midwives signpost individuals toward health promotion sources to protect and inform but this raises issues about the reliability of information, where clients find this information and how they filter effectively to meet their own needs. Midwives routinely signpost people to information, but a lack of discussion around what this information comprises can be problematic for women who are incorporating new concepts or encountering information which is opposed to previously held beliefs. The client's own health literacy also plays a part in the way in which information is sourced and discussed.

Individualised information is key for people to make informed choices which support their wishes for birth and parenting, yet many maternity public health messages are aimed at the general maternity population, leaving it to the individual midwife to signpost to appropriate information beyond the mainstream messages. This may mean that individuals have bespoke information tailored to them, however when individuals then discuss with their wider communities and networks, the information provided for one person will not be the same for the next. The Muslim Women's network survey (2022) identified that although there is known risk of gestational diabetes in women from South Asian communities this was not always discussed in antenatal care. This can lead to confusion when women discuss with their social support networks and pregnant friends who may have been given alternative or conflicting sources. This at its worst can lead to a mistrust in professional abilities to cater for individuals, or lead women to question midwifery knowledge, making it important to follow up on information-giving at subsequent antenatal or postnatal contacts and evaluating how health messages were received. Midwives have a responsibility to check the information they provide to women, to ensure that it is fit for purpose and applicable to the individual's situation, evidence-based and current (RCM, 2023). This can be a challenge as written trust guidelines are not always updated as evidence emerges which calls for further discussion from individual midwives to ensure health messages are explored antenatally.

REFLECTIVE ACTIVITY

- When sourcing information yourself as midwife, where do you begin accessing information from?
- Find health promotion information related to heath issues e.g., weight management in pregnancy or flu vaccination or smoking.
- What is the range of sources (leaflets, video, and infographics) and how inclusive are they?

- What drew you to these sources? Are they your usual sites for information, government or WHO or charity sources, or first on a google search?
- As a midwife how do you know they are reputable and trustworthy?
- Have you been able to find information which has fully answered your query?
- Do you notice a difference in the quality of them and would your clients notice the same?

INFORMATION SHARING

Health literacy is considered by the WHO as one of the three key pillars toward the United Nations Sustainable Development Goals (WHO, 2017). However, levels of health literacy can vary widely and so meeting specific patient-related information needs will depend on certain aspects which may not be ordinarily considered such as language barriers, differences in minority cultural and linguistic backgrounds, people with low socioeconomic status who can struggle to access care, people with neurodivergence and individuals with specific learning disabilities (Creedy et al, 2021; Rayment-Jones et al, 2023; Viveiros & Darling, 2019).

Midwives hold a unique role in being able to discuss issues face to face, an element women report to want more of (Wilmore et al, 2015) as the format of information becomes increasingly important with the ever-expanding range outside the health providers relationship with the maternity population. However, Creedy et al. (2021) found that midwives needed further training and skill in assessing people's understanding of health information, particularly when experiencing pressures on time and resources (Mackley et al, 2016). Health promotion can be overwhelming for the client so pacing information-giving across the process of pregnancy and postnatally is important to ensure that messages are understood and contextualised (Nicholls et al, 2019). This may mean the midwife revisiting discussions about alcohol consumption, nutrition, feeding choices, mode, and place of birth at regular intervals. Some topics may be more challenging for individuals such as how to manage weight gain, perinatal mental health due to stigma and financial situation. The order of information giving is important to avoid overload, and navigating so many messages can become overwhelming, therefore targeted information giving by the midwife is important at each contact.

Wilmore et al (2015) suggest that estimates of health literacy are often incorrect, and healthcare professionals can overestimate peoples' ability to comprehend and enact advice (Dickens et al, 2013; Mackley et al, 2016). Relational care models like continuity of carer can assist with this, with women reporting higher rates of satisfaction as well as improved outcomes for mothers and infants (Sandall et al, 2016). This model enables midwives to follow through on health information and health promotion topics over a series of visits and consultations rather than trying to provide all information and assess understanding within one short appointment. If this is not possible, then midwives may plan touch points throughout the pregnancy journey to introduce and reiterate health messages and information, layering knowledge so as not to overwhelm individuals across the schedule of care, aligning healthcare messages to the stage of pregnancy. This can then be continued regardless of caregiver to ensure a streamlined experience throughout the antenatal and postnatal periods.

FAKE NEWS AND EVALUATING INFORMATION

Media sources, including television, advertising and the internet, are rife with information about pregnancy and childbirth, with much debate about how influential these are on particularly first-time parents (Luce et al, 2017). Visual representations of birth on television are portrayed as risky, dramatic and often depict painful experiences, potentially fueling prospective parents' fear about childbirth (Roberts et al, 2021). Midwifery specific jargon is often used across maternity documents, and on social media platforms, causing further potential for confusion and impacting levels of health literacy. Jargon, although useful between healthcare professionals in certain situations, can create barriers with clients with the use of acronyms, unclear language and can disempower individuals by compromising their ability to make fully informed decisions and influence levels of satisfaction (Marsh, 2019).

REFLECTIVE ACTIVITY

- How do you feel about representations of midwifery across media formats?
- How do you think birth is portrayed on social media and television?
- What narratives have you encountered which may influence the societal perceptions of birth?
- How do you choose to engage with representations of childbearing on the internet or do you avoid these and if so, why?

Fake news, misinformation or disinformation include stories, messages and opinions which are spread through social networks or via different media formats online (Wang et al, 2019). There is a difference between misinformation which does not have the intention of causing harm to the information receiver, whereas disinformation means the communicator is aware of the inaccuracy of the information and is purposefully using it to cause harm (Wardle & Derakhshan, 2017). As midwives, we need to have an understanding about how misinformation and disinformation are being used and shared – is information associated with the original or primary messages or has it been altered by being taken out of context, and how does this feed into the notion of fake news? How can individuals sift the information to make informed decisions if they are working with numerous iterations of a possible initial message? Wardle and Derakhshan describe fake news as a type of 'information pollution' (2017, p. 5) arguing that the term fake news is inadequate to describe such a complicated social phenomenon. However, because of its familiarity across social media, this may be a positive initial way of engaging in conversations with people about what they are sourcing, particularly from the internet, examining accuracy of information sources and how it is perceived by clients.

Midwives have an opportunity to engage in the media, becoming increasingly tech-savvy, and some academics have argued that only by engaging further with media and specifically social media will the profession be able to harness its power and perhaps understand more fully the motivations behind where the messages come from (Luce et al, 2017). People may encounter internet 'trolls' whose mission can be to create chaotic and confusing contradictions about health information, with a goal to destabilise people's views and thrive on people becoming emotionally invested in a debate after taking the bait. The difference between this type of debating and evidence-based academic discussion is that the latter is ordinarily done with a professional and respectful tone, neither of which is present from the trolls operating in the childbirth and pregnancy arena online (Brown, 2019).

Anti-vaccination campaigns are a frequent source of anxiety for maternity clients. Vaccine hesitancy towards COVID-19 and flu vaccines in clients and in health professionals has potential to lower uptake (Marcell et al 2022). There is now strong evidence with longitudinal follow up to the age of 5 that flu vaccines in pregnancy are not harmful to the baby (Walsh et al, 2019). Therefore, the research and evidence literacy of midwives is essential to counter the fake news. The stories that circulated on social media during the COVID-19 pandemic used pseudoscience to convince the reader that facts were being presented, when, in reality, much of the presentation was based on supposition and conjecture and lacked any objective scientific data (Vilar-Compte et al, 2021). These can be exacerbated by the presence of algorithms and bots.

Algorithms influence what is looked at by seeking out patterns of searching and showing more of the types of pages which have been previously accessed, therefore filtering the information users are accessing a little more each day. Bots can replicate human interactions and can be used to spread positive health messages. However, these can also be used to spread misinformation and may, in the case of vaccine discussions, use various techniques like reposting, following and specific content generation to influence and create the illusion that someone has more 'followers' than they actually do (Broniatowski et al, 2018). Bots can be programmed to find specific words and phrases as well as source articles associated online and then reframe these to generate further debate. This in turn makes them appear more reliable but these nuances are often lost by the general social media consumer (Brown, 2019. See Chapter 18 on vaccinations and pregnancy.).

Examples from social media include emotive stories about breast-fed babies being allowed to starve due to midwives' strong position on breastfeeding which can portray midwifery in a negative light (Luce et al, 2016). People's experiences shared online offer a frequently polarised position of birth, and the role of the midwife, such as examples of birth stories of trauma that are anti-midwifery in tone (Luce et al, 2017). These stories are often compelling and emotional. The convincing nature of these and the comments in support make them seem highly plausible. However true the heart of the story is, the lack of any balanced or alternative perspective means that critical appraisal is impossible. Therefore, with family, friends and online 'experts' also contributing their own views and opinions with the range of ever-expanding risks and benefits this makes information a mine field for the lay person. The number of decisions which must be made and the pace at which these compete for prioritisation can make the journey of pregnancy an anxiety provoking one, with women making decisions steered by societal norms, informed by what they view and see on television and the internet (Morris & McInerney, 2010).

Midwives can be instrumental in the process of myth-busting and de-bunking misinformation, but this requires a relationship of sharing and trust between professionals and clients so that women do not feel patronised or unable to share their findings with professionals (Chatwin et al, 2021). Midwives need to discuss with women how to critically appraise what is presented as factual information about pregnancy, childbirth, and parenting, as well as providing accurate alternatives and correcting understanding when encountering sources which include misinformation (Krishna & Thompson, 2019; Rolls & Massey, 2019). Misinformation or disinformation can reduce a client's ability to achieve health literacy and creates challenges to decision-making being uninformed or ill advised.

The difficulty for maternity clients and for health professionals is in sorting fake news and real news. This may become more difficult and part of the role of the midwife may be to enable clients to use them as fact checkers. This is something for which health professionals have not been trained (Wang et al, 2019). Therefore, the role of the midwife is to understand where to find reliable and usable information to support discussions on common topics. Fact checking can be part of the midwifery contact starting with an understanding at initial booking contact of what women are accessing and how they feel about what they are seeing. Women may use midwives in the triangulation of data sources (Yuil et al, 2020), needing to check information or confirm with other sources like family, friends, and the internet that what they have found is true. We must examine the way that we as midwives suggest, advise and offer professional judgement and how explicit we make this to clients. This shared decision-making process is important to examine to facilitate the transition for clients from initial decisions to an informed position in which decisions are made.

HEALTHY DEBATE

Approaches to health and illness will vary with risk management strategies, protocols, and guidelines driving practitioners' decision-making processes and influencing the way that options and choices are facilitated (Eri et al, 2020). Our ideas as professionals may be different from the people we care for, yet consensus can be reached through a process of evaluation, deliberation and consideration of each individual's needs and preferences. Some researchers have suggested that increasing client's autonomy is a complex process which may involve certain "trade-offs" (Yuill et al, 2020, p. 2), due to the range of service provision rather than individual clinician's assessments. Pregnant people may make decisions which diverge from practitioners own, especially if this is couched within a context of recommended or standard care practices. Social media and news reports have documented where women's right to decline care has not been respected and consequently, eroded (Jenkinson et al, 2016). If women cannot find the support that they require within the professional sphere, they will seek for it outside, accessing informal information sources to inform their choices and which may result in disengagement from services if not appropriately supported.

The Code (Nursing & Midwifery Council [NMC], 2018; International Confederation of Midwives [ICM], 2019) states it is the midwife's duty to uphold human rights and promote client choice, and that as practitioners we must acknowledge that some people will make choices outside recommended guidelines. Declining professional recommendations can be a challenging decision for individuals but an essential aspect of facilitating woman-centred care. Non-normative decisions must be respected, otherwise consent becomes coercive with decisions being made which people may find compromise their body autonomy and self-actualisation. More detail can be necessary if women have not met care providers before and trust in the attending professional was suggested in recent research as being more important and influential than the detail of what is discussed (Nicholls et al, 2019). Individuals who withhold consent or do not wish to uptake standard recommendations can be deemed by professionals as 'difficult' giving rise to challenging conversations particularly around risk, safety, and choice potentially leading to adversarial behaviour or conflict between the client and the professional caring for them. Understanding women's reasons for specific choices in these instances is key and may arise from unknown aspects such as the desire to find psychological safety. Careful and sensitive discussion in a non-challenging manner can lead to a broader acknowledgement of people's needs and added insight of the context of biopsychosocial factors influencing their choices.

PRACTICE POINTS

- Ensure that you give full and balanced information using evidence where possible.
- Confirm the client has understood the information.
- Use a range of communication skills and formats in conversation with clients to meet individual needs.
- Be open to people who have a different viewpoint on the health promotion advice being given.

SUMMARY

- It is necessary for midwives to examine their own biases, psychological safety and cultural safety, and competence to enable women and birthing people to make the right choices for themselves through discussion, facilitation and information-sharing processes.
- Informed choice and support can then be generated in a collaborative way via a journey of exploration with individuals, by gaining trust and mutual respect between midwives and the women and families in their care.
- Midwives need to be aware of the information available and be able to direct clients away from those specialising in disinformation.

REFERENCES

Atmuri, K., Sarkar, M., Obudu, E., & Kumar, A. (2022). Perspectives of pregnant women during the COVID-19 pandemic: A qualitative study. *Women and Birth.* 35: 280–288.

Baron, R., Heesterbeeka, Q., Manniëna, J., Huttona, E.K., Johannes Brug, J., & Westermand, M.J. (2017). Exploring health education with midwives, as perceived by pregnant women in primary care: A qualitative study in the Netherlands. *Midwifery.* 46: 37–44.

Broniatowski, D., Jamison, A., Qi, S., AlKulaib, L., Chen, T., Benton, A., Quinn, S., & Dredze, M. (2018). Weaponized health communication: Twitter bots and Russian trolls amplify the vaccine debate. *American Journal of Public Health.* 108(10): 1378–1384.

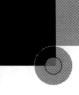

Brown, A. (2019). *Informed Is Best. How to Spot Fake News about Your Pregnancy, Birth and Baby.* Pinter & Martin UK.

Chatwin, J., Butler, D., Jones, J., James, L., Choucri, L., & McCarthy, R. (2021). Experiences of pregnant mothers using social media based antenatal support service during the COVID-19 lockdown in the UK: Findings from a user survey. *BMJ Open.* 11:e040649. https://doi.org/10.1136/bmjopen-2020-040649

Creedy, D., Gamble, J., Boorman, R., & Allen, J. (2021). Midwives' self-reported knowledge and skills to assess and promote maternal health literacy: A national cross-sectional survey. *Women and Birth.* 34:e188–e195.

De Leo, A., Bayes, S., Geraghty, S., & Butt, J. (2019). Midwives' use of best available evidence in practice: An integrative review. *Journal of Clinical Nursing.* 28(23–24): 4225–4235. https://doi.org/10.1111/jocn.15027

Department of Health. (**2013**). *The NHS Constitution: The NHS Belongs to Us All.* London. The NHS Constitution the NHS belongs to us all (publishing.service. gov.uk)

Department of Health & Social Care. (2022). Women's health strategy for England. Policy paper. Presented to Parliament by the Secretary of State for Health and Social Care. CP 736 ISBN 978-1-5286-3665-0

Dickens, C., Lambert, B.L., Cromwell, T., & Piano, M.R. (2013). Nurse overestimation of patients' health literacy. *Journal of Health Communication.*18: 62–69. http://doi. org/10.1080/10810730.2013.825670.

Eri, T., Berg, M., Dahl, B., Gottfredsdottir, H., Sommerseth, E., & Prinds, C. (2020). Models for midwifery care: A mapping review. *European Journal of Midwifery.* 4(30), 1–17.

Esegbona-Adeigbe, S. (2023). *Transcultural Midwifery Practice Concepts, Care and Challenges.* London: Elsevier.

Filby, A., McConville, F., & Portela, A. (2016). What prevents quality midwifery care? A systematic mapping of barriers in low and middle income countries from the provider perspective. *PLoS ONE.* 11(5): e0153391. http://doi.org/10.1371/journal. pone.0153391

Foronda, C., MacWilliams, B., & McArthur, E. (2016). Interprofessional communication in healthcare: an integrative review. *Nurse Education in Practice.* 19: 36–40. https://doi.org/10.1016/j.nepr.2016.04.005

Giger, J., & Haddad, L. (2021). *Transcultural Nursing. Assessment and Intervention* (8th ed.). London: Elsevier.

Independent Review Group. (2022). Ockenden Report. London: Independent Review Group.

International Confederation of Midwives. (2019). *Essential Competencies for Midwifery Practice.* Essential Competencies for Midwifery Practice | International Confederation of Midwives (internationalmidwives.org)

Jenkinson, B., Kruske, S., Stapleton, H., Beckmann, M., Reynolds, M., & Kilda, S. (2016). Women's, midwives' and obstetricians' experiences of a structured process to document refusal of recommended maternity care. *Women and Birth.* 29: 531–541.

Krishna, A., & Thompson, T. (2019). Misinformation about health: A review of health communication and misinformation scholarship. *American Behavioural Scientist.* 65(2): 316–332.

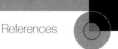

Lagan, B., Sinclair, M., & Kernohan, W.G. (2010). Internet use in pregnancy informs Women's decision making: A web-based survey. *Birth*. 37(2): 106–115.

Larsson, M.A. (2009). Descriptive study of the use of the internet by women seeking pregnancy-related information. *Midwifery*. 25(1): 14–20.

Lewis, A. (2019). Communication skills in promoting health. In K. Norman (Ed.), *Communication Skills for Nursing and Healthcare Students*. Banbury: Lantern Publishing Limited.

Lippke, S., Derksen, C., Keller, F.M., Kötting, L., Schmiedhofer, M., & Welp, A. (2021). Effectiveness of communication interventions in obstetrics—A systematic review. *International Journal Environment Research and Public Health*. 18: 2616. https://doi.org/10.3390/ijerph18052616

Luce, A., Cash, M., Hundley, V., Cheyne, H., van Teijlingen, E., & Angell, C. (2016). "Is it realistic?" the portrayal of pregnancy and childbirth in the media. *BMC Pregnancy Childbirth*. 16: 40. https://doi.org/10.1186/s12884-016-0827-x

Luce, A., Hundley, V., & van Teijlingen, E. (2017). *Midwifery Childbirth and the Media*. London: Palgrave Pivot.

McCarthy, R., Byrne, G., Brettle, A., Choucri, L., Ormandy, P., & Chatwin, J. (2020). Midwife-moderated social media groups as a validated information source for wone during pregnancy. *Midwifery*. 88: 102710.

Mackley, A., Winter, M., Guillen, U., Paul, D.A., & Locke, R. (2016). Health literacy among parents of newborn infants. *Advanced Neonatal Care*. 16(4): 283–288.

Madeley, A.M., Earle, S., & O'Dell, L. (2023). Challenging norms: Making non-normative choices in childbearing. Results of a meta ethnographic review of the literature. *Midwifery*. 116: 103532.

Marcell, L., Dokania, E., Navia, I., Baxter, C., Crary, I., Rutz, S., Soto Monteverde, M.J., Simlai, S., Hernandez, C., Huebner, E.M., Sanchez, M., Cox, E., Stonehill, A., Koltai, K., & Adams Waldorf, K.M. (2022). One vax two lives: A social media campaign and research program to address COVID-19 vaccine hesitancy in pregnancy. *American Journal of Obstetrics Gynecology*. 23;227(5): 685–695.e2. https://doi.org/10.1016/j.ajog.2022.06.022.

Marsh, A. (2019). The importance of language in maternity services. *British Journal of Midwifery*. 27(5): 320–323.

Morris, T., & McInerney, K. (2010). Media representations of pregnancy and childbirth: An analysis of reality television programs in the United States. *Birth*. 37(2): 134–140.

Muslim Woman's Network UK. (2022). *Invisible Maternity Experiences of Muslim Women from Racialised Minority Communities*. https://www.mwnuk.co.uk/go_files/resources/maternity_report_120722.pdf

National Maternity Review. (2016). *Better Births: Improving Outcomes of Maternity Services in England*. London: NHS England.

NHS England Patient and Public Participation and Insight Group. (2016). *NHS England Accessible Information and Communication Policy*. Leeds: NHS England.

Nicholls, J., David, A., Iskaros, J., & Lanceley, A. (2019). Consent in pregnancy: A qualitative study of the views and experiences of women and their healthcare professionals. *European Journal of Obstetrics & Gynecology and Reproductive Biology*. 238: 132–137.

Nursing and Midwifery Council. (2018). *The Code: Professional Standards of Practice and Behaviour for Nurses and Midwives*. London: NMC.

Rayment-Jones, H., Dalrymple, K., Harris, JM., Parslow, E., Georgi, T., & Sandal, J. (2023). Project20: Maternity care mechanisms that improve access and engagement for women with social risk factors in the UK – A mixed-methods, realist evaluation. *BMJ Open.* 13: e064291. https://doi.org/10.1136/ bmjopen-2022-064291

Redshaw, M., Martin, C.R., Savage-McGlynn, E., & Harrison, S. (2019). Women's experiences of maternity care in England: Preliminary development of a standard measure. *BMC Pregnancy Childbirth.* 19: 167 https://doi.org/10.1186/ s12884-019-2284-9.

Regan, M., McElroy, K., & Moore, K. (2013). Choice? Factors that influence women's decision making for childbirth. *Journal Perinatal Education.* 22(3): 171–180.

Roberts, J., Bennett, B., Slack, H., Borrelli, S., Spiby, H., Walker, L., & Jomeen, J. (2021). Midwifery students' views and experiences of birth on mainstream factual television. *Midwifery.* 92. https://doi.org/10.1016/j.midw.2020.102859.

Rolls, K., & Massey, D. (2019). Social media is a source of health-related misinformation. *Evidence Based Nursing.* 24(2): 46.

Royal College of Midwives. (2023). Informed decision making. https://www.rcm.org. uk/media/6007/informed-decision-making_0604.pdf.

Sandall, J., Soltani, H., Gates, S., Shennan, A., & Devane, D. (2016). Midwife-led continuity models versus other models of care for childbearing women. *Cochrane Database System Review.* 28;4(4): CD004667. https://doi.org/10.1002/14651858.

Sanders, J., Hunter, B., & Warren, L. (2016). A wall of information? Exploring the public health component of maternity care in England. *Midwifery.* 34: 253–260.

Sanders, R., & Crozier, K. (2018). How do informal information sources influence women's decision-making for birth? A meta-synthesis of qualitative studies. *BMC Pregnancy and Childbirth.* 18: 21.

Song, F., West, J., Lundy, L., & Dahmen, N. (2012). Women, pregnancy and health information online: The making of informed patients and ideal mothers. *Gender & Society.* 26(5): 773–798.

Vilar-Compte, M., Gaitán-Rossi, P., Rhodes, E.C., Cruz-Villailba., & Pérez-Escamilla, R. (2021). Breastfeeding media coverage and beliefs during the COVID-19 pandemic in Mexico: implications for breastfeeding equity. *International Journal of Equity Health.* 20: 260. https://doi.org/10.1186/s12939-021-01588-y

Viveiros, C., & Darling, E. (2019). Perceptions of barriers to accessing perinatal mental health care in midwifery: A scoping review. *Midwifery.* 70: 106–118.

Walsh, L.K., Donelle, J., Dodds, L., Hawken, S., Wilson, K., Benchimol, EI., Chakraborty, P., Guttmann, A., Kwong, J.C., MacDonald, N.E., Ortiz, J.R., Sprague, A.E., Top, K.A., Walker, M.C., Wen, S.W., Fell, D.B., Deshayne, B. (2019). Health outcomes of young children born to mothers who received 2009 pandemic H1N1 influenza vaccination during pregnancy: Retrospective cohort study. *British Medical Journal.* 366: l4151. http://doi.org/10.1136/bmj.l415

Wang, Y., McKee, M., Torbica, A., & Stuckler, D. (2019). Systematic literature review on the spread of health-related misinformation on social media. *Social Science and Medicine.* 240: 112552.

Wardle, C., & Derakhshan, H. (2017). Information disorder: An interdisciplinary framework. Retrieved 4 March 2023, from first draft news website. https:// firstdraftnews.org:443/coe-report/

Wilmore, M., Rodger, D., Clifton, C., Flabouris, M., & Skuse, A. (2015). How midwives tailor health information used in antenatal care. *Midwifery.* 31: 74–79.

World Health Organisation. (2017). *World Health Statistics 2017: Monitoring Health for the SDGs, Sustainable Development Goals.*

World Health Organisation. (2022). Using e-health and information technology to improve health [Online]. Retrieved 15 February 2023, from https://www.who.int/westernpacific/activities/using-e-health-and-information-technology-to-improve-health

Yuill, C., McCourt, C., Cheyne, H., & Leister, N. (2020). Women's experience of decision-making and informed-choice about pregnancy and birth care: A systematic review and meta-synthesis of qualitative research. *BMC Pregnancy and Childbirth.* 20: 343. https://doi.org/10.1186/s12884-020-03023-6

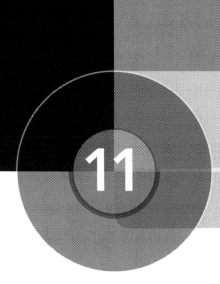

Smoking Cessation in Pregnancy

11

TOMASINA STACEY AND
CHELSEA LEADLEY

INTRODUCTION

The purpose of this chapter is to explore evidence related to cigarette smoking in pregnancy and review strategies that midwives can utilise to help support women and birthing people be smoke free during the peripartum period and beyond. This chapter will not address other forms of tobacco consumption, nor the frequent combination of tobacco and marijuana use. Evidence has shown that although it is ideal to start pregnancy smoke free, if a woman is able to stop smoking by 16 weeks' gestation, most of the adverse outcomes to the baby can be avoided (Diamanti et al., 2019). There is therefore an opportunity to make a difference to perinatal outcomes during pregnancy itself. In addition, although smoking can reduce life expectancy by ten years, if a person is able to stop smoking permanently by the age of 40, they can expect an almost normal lifespan (Doll et al., 2004). Midwives play a key role in public health and health promotion; stopping smoking before or during pregnancy is one of the most beneficial health behaviour changes that a childbearing woman can make.

This chapter outlines the effect of smoking tobacco in pregnancy, the association with health inequalities and the complexity of why it is so difficult to quit smoking. It will then examine current evidence on what works for whom and when and outline recommendations for midwifery practice.

DOI: 10.4324/9781003350071-11

Table 11.1 Carbon monoxide monitoring

- CO is a poisonous gas contained within cigarettes. It impacts on oxygen transport, which reduces the oxygen available for the developing fetus.
- CO monitoring is a quick, non-invasive test. The woman holds her breath for 15 seconds to allow the CO in the blood to pass into the air in her lungs. She then blows into the machine until it indicates enough breath has been expelled. The recommended cut off for detecting smoking in pregnant women is four parts per million (4 ppm).
- CO is also present in exhaust fumes and faulty gas appliances (i.e. boilers). There have been documented cases of a faulty boiler being identified due to routine antenatal CO monitoring.

EFFECT OF SMOKING IN PREGNANCY

Cigarettes contain a complex mixture of harmful chemicals, including carbon monoxide (CO), nicotine, tar, hydrogen cyanide, formaldehyde, and tobacco-specific nitrosamines (TSNAs) (Engstrom & Schnoll, 2003). Around 60 of these elements are known to be carcinogenic. These chemicals can have a profound and lasting effect not only on the smoker themselves, but on those around who inhale the second-hand smoke, and importantly in pregnancy, on the growing fetus. CO, which is a product of incomplete combustion, competes with oxygen by binding haemoglobin in the blood, preventing the cells and tissues in the body from getting the oxygen that they need. In pregnancy, CO crosses the placenta where the effect can be even more damaging as fetal haemoglobin binds CO 2.5 to 3-fold stronger than maternal haemoglobin (Culnan et al., 2018) (Table 11.1).

Smoking in pregnancy increases the risk of preterm birth by more than 60% and doubles the chance of a baby being born small for gestational age (Diamanti et al., 2019). In addition, it is associated with an increased risk of miscarriage, stillbirth, and neonatal mortality (Diamanti et al., 2019; Flenady et al., 2011). It is the single most important modifiable risk factor for all adverse perinatal outcomes. The negative consequences linked with maternal smoking during pregnancy also extend beyond birth through childhood. Children exposed to tobacco in utero are at an increased risk of experiencing respiratory infections; asthma; problems of ear, nose and throat, such as "Glue" ear; psychological and behavioural difficulties (Ekblad et al., 2010) obesity (Oken et al., 2008); and early onset of adult diabetes and high blood pressure (Montgomery & Ekbom, 2002).

SMOKING AND INEQUALITY

In high-income countries, smoking is strongly associated with poverty. In the UK, women who live in the most deprived areas are more than twice as likely to have smoked in the 12 months before conception and are less likely to quit before conception or in early pregnancy compared to their less deprived counterparts (19% vs 41%) (Schoenaker et al., 2021). The reasons for this are likely to be multifactorial and include not only cultural norms and expectations, but also the effect of a number of environmental, social, and psychological factors that are associated with social and economic deprivation (Madureira et al., 2020). In general, women who experience socioeconomic disadvantages, problems in their interpersonal relationships, stress or depression have been found to be more likely to smoke during pregnancy than those that do not have these challenges (Miyazaki et al., 2015; Rodriguez et al., 2000).

Smoking in pregnancy is a complex issue, influenced by a combination of social, emotional, and physical factors. Research suggests that pregnant women generally do want to stop smoking but often do not feel that they have the necessary support, confidence or self-efficacy to do so (Fletcher et al., 2022; Stacey et al., 2022). Those attempting to quit need a high level of social, behavioural, and pharmacological support in order to be successful. The following interventions have been found to have some degree of efficacy in promoting cessation of smoking in pregnancy. They can be broadly grouped into behavioural interventions (which include a wide range of strategies including counselling, financial incentives, and biofeedback) and pharmacological treatments. It is somewhat unclear whether one intervention is more effective than the other, although financial incentives and intensive counselling are currently considered to be the two most effective (Chamberlain et al., 2017).

BEHAVIOURAL INTERVENTIONS

Behavioural interventions or behavioural change techniques (BCTs) refer to strategies that do not use pharmacological treatments but provide motivation and support to smokers wishing to quit through cognitive-behavioural, motivational and supportive therapies (Chamberlain et al., 2017). These include incentives, psychological support, health education and risk perception, social and peer support, and biofeedback, amongst others (for a comprehensive list, see Robert West's and colleagues' exploration of behaviour change techniques used by the English Stop Smoking Services (West et al., 2010).

FINANCIAL INCENTIVES

Financial incentives involve a process of providing financial reward for ongoing smoking cessation and have been found to be a cost effective and successful intervention in promoting smoking cessation in pregnant women particularly for those who live in poorer areas (Tappin et al., 2015). This approach has been supported by the Smoking in Pregnancy challenge group, and in 2021, the provision of financial incentives was recommended as a national strategy in the UK by the All-Party Parliamentary Group (APPG) on Smoking and Health.

Incentives are thought to use the same neurobiological reward and conditioning processes that are the basis of gaining and maintaining unhealthy behaviour to promote healthy behaviour (Higgins et al., 2022). Additionally, incentives may also overcome, in part, the issue of poor engagement with stop smoking services, with women receiving incentives engaging more and feeling motivated by the feedback and monitoring of their progress (Mantzari et al., 2012).

PSYCHOLOGICAL SUPPORT

Psychological support includes different forms of counselling, cognitive behavioural therapy (CBT) and psychotherapy. Intensive behavioural support is typically delivered by a trained, dedicated stop-smoking advisor, and consists of advice, discussion and targeted activities that aim to minimise a smoker's motivation to smoke, facilitate relapse prevention and coping and optimise the use of smoking cessation medications and social support (West & Stapleton, 2008). The Cochrane review from 2017 found high-quality evidence from 48 studies that counselling can lead to a 44% increase in smoking cessation (Chamberlain et al., 2017). The specific effect of different forms of counselling (such as psychotherapy or CBT specifically) is unclear. However, counselling has been found to be most effective when it is intensive and when women have the desire to quit when they start and when a positive therapeutic relationship has been established (Diamanti et al., 2019).

HEALTH EDUCATION AND RISK PERCEPTION

Health education and risk perception refers to the provision of evidence relating to the impact of smoking on both the individual smoker and the baby. Pregnancy is seen as a 'window of opportunity' for positive behavioural change, but if women are not aware of, or do not believe in, the full risks associated with smoking during pregnancy then there is less likely to be a motivation for change (Bell et al., 2018). Lack of education and knowledge surrounding the impact of smoking during pregnancy may be one of the first obstacles to cessation, with a high level of knowledge about the harms of smoking being related to increased intentions to quit (Ferguson & Hansen, 2012). The current evidence suggests that health education and risk advice alone is insufficient in promoting smoking cessation (Chamberlain et al., 2017); however, it may be an important element in a package of care and may influence motivation and the readiness to quit (Bell et al., 2018). Evidence suggests that women have a mixed level of understanding and awareness of the impact of smoking on the health of the baby (Stacey et al., 2022). Midwives have the opportunity to play a crucial role in providing health education and raising awareness in a supportive and non-judgemental manner.

SOCIAL AND PEER NETWORK-BASED INTERVENTIONS

An important facilitator for successful smoking cessation is a supportive social network, particularly supportive partners. Women who have support to quit from close friends and partners are more likely to be successful (Flemming et al., 2015). Other interventions that involve support from friends, volunteer or paid lay person, or a trained health care professional to promote smoking cessation have not been well researched to date, although they have been suggested as potentially important by women themselves and show potential in initial small-scale studies (Chamberlain et al., 2017). Unsurprisingly, women find it more difficult to quit if people close to them smoke, therefore, for smoking cessation initiatives in pregnancy to be more successful, it is best to adopt a whole family approach (Koshy et al., 2010).

BIOMARKER FEEDBACK

Biofeedback includes CO monitoring, ultrasound feedback and cotinine measurements. For pregnant women, CO monitoring was highlighted as a visual indicator of the risk to the baby and viewed as a motivational tool by both them and healthcare professionals (Bauld et al., 2017). It can also track a reduction or abstinence of smoking. Routine CO monitoring (alongside an opt-referral process) is a key element of the NHS Saving Babies Lives Care Bundle v2. However, evidence supporting biomarker feedback efficacy in smoking cessation is limited and more research is required. The literature is less clear on the impact of other behavioural facilitators to smoking cessation, although increased self-efficacy, motivation to quit and the relationship with health care professionals (in particular their midwife) are all of relevance.

PHARMACOLOGICAL TREATMENTS

Pharmacotherapy is particularly recommended for pregnant women who are heavy smokers and have previously been unable to quit without medication (Claire et al., 2020).

NICOTINE REPLACEMENT THERAPY

Nicotine replacement can come in various forms (patches, gum, lozenge, or inhaler) and is a key element of smoking cessation support for the non-pregnant population. Some have expressed concern about the use of nicotine replacement therapy (NRT) in pregnancy; however NRT provides lower levels of nicotine than cigarette smoking and it does not emit CO and other toxins present in cigarettes. In the most recent systematic review available, it was found that NRT may increase smoking cessation rates in late pregnancy, but there was low certainty in this evidence (Claire et al., 2020). Current advice from NICE is to consider offering NRT at the earliest opportunity in pregnancy, alongside behavioural therapy to help support women stop smoking (NICE, 2021) (Table 11.2).

Table 11.2 Summary of NICE guidance

Summary of NICE Guidance

Tobacco: Preventing uptake, promoting quitting, and treating dependence [NG 209] [2021].

1. Identify pregnant women who smoke and refer them for stop-smoking support (SSS)
   Routine CO monitoring at booking and 36 weeks for all women and at every appointment for women who smoke or who have recently quit. Provide referral to stop smoking support.
2. Follow up women who have been referred to stop smoking support.
   Provide information on risks (to her and her baby) of smoking in pregnancy.
   Consider factors that may prevent women from accessing SSS, such as self-efficacy, knowledge about the service, access to childcare.
3. Provide support to stop smoking
   Provide ongoing support throughout pregnancy and beyond
   Consider NRT alongside behavioural therapy support

ELECTRONIC CIGARETTES AND VAPING

The number of e-cigarette users in the UK has increased considerably over the last decade, with approximately 4.3 million in 2022 compared to 700,000 users in 2012 (Action on Smoking and Health, 2023). The increasing popularity of e-cigarettes, both in the general population and in pregnancy, is generally thought to be a result of its perceived safety in comparison to conventional cigarettes (Noël et al., 2023). One study found that compared to nicotine patches, e-cigarettes were effective in helping women quit, but the safety and efficacy of these remain unknown (Hajek et al., 2019). In the UK, the NHS state that e-cigarettes are less risky than cigarette smoking, and that nicotine alone is relatively harmless. Despite this, there is insufficient evidence surrounding the effects of e-cigarettes on fetal development and pregnancy outcomes. The most recent report for the Office for Health Improvement and Disparities in England states only a single paper was identified that had researched the effect of e-cigarettes on pregnancy outcome, which found vaping had little to no effect on birth weight (McNeill et al., 2022). However, studies using rats and mice suggest in-utero exposure to e-cigarettes may result in decreased respiratory health and brain development (Noël et al., 2023) (Orzabal et al., 2019). Ingredients from e-cigarettes, in addition to nicotine, have also been found to be toxic to human placenta cells through modifying biomarkers key to placental and fetal development (Potter et al., 2022). The use of e-cigarettes in pregnancy is under-researched, and there are currently no high-quality trials on the safety and efficacy of e-cigarettes as a tool for smoking cessation (Claire et al., 2020). This is an area that still needs further research, particularly outside of animal studies.

LEARNING ACTIVITY

Prior to reading the next section, consider what the enablers and barriers might be for midwives supporting pregnant smokers to stop smoking.

DIFFICULTIES IN QUITTING

Although the above interventions have been identified as being successful in clinical trials, it is clear from the persistently high rates of smoking amongst some groups of women that there are challenges to the implementation of these interventions in practice. One of the biggest issues faced by smoking cessation interventions or programmes is the low engagement and high drop-out rates. There is a significant difference in the number of women who are interested in these services and those who actually engage with them (Naughton et al., 2019). There is therefore a need to understand better the barriers to accessing support and how to encourage women to engage with the available services. An important factor in the success of specific interventions is the motivation of women to quit: desire and motivation are rarely considered in randomised trials of interventions (as those women who do not want to quit are less likely to agree to be part of the study) and this may contribute to inconsistency when the interventions are incorporated into standard care.

Cigarette smoking is notoriously addictive. Nicotine, the second most abundant constituent of tobacco smoke is not, of itself, particularly harmful, but it is responsible for the physically addictive nature of tobacco. However, smoking is not just physically addictive but also psychologically addictive. Most smokers start in early life, and it can become integral to their sense of self – associated with how they identify themselves.

SELF-EFFICACY

Levels of self-efficacy and belief in ability to stop smoking have been found to be linked with motivation to quit (Bauld et al., 2017). High self-efficacy is a predictor of smoking cessation during pregnancy, whilst lower self-efficacy has been associated with lowered effectiveness of cessation and higher rates of post-partum smoking relapse (Emery et al., 2017). Women who wanted to quit or were successful spoke about having a 'focus' and strong desire to quit for the health of the baby (Bauld et al., 2017). Self-efficacy can be increased through understanding the circumstances likely to lead to smoking or temptation to smoke (Abrahamsson et al., 2005) as well as through a positive feedback loop. Health care professionals felt that as a motivational tool, the use of CO monitoring was somewhat effective; however, there were concerns that there was a need for improved training for midwives of how to discuss it (Bauld et al., 2017).

PERCEIVED STRESS AND MENTAL HEALTH

Daily stressors and poor mental health are strongly associated with smoking in pregnancy (Paarlberg et al., 1999). It is important for midwives to understand the social situation and psychosocial characteristics of each person to provide interventions that are tailored to the individual and aid in smoking cessation (Boucher & Konkle, 2016). Evidence suggests that women want empathy and recognition of their personal circumstances and barriers and facilitators to cessations (Stacey et al., 2022). When health care professionals (HCPs) understand the reasons that women smoke and appreciate why this makes quitting more of a challenge, they can be more supportive and empathetic (Flemming et al., 2016).

REFLECTION ACTIVITY

Consider a time when you have discussed smoking with a pregnant woman.

- Did you feel able to give all of the information on the effects of smoking in pregnancy (for her and her baby)?
- Did you offer further help to quit smoking? Was this taken up? If no, could you have done anything differently?
- Do you feel as comfortable discussing smoking cessation as you do with discussing dietary choices in pregnancy? If not, consider the reasons why.

THE ROLE OF THE MIDWIFE AND IMPLICATIONS FOR PRACTICE

Whilst the social influence of friends, family and partners has considerable influence on women's intention and commitment to quitting, for some women support from a midwife is even more important than support from their social network (Ashwin & Watts, 2010). Midwives often fear that discussion of smoking cessation might damage their relationship with the women in their care (Kalamkarian et al., 2023); however if the approach is non-judgemental, supportive and well-informed, it can have a positive impact both on the relationship and the successful smoking cessation (McLeod et al., 2003). Midwives can best assist women by providing both support and understanding in addition to referral to professional support (Bauld et al., 2017).

Although health care professionals recognised that supporting smoking cessation was a key part of their job (Flemming et al., 2016), midwives often hold a negative view with regards to providing stop smoking advice, feeling it was difficult or challenging to do so, and that the topic of smoking during pregnancy was sensitive and potentially intrusive. A lack of training was commonly cited by health care professionals as a barrier to providing adequate smoking cessation advice (Bauld et al., 2017). Midwives and other health care professionals need confidence to implement smoking cessation interventions (through familiarity, training, experiences, and access to resources) in order to adequately support pregnant smokers to quit (Passey et al., 2020). One of the key elements of this is knowing how to bring up the topic of smoking cessation in the first place, and how to follow on from these first discussions, the most important aspect being the need to approach the topic in a non-judgemental and supportive way, that appreciates the individual situation (Flemming et al., 2016). (Please see Chapter 10 of this manuscript).

In order to frame these conversations, it has been found to be helpful to have a structured approach such as the Very Brief Advice approach (Figure 11.1) which has

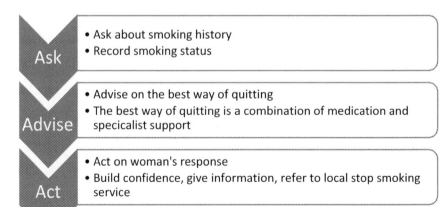

Figure 11.1 Very brief advice.

Source: Adapted from https://www.ncsct.co.uk/index.php

been developed by the National Centre for Smoking Cessation Training (NCSCT) in the UK and has been adopted as standard by the NHS.

Health care professionals generally favour shorter interactions that briefly engage women and put them at the centre of the decision to quit, viewing them as responsible for the change (Flemming et al., 2016). This also includes helping women to understand how smoking could negatively impact their baby, using both written and visual images.

As mentioned earlier, key barriers to midwives providing stop smoking advice is a lack of knowledge and training, alongside a lack of belief in their ability to deliver the advice (self-efficacy) in a supportive and non-judgemental way (Flemming et al., 2016). It may be the case that the current focus on the medical issues surrounding pregnancy means that limited time is given to midwifery curricula to teaching communication skills and increasing knowledge on issues such as smoking cessation. Indeed, significant gaps have been identified in the current curricula of UK midwifery, nursing, and medical schools regarding the teaching of issues related to smoking and smoking cessation (Richards et al., 2014). In addition, midwives felt there were so many other things to do that discussing smoking cessation was not a priority, particularly when they felt most women would not quit (Flemming et al., 2016).

SUMMARY

- Smoking in pregnancy is the single most important modifiable risk factor for poor perinatal outcome.
- Women should be supported with quitting as early as possible in pregnancy.
- Women who stop smoking before 16 weeks' gestation have a similar risk of preterm birth and small for gestational age baby as that of a non-smoker.
- Smoking in pregnancy exacerbates existing health inequalities.
- Some women will be able to stop smoking on their own when they find out that they are pregnant, but for many there are complex psychological and physical barriers affecting motivation, capability, and opportunity to stop.
- Women are four times more likely to stop smoking if they receive support from a trained stop smoking practitioner.
- For women who struggle with smoking during pregnancy, they need non-judgemental, individual, ongoing support.
- Ideally this support would be provided by a midwife that they know and trust.

ONLINE RESOURCES

National Centre for smoking cessation and training: https://www.ncsct.co.uk/index.php

NHS advice on smoking cessation in pregnancy: https://www.nhs.uk/pregnancy/keeping-well/stop-smoking/

Royal College of Midwives (RCM) position statement on smoking cessation: https://www.rcm.org.uk/media/3394/support-to-quit-smoking-in-pregnancy.pdf

Royal College of Obstetrics and Gynaecology (RCOG) support and information: https://www.rcog.org.uk/for-the-public/browse-our-patient-information/smoking-and-pregnancy-patient-information-leaflet/

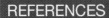

REFERENCES

Abrahamsson, A., Springett, J., Karlsson, L., & Ottosson, T. (2005). Making sense of the challenge of smoking cessation during pregnancy: A phenomenographic approach. *Health Education Research*, 20(3), 367–378.

Action on Smoking and Health. (2023). *Fact Sheet: Use of e-cigarettes (vapes) among adults in Great Britain.* Action on Smoking and Health. Use-of-e-cigarettes-among-adults-in-Great-Britain-2023.pdf (ash.org.uk)

Ashwin, C., & Watts, K. (2010). Women's use of nicotine replacement therapy in pregnancy – A structured review of the literature. *Midwifery,* 26(3), 304–310. https://doi.org/10.1016/j.midw.2008.08.002

Bauld, L., Graham, H., Sinclair, L., Flemming, K., Naughton, F., Ford, A., McKell, J., McCaughan, D., Hopewell, S., Angus, K., Eadie, D., & Tappin, D. (2017). Barriers to and facilitators of smoking cessation in pregnancy and following childbirth: Literature review and qualitative study. *Health Technology Assessment,* 21(36). https://www.journalslibrary.nihr.ac.uk/hta/hta21360#/full-report

Bell, R., Glinianaia, S. V., Waal, Z. V. D., Close, A., Moloney, E., Jones, S., Araújo-Soares, V., Hamilton, S., Milne, E. M., Shucksmith, J., Vale, L., Willmore, M., White, M., & Rushton, S. (2018). Evaluation of a complex healthcare intervention to increase smoking cessation in pregnant women: interrupted time series analysis with economic evaluation. *Tobacco Control,* 27(1), 90–98. https://doi.org/10.1136/tobaccocontrol-2016-053476

Boucher, J., & Konkle, A. T. (2016). Understanding inequalities of maternal smoking—Bridging the gap with adapted intervention strategies. *International Journal of Environmental Research and Public Health,* 13(3), 282.

Chamberlain, C., O'Mara-Eves, A., Porter, J., Coleman, T., Perlen, S. M., Thomas, J., & McKenzie, J. E. (2017). Psychosocial interventions for supporting women to stop smoking in pregnancy. *Cochrane Database of Systematic Reviews,* 2, CD001055. https://doi.org/10.1002/14651858.CD001055.pub5

Claire, R., Chamberlain, C., Davey, M. A., Cooper, S E., Berlin, I., Leonardi-Bee, J., & Coleman, T. (2020). Pharmacological interventions for promoting smoking cessation during pregnancy. *Cochrane Database of Systematic Reviews,* (3), CD010078. https://doi.org/10.1002/14651858.CD010078.pub3

Culnan, D. M., Craft-Coffman, B., Bitz, G. H., Capek, K. D., Tu, Y., Lineaweaver, W. C., & Kuhlmann-Capek, M. J. (2018). Carbon monoxide and cyanide poisoning in the burned pregnant patient: An indication for hyperbaric oxygen therapy. *Annals of Plastic Surgery,* 80(3 Suppl 2), S106–S112. https://doi.org/10.1097/sap.0000000000001351

Diamanti, A., Papadakis, S., Schoretsaniti, S., Rovina, N., Vivilaki, V., Gratziou, C., & Katsaounou, P. A. (2019). Smoking cessation in pregnancy: An update for maternity care practitioners. *Tobacco Induced Diseases,* 17, 57. https://doi.org/10.18332/tid/109906

Doll, R., Peto, R., Boreham, J., & Sutherland, I. (2004). Mortality in relation to smoking: 50 years' observations on male British doctors. *BMJ,* 328(7455), 1519. https://doi.org/10.1136/bmj.38142.554479.AE

Ekblad, M., Gissler, M., Lehtonen, L., & Korkeila, J. (2010). Prenatal smoking exposure and the risk of psychiatric morbidity into young adulthood. *Archives of General Psychiatry,* 67(8), 841–849. https://doi.org/10.1001/archgenpsychiatry. 2010.92

Emery, J. L., Sutton, S., & Naughton, F. (2017). Cognitive and behavioral predictors of quit attempts and biochemically-validated abstinence during pregnancy. *Nicotine & Tobacco Research,* 19(5), 547–554. https://doi.org/10.1093/ntr/ntw242

Engstrom, P. F., Clapper M. L., & Schnoll, R. A. (2003). Physiochemical composition of tobacco smoke. In Pollack, R. E., Kufe, D. W., Weichselbaum, R. R., et al. (ed.), *Holland-Frei Cancer Medicine.* 6th edition. https://www.ncbi.nlm. nih.gov/books/NBK13173/

Ferguson, S. G., & Hansen, E. C. (2012). A preliminary examination of cognitive factors that influence interest in quitting during pregnancy. *Journal of Smoking Cessation,* 7(2), 100–104.

Flemming, K., Graham, H., McCaughan, D., Angus, K., Sinclair, L., & Bauld, L. (2016). Health professionals' perceptions of the barriers and facilitators to providing smoking cessation advice to women in pregnancy and during the post-partum period: A systematic review of qualitative research. *BMC Public Health,* 16(1), 290. https://doi.org/10.1186/s12889-016-2961-9

Flemming, K., McCaughan, D., Angus, K., & Graham, H. (2015). Qualitative systematic review: Barriers and facilitators to smoking cessation experienced by women in pregnancy and following childbirth. *Journal of Advanced Nursing,* 71(6), 1210–1226. https://doi.org/10.1111/jan.12580

Flenady, V., Koopmans, L., Middleton, P., Frøen, J. F., Smith, G. C., Gibbons, K., Coory, M., Gordon, A., Ellwood, D., McIntyre, H. D., Fretts, R., & Ezzati, M. (2011). Major risk factors for stillbirth in high-income countries: A systematic review and meta-analysis. *The Lancet,* 377(9774), 1331–1340. https://doi.org/10.1016/ S0140-6736(10)62233-7

Fletcher, C., Hoon, E., Gialamas, A., Dekker, G., Lynch, J., & Smithers, L. (2022). Isolation, marginalisation and disempowerment – Understanding how interactions with health providers can influence smoking cessation in pregnancy. *BMC Pregnancy Childbirth,* 22(1), 396. https://doi.org/10.1186/s12884-022-04720-0

Hajek, P., Phillips-Waller, A., Przulj, D., Pesola, F., Smith, K. M., Bisal, N., Li, J., Parrott, S., Sasieni, P., & Dawkins, L. (2019). E-cigarettes compared with nicotine replacement therapy within the UK Stop Smoking Services: The TEC RCT. *Health Technology Assessment (Winchester, England),* 23(43), 1.

Higgins, S. T., Nighbor, T. D., Kurti, A. N., Heil, S. H., Slade, E. P., Shepard, D. S., Solomon, L. J., Lynch, M. E., Johnson, H. K., Markesich, C., Rippberger, P. L., Skelly, J. M., DeSarno, M., Bunn, J., Hammond, J. B., Roemhildt, M. L., Williams, R. K., O'Reilly, D. M., & Bernstein, I. M. (2022). Randomized controlled trial examining the efficacy of adding financial incentives to best practices for smoking cessation among pregnant and newly postpartum women. *Preventive Medicine,* 165, 107012. https://doi.org/10.1016/j. ypmed.2022.107012

Kalamkarian, A., Hoon, E., Chittleborough, C. R., Dekker, G., Lynch, J. W., & Smithers, L. G. (2023). Smoking cessation care during pregnancy: A qualitative exploration of midwives' challenging role. *Women and Birth,* 36(1), 89–98. https://doi.org/10.1016/j.wombi.2022.03.005

Koshy, P., Mackenzie, M., Tappin, D., & Bauld, L. (2010). Smoking cessation during pregnancy: The influence of partners, family and friends on quitters and non-quitters. *Health & Social Care in the Community,* 18(5), 500–510.

Madureira, J., Camelo, A., Silva, A. I., Reis, A. T., Esteves, F., Ribeiro, A. I., Teixeira, J. P., & Costa, C. (2020). The importance of socioeconomic position in smoking, cessation and environmental tobacco smoke exposure during pregnancy. *Scientific Reports,* 10(1), 15584. https://doi.org/10.103/s41598-020-72298-8

Mantzari, E., Vogt, F., & Marteau, T. M. (2012). The effectiveness of financial incentives for smoking cessation during pregnancy: Is it from being paid or from the extra aid? BMC *Pregnancy and Childbirth,* 12(1), 24. https://doi.org/10.1186/1471-2393-12-24

McLeod, D., Benn, C., Pullon, S., Viccars, A., White, S., Cookson, T., & Dowell, A. (2003). The midwife's role in facilitating smoking behaviour change during pregnancy. *Midwifery,* 19(4), 285–297. https://doi.org/10.1016/S0266-6138(03)00038-X

McNeill, A., Simonavičius, E., Brose, L., Taylor, E., East, K., Zuikova, E., Calder, R., & Robson, D. (2022). *Nicotine vaping in England: An evidence update including health risks and perceptions, 2022.* A report commissioned by the Office for Health Improvement and Disparities, King's College London. Available at: www.gov.uk/government/publications/nicotine-vaping-in-england-2022-evidence-update.

Miyazaki, Y., Hayashi, K., & Imazeki, S. (2015). Smoking cessation in pregnancy: psychosocial interventions and patient-focused perspectives. *International Journal of Women's Health,* 7, 415–427. https://doi.org/10.2147/IJWH.S54599

Montgomery, S. M., & Ekbom, A. (2002). Smoking during pregnancy and diabetes mellitus in a British longitudinal birth cohort. *BMJ,* 324(7328), 26–27. https://doi.org/10.1136/bmj.324.7328.26

Naughton, F., Vaz, L. R., Coleman, T., Orton, S., Bowker, K., Leonardi-Bee, J., Cooper, S., Vanderbloemen, L., Sutton, S., & Ussher, M. (2019). Interest in and use of smoking cessation support across pregnancy and postpartum. *Nicotine & Tobacco Research,* 22(7), 1178–1186. https://doi.org/10.1093/ntr/ntz151

NICE. (2021). *Tobacco: Preventing uptake, promoting quitting and treating dependence.* [NG 209]. https://www.nice.org.uk/guidance/ng209

Noël, A., Yilmaz, S., Farrow, T., Schexnayder, M., Eickelberg, O., & Jelesijevic, T. (2023). Sex-specific alterations of the lung transcriptome at birth in mouse offspring prenatally exposed to vanilla-flavored E-cigarette aerosols and enhanced susceptibility to asthma. *International Journal of Environmental Research and Public Health,* 20(4), 3710.

Oken, E., Levitan, E. B., & Gillman, M. W. (2008). Maternal smoking during pregnancy and child overweight: Systematic review and meta-analysis. *International Journal of Obesity,* 32(2), 201–210. https://doi.org/10.1038/sj.ijo.0803760

Orzabal, M. R., Lunde-Young, E. R., Ramirez, J. I., Howe, S. Y., Naik, V. D., Lee, J., Heaps, C. L., Threadgill, D. W., & Ramadoss, J. (2019). Chronic exposure to e-cig aerosols during early development causes vascular dysfunction and offspring growth deficits. *Translational Research,* 207, 70–82.

Paarlberg, K. M., Vingerhoets, A. J. J. M., Passchier, J., Heinen, A. G. J. J., Dekker, G. A., & van Geijn, H. P. (1999). Smoking status in pregnancy is associated with daily stressors and low well-being. *Psychology & Health*, 14(1), 87–96. https://doi.org/10.1080/08870449908407316

Passey, M. E., Longman, J. M., Adams, C., Johnston, J. J., Simms, J., & Rolfe, M. (2020). Factors associated with provision of smoking cessation support to pregnant women–a cross-sectional survey of midwives in New South Wales, Australia. *BMC Pregnancy and Childbirth*, 20, 1–10.

Potter, N. A., Arita, Y., Peltier, M. R., & Zelikoff, J. T. (2022). Ex vivo toxicity of E-cigarette constituents on human placental tissues. *Journal of Reproductive Immunology*, 154, 103737. https://doi.org/10.1016/j.jri.2022.103737

Richards, B., McNeill, A., Croghan, E., Percival, J., Ritchie, D., & McEwen, A. (2014). Smoking cessation education and training in UK nursing schools: A national survey. *Journal of Nursing Education and Practice*, 4(8), 188.

Rodriguez, A., Bohlin, G., & Lindmark, G. (2000). Psychosocial predictors of smoking and exercise during pregnancy. *Journal of Reproductive and Infant Psychology*, 18(3), 203–223. https://doi.org/10.1080/713683039

Schoenaker, D., Stephenson, J., Godfrey, K., Barker, M., & Alwan, N. (2021). OP69 Socio-demographic differences in smoking status and cessation before and during early pregnancy among women in England: An analysis of the national maternity services dataset. *Journal of Epidemiology and Community Health*, 75(Suppl 1), A32–A33. https://doi.org/10.1136/jech-2021-SSMabstracts.69

Stacey, T., Samples, J., Leadley, C., Akester, L., & Jenney, A. (2022). 'I don't need you to criticise me, I need you to support me'. A qualitative study of women's experiences of and attitudes to smoking cessation during pregnancy. *Women and Birth*, 35(6), e549–e555. https://doi.org/10.1016/j.wombi.2022.01.010

Tappin, D., Bauld, L., Purves, D., Boyd, K., Sinclair, L., MacAskill, S., McKell, J., Friel, B., McConnachie, A., de Caestecker, L., Tannahill, C., Radley, A., & Coleman, T. (2015). Financial incentives for smoking cessation in pregnancy: Randomised controlled trial. *BMJ: British Medical Journal*, 350, h134. https://doi.org/10.1136/bmj.h134

West, R., Walia, A., Hyder, N., Shahab, L., & Michie, S. (2010). Behavior change techniques used by the English stop smoking services and their associations with short-term quit outcomes. *Nicotine & Tobacco Research*, 12(7), 742–747. https://doi.org/10.1093/ntr/ntq074

West, R., & Stapleton, J. (2008). Clinical and public health significance of treatments to aid smoking cessation. *European Respiratory Review*, 17(110), 199–204. https://doi.org/10.1183/09059180.00011005

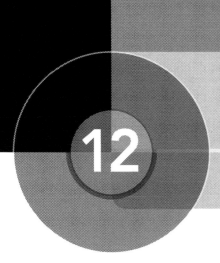

Breastfeeding Matters: A Multifaceted Perspective on Health Promotion

12

ZENI KOUTSI AND SARAH JOHNSON

INTRODUCTION

WHY BREASTFEEDING MATTERS: A MULTIFACETED PERSPECTIVE ON HEALTH PROMOTION

Breastfeeding matters; it plays a crucial role in various aspects of life, spanning not only individual wellbeing but also wider societal health and sustainability. Understanding the significance of breastfeeding in the early stages of infancy and beyond is paramount. Its relevance is vital for making informed choices for the health and sustainability of the mother, infant, and society. An increasing body of research is highlighting the significant correlations between early nutrition and lifelong health implications. Therefore, underscoring the essential significance of breastfeeding in fostering holistic physiological development (Pérez-Escamilla et al., 2023).

This is especially clear during times of global crises like pandemics, financial instability, wars, and famines. Human milk is a self-sustaining nutritional source, uncontaminated and tailored to the needs of the infant/child. It eases the healthcare burden during economic downturns, providing a buffer against the financial strains of families (Pérez-Escamilla et al., 2023). In addition, breastfeeding is an environmentally sustainable choice; leaving a minimal carbon footprint, as it requires no production processes that harm the environment.

Implementing multilevel interventions and policies across the socio-ecological model and settings can contribute to improving breastfeeding practices at a population level, thereby elevating global health (Victora et al., 2016). The act of breastfeeding holds significant influence in determining positive health outcomes for both individuals and society. It establishes a solid foundation for mothers and babies, promoting the best possible health outcomes, cultivating meaningful connections, and supporting

DOI: 10.4324/9781003350071-12

cognitive growth. The impact is multigenerational, significantly improving intelligence, and thereby uplifting communities through better educational outcomes and career prospects (Pérez-Escamilla et al., 2023). Breastfeeding transcends being a mere feeding option; it embodies a commitment to a more sustainable, healthier, and resilient future.

The diverse aspects and exceptional value of human milk are examined in this chapter. Furthermore, it will explore the factors which influence the choices of infant feeding and their impact on the breastfeeding rates and policy initiatives in the UK. In addition, the chapter will introduce emerging technologies and recent evidence, such as epigenetics and the microbiome.

IMPACT OF BREASTFEEDING

SOCIETY

Breastfeeding plays a crucial role in establishing a healthy society. It helps to decrease healthcare burdens by reducing the incidences of illnesses and diseases in both children and mothers, leading to a healthier population. Table 12.1 highlights some of the substantial health benefits breastfeeding offers to both mothers and babies, underscoring the profound impact it has on public health. Promoting breastfeeding as an equaliser in society, as it offers every child, regardless of their socio-economic background, a healthy start in life. Breastfeeding requires a collective societal approach that considers gender inequities, and not the sole responsibility of women.

HEALTH BENEFITS

Table 12.1 Health benefits of breastfeeding

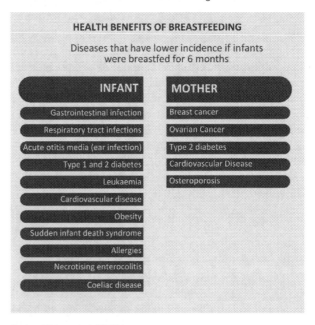

Source: Victora et al. (2016).

ENVIRONMENTAL PERSPECTIVE

Breastfeeding has a positive impact on our climate and environment; it contributes to the prevention of global warming, protects biodiversity and conserves natural resources (Joffe et al., 2019). Powdered commercial milk formula (CMF) sales in North America have a carbon footprint of 2.8 billion car miles per year; the equivalent of driving around Earth's equator over 114,000 times (Cadwell et al., 2020). These figures focus on powdered CMF within one continent and do not account for the environmental cost of plastic packaging, utensils and ready-made formula.

EPIGENETICS

Advances in epigenetics offer insights into the extensive consequences of infant nutrition and development that can transcend generations. Epigenetics provides insights into the impact of hormonal fluctuations during breastfeeding on gene expression.

To make these complex terms clearer, it is helpful to draw a parallel with editing photos (Figure 12.1).

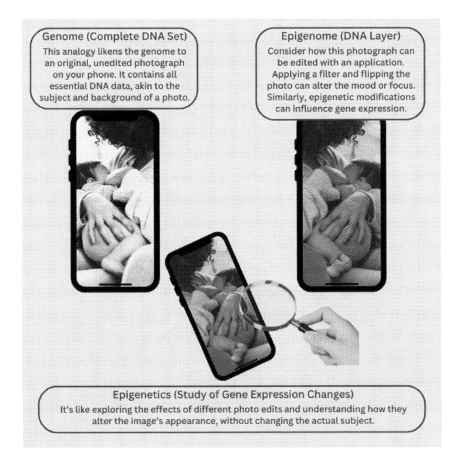

Figure 12.1 Epigenetics analogy.

Source: Authors.

The provision of nutrition that is tailored to an individual's genetic predispositions and preferences can lead to improved health outcomes (Alvarez-Pitti et al., 2020). Grandparents' habits, such as smoking or poor diet, may affect their grandchildren's health (Arshad et al., 2018). This discovery paves the way for more research into the potential correlation between breastfeeding and long-term health effects.

MICROBIOME

The development of the body and immune system holds utmost importance during the 1,001-day period, spanning from conception to two years of age. They play a fundamental role in shaping long-term health and mitigating the occurrence of common diseases throughout the lifespan of the infant (Çavdar et al., 2019). The microbiome is a complex ecosystem of bacteria, fungi, and viruses, influencing human health. Several factors can influence microbiome, such as maternal lifestyle, diet, birth method and antibiotic use, leading to negative consequences (Fasano, 2018).

UNDERSTANDING HUMAN MILK AND CMF

Beyond its nutritional value, human milk serves a purpose of greater significance. Breast milk enriches the defensive mechanism through essential nutrients and immune support during the extra-uterine transition and caters to the developing needs of the infant (Azad et al., 2020). The innate immune system present in human

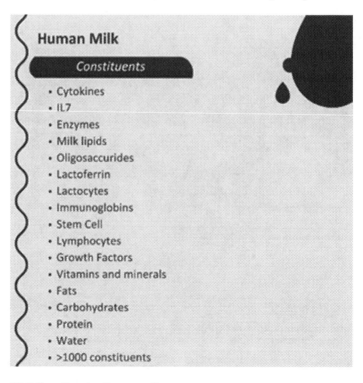

Figure 12.2 Constituents of human milk.

Source: Christian et al. (2021).

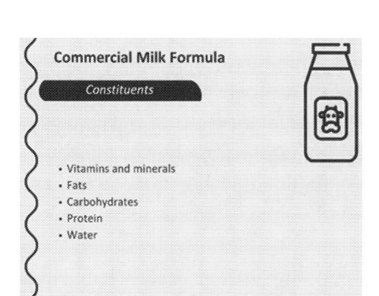

Figure 12.3 Constituents of commercial milk formula.

Source: Beck et al. (2015).

milk plays a crucial role as the primary defence mechanism against pathogens in infants (Wedekind & Shenker, 2021).

Significant variations can be observed between human breast milk and CMF in terms of their impact on immunity and nutritional content. Human milk has unique components and is a complex living biodiverse fluid tailored to a baby's individual needs (Figures 12.2 and 12.3).

CMF, though nutritionally adequate, cannot replicate the range and functionality of components in human milk. For instance, the proteins in CMF are larger and not easily absorbed. Formula companies claim their products are close to breast milk. However, specific components, such as stem cells, transfer factors, and specific growth factors, are exclusively present in human milk, making it particularly advantageous for premature infants. Thus, while both can nourish, breast milk offers a more comprehensive range of benefits tailored to a baby's growth and development (Wedekind & Shenker, 2021).

PREVALENCE, INITIATION, AND DURATION

Optimising the growth and development of children and ensuring they thrive and not just survive (United Nations [UN], 2015) has been at the forefront of the global Public Health agenda. Human milk is widely recognised as an invaluable resource in the effort to reduce mortality and morbidity among children under the age of five (Victora et al., 2016), as well as to promote food security in infants and young children. This aligns with the Sustainable Development Goals (SDGs) outlined in the United Nations' 2030 Agenda (Tomori, 2023). SDGs are yet to be achieved, low rates of breastfeeding are attributed as a factor for this due to lack of policy engagement and investment (Global Breastfeeding Collective, 2017).

The World Health Organization (WHO) and UNICEF recommend initiation of breastfeeding within the first hour of birth, exclusive breastfeeding for the first six

LEARNING ACTIVITY

Select two SDGs and create a detailed mind map linking breastfeeding to their targets for improvement.

months of life and continuing breastfeeding until two years of age or beyond alongside nutritionally adequate, safe and appropriate complementary foods (WHO, 2003). Anthropological and evolutionary literature suggest the norm for human breastfeeding is 2.5–7 or 2–3 years when socio-cultural factors are considered (Tsutaya & Mizushima, 2023). Globally, only 48% of infants are exclusively breastfed at six months. Furthermore, only 40 countries have exclusive breastfeeding rates above 50%–70% (Table 12.2) according to the Global Breastfeeding Collective (2022).

The rates of breastfeeding in the UK present even more significant challenges. The national Infant Feeding Survey (IFS), decommissioned more than a decade ago, reveals in its report, 81% of mothers initiated breastfeeding (McAndrew et al., 2012) (Table 12.3). Subsequently, the rates significantly decreased (Table 12.4), positioning this as one of the most minimal breastfeeding rates on a worldwide scale (Victora et al., 2016).

Table 12.2 Current global prevalence of breastfeeding and 2030 targets

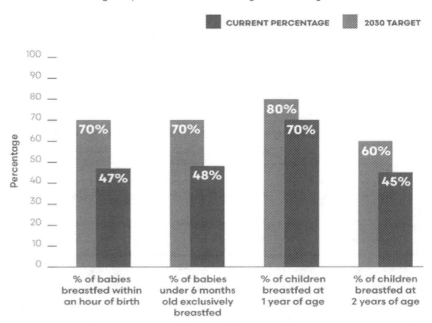

Source: Global Breastfeeding Collective (2022).

Table 12.3 Incidence of breastfeeding (any human milk from birth, including one feed)

	2005 (%)	2010 (%)
England	78	83
Scotland	70	74
Wales	67	71

Source: Adapted from McAndrew et al. (2012).

Table 12.4 Duration of breastfeeding (any breastfeeding occurring, including alongside formula milk)

Time	UK total in 2005(%)	UK total in 2010(%)
Birth	76	81
One week	63 (decrease of 13%)	69 (decrease of 12%)
six week	48 (decrease of 28%)	55 (decrease of 26%)
six months	25 (decrease of 51%)	34 (decrease of 47%)

Source: Adapted from McAndrew et al. (2012).

The IFS was replaced by a local quarterly report that specifically outlines the prevalence of breastfeeding during the six-to-eight-week postnatal period. Local authorities have observed discrepancies in data collection and inaccuracies, which have hindered the comprehension of breastfeeding rates, effectiveness of support, and implementation of public health priorities. A considerable difference in breastfeeding rates can be observed among different regions in England. In the North-East, 32% of babies receive breastmilk, whereas in certain areas of London, the figure exceeds 80% at six to eight weeks.

The Scottish Maternal and Infant Nutrition Survey (Scottish Government, 2018) presents promising results, indicating significant progress in breastfeeding rates. From 2010 to 2017, the proportion of breastfeeding at six months increased from 32% to 43%. The outcomes show the favourable impact of implementing a nationwide strategy for infant feeding, which notably facilitates the attainment of Baby Friendly Initiative (BFI) accreditation by all maternity and community services in Scotland. This development can have far-reaching effects across the entire UK. The Office for Health Improvement and Disparities (OHID) has re-commissioned the IFS (OHID, 2023).

BREAST IS NOT BEST – IT IS THE BIOLOGICAL NORM

The slogan 'breast is best' was first introduced with good intentions (Stanway & Stanway, 1978). In the realm of infant feeding, numerous perspectives that criticise the phrase. Some individuals perceive it as endorsing the superiority of breastfeeding, while recognising CMF is an acceptable alternative. Conversely, individuals interpret the term 'best' negatively, considering it to be hierarchical and implying it can only be achieved by a privileged minority, rather than accepting it as the biological norm (Cassidy et al., 2018). The use of this expression unintentionally intensified feelings of shame and guilt among mothers, resulting in a considerable backlash. This is particularly relevant for mothers who have not met their breastfeeding targets, are medically unable to breastfeed, or have chosen not to breastfeed. Mothers deserve support and understanding, not judgment or feelings of failure, for their parenting choices. Avoidance of creating these divisions is of utmost importance (McIntyre et al., 2018). Language carries significant importance, given that conversations about infant feeding profoundly influence public perception, policy development and women's lived experiences.

THE UK'S INFANT FEEDING CULTURE

When considering the factors influencing infant feeding in the UK and seeking solutions to the decline in breastfeeding rates, essential to examine the culture of CMF and explore potential strategies and health promotion initiatives.

To evaluate these factors, please review the case study below.

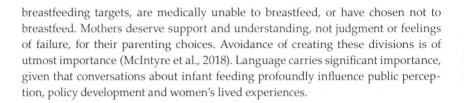

REFLECTIVE ACTIVITY

Ameena and her partner are expecting their first baby. She receives universal care in her community, seeing a different midwife for each antenatal appointment. Breastfeeding is strongly advised by a midwife as the best feeding choice. Ameena is unable to attend antenatal classes due to work, but breastfeeding leaflets are available. Ameena opts on a BFI Stage 1 accredited regional hospital as her birthplace.

Throughout Ameena's pregnancy, she is presented with a range of messages from television and social media. Topics such as bottles, infant formula, breastfeeding challenges, and sleep deprivation are frequently discussed by influencers in their advertisements, reels, and stories. Some narratives are sponsored by the CMF industry. Ameena is fortunate to have support from her partner and family, who will help with feeding.

Ameena required an induction of labour, and the circumstances necessitated a forceps birth. Within the first hour of birth, Baby Aamin is breastfed. Ameena feels overwhelmed in the busy maternity ward due to understaffing and conflicting advice. Ameena ultimately opts to supplement with formula because of her concerns regarding her milk supply. At home, she combines breastfeeding and formula feeding, reporting Aamin seems satisfied with the bottle.

Take a moment to reflect:

- Can you pinpoint certain elements that might support or hinder Ameena's breastfeeding journey?

What alterations would you propose in this narrative to enhance the likelihood of Ameena meeting her breastfeeding goals?

WOMEN'S EXPERIENCES

The individual breastfeeding experiences of women influence their perceptions and intentions regarding infant feeding. Breastfeeding challenges, like pain, ineffective attachment and perceived milk insufficiency, can lead to early cessation or formula use

(Roberts et al., 2023). Women have limited access to specialised support for maternal care and breastfeeding. Confidence enhancement, reassurance provision, motivation, and practical support are regarded as crucial elements by mothers, particularly in low socio-economic and culturally diverse communities (Cook et al., 2021).

The lack of support was further exacerbated during the COVID-19 pandemic (Turner et al., 2023). The impact is more significant for mothers belonging to diverse racial groups, those facing challenging living circumstances, and lower educational attainment (Brown & Shenker, 2021). This exposes the systemic gap in infant feeding and mental health support (Constantini et al., 2021). It is imperative to establish targeted public health initiatives in order to meet the needs of families.

PERINATAL MENTAL HEALTH AND INFANT FEEDING

In recent years, the public health agenda has placed emphasis on acknowledging the equal importance of mental and physical health (Garratt, 2023). Although the relationship between perinatal mental health and breastfeeding is still unclear, recent evidence indicates that exclusive breastfeeding promotes maternal mental wellbeing (Dagla et al., 2021). Furthermore, it contributes to the improvement of multiple physical factors, including the role of oxytocin in stress and inflammatory response systems (Gómez et al., 2021), and emotional factors such as maternal self-efficacy (Lau et al., 2018).

When mothers face difficulties and stop breastfeeding before planned, they experience elevated levels of PTSD symptoms and postnatal depression (Gianni et al., 2019). The duration of breastfeeding is influenced by maternal mental health (Krol & Grossmann, 2018). The presence of emotions, such as internalised blame, grief, guilt, regret and anger has been described within the context of breastfeeding grief and trauma (Brown, 2019). Women and parents who formula feed describe similar feelings and frustration with the absence of support and the quality of infant feeding care (Jackson et al., 2021).

Trauma-informed care must be adopted as the benchmark for all healthcare provision and health promotion initiatives. It is imperative to acknowledge and comprehend the emotions, circumstances and sentiments of women in relation to their infant feeding experience, choices or necessities. When interpreting this understanding, it is important to consider the broader cultural context of child rearing and nutrition, as it can lead to the establishment of a more diverse culture and system promotes and safeguards breastfeeding (Brown, 2018).

PARTNERS AND FAMILY

The UN (2018) has emphasised the role of the intimate partner, typically the father, regarding child and maternal health, wellbeing and food security, urging them to adopt a more proactive approach. Few partners had satisfactory knowledge about breastfeeding and were unfamiliar with its benefits and technicalities, while most had a positive perspective on it (Chang et al., 2021). Fathers were informed about breastfeeding obstacles, despite the assumption of it being 'easy and natural'. It was recognised, fathers provided support, although there were occasions when their help was perceived as being rejected. Additionally, they acknowledged and attached importance to the maternal-child bond. Bottle-feeding, whether with expressed human milk or formula, was regarded as an intimate act that fostered bonding (Merritt et al.,

2019). To recognise their parenting capabilities, men require education, practical assistance and breastfeeding integration. This includes promoting skin-to-skin contact, emphasising the importance of emotional bonding, and offering support to the new mother. There is a correlation between implementing extended shared parental leave and a lengthened period of breastfeeding (Grandahl et al., 2020).

As society becomes more inclusive, there is a notable increase in research centred on non-'traditional' family structures. Same-sex female partners exhibit receptiveness towards the notion of co-breastfeeding and express a strong commitment to fostering the wellbeing of their breastfeeding partner (Chang et al., 2021). The feasibility of inducing lactation in a non-gestational parent is supported by various case studies, anecdotal evidence, and existing clinical protocols (Reisman & Goldstein, 2018; Schnell, 2022). Parental motivation and support from both the family and professionals are crucial for enabling adoptive non-gestational mothers to induce lactation for their infants (Mohd et al., 2021). It is essential to acknowledge, gay fathers have a strong desire for increased education and support in relation to CMF feeding, as well as more inclusive parenting support (Fantus, 2020). Considering the evolving landscape of chest/breastfeeding within the transgender and gender-diverse community, it is necessary to adopt a more nuanced approach to support. This will facilitate the promotion of human milk utilisation and human milk among these parents (Yang et al., 2023).

HARNESSING THE DIGITAL REALM

Engaging with the internet and digital solutions, like mobile apps, social media and games, is the norm for many individuals, especially younger generations. Breastfeeding groups on social media moderated by mothers or trained lactation specialists are highly valued by mothers, whether local, national or international. These services bridge a service gap, providing convenience and facilitating connections for parents that persist throughout the toddler stage (Morse & Brown, 2021). Additionally, they contribute to improved outcomes, specifically in terms of exclusive breastfeeding duration and support for breastfeeding difficulties (Almohanna et al., 2020). This approach is consistent with the NHS Digital Transformation Strategy. Social media, virtual clinics, and digital resources played a significant role during COVID-19 and continue to be essential for public communication, health initiatives, and education (Constantini et al., 2021).

The adoption of augmented reality (AR) or virtual reality (VR) solutions has initiated in the field of midwifery education and clinical practice. The enhancement of education and practice is thought to be facilitated by the development and proficient utilisation of various modalities, including chat bots, conversational robotics, and AR/VR simulation or gaming (Ryan et al., 2022). Machine learning may enable the prediction of breastfeeding initiation and duration, facilitating the development of policies and health initiatives for better infant feeding outcomes (Oliver-Roig et al., 2022).

MIDWIVES' EXPERIENCES

Midwives, being fundamental advocates and practitioners of breastfeeding, play an essential role in the promotion and preservation of breastfeeding through collaborative efforts with healthcare professionals. Considering the diverse perspectives, influences, and experiences present within the maternity workforce, it becomes necessary for midwives to engage in self-reflection. This includes evaluating the potential impact of their own beliefs and attitudes on decision-making and actions related to breastfeeding.

Service users have expressed concerns regarding the insufficient, untimely, and inconsistent provision of infant feeding support from midwives and other healthcare professionals. Midwives encounter obstacles such as staffing shortages and time constraints, along with the perception that breastfeeding support is incompatible with healthcare system demands (Byrom et al., 2021). To achieve system harmonisation, validated standards should be adopted in practice and education for all healthcare professionals. The purpose of this is to ensure discussions about breastfeeding with new mothers are based on information and objectivity, without coercion or undue pressure (UNICEF UK, 2017). Healthcare professionals must incorporate active listening, validation, and open communication into their daily practice (UNICEF UK, 2018a).

LEARNING ACTIVITY

How you could rephrase the following questions into a more active listening and meaningful communication style:

1. Would you like to breast or bottle feed your baby?
2. Let me put the baby on the breast.

Here is a bottle preparation leaflet.

FACTORS SHAPING UK'S BOTTLE-FEEDING CULTURE

- Societal misperception of the 'equal' value and easiness of formula bottle-feeding vs breastfeeding
- Varied policy implementation at local and national level/ lack of public funding
- Family and societal norms
- Lack of systematic and consistent professional support
- Advertising and marketing of human milk substitutes and related products such as bottles and dummies (UK's law is not in full alignment with the WHO Code)
- Digital marketing, social media influencers and algorithms, unregulated online groups, web resources sharing non-evidence based or incorrect information
- Women's emancipation and employment; associated workforce regulation and law (inc. parental leave duration and remuneration)
- Social and health inequalities
- The ability to manufacture bottles and teats, breast pumps, and other relevant items/ gadgets
- Medical control of childbirth and making infant feeding 'scientific'/ 'medical'

UNICEF UK, BFI STANDARDS

The BFI standards are a comprehensive accreditation program, significantly enhanced in 2012 to incorporate relationship-building components. These standards

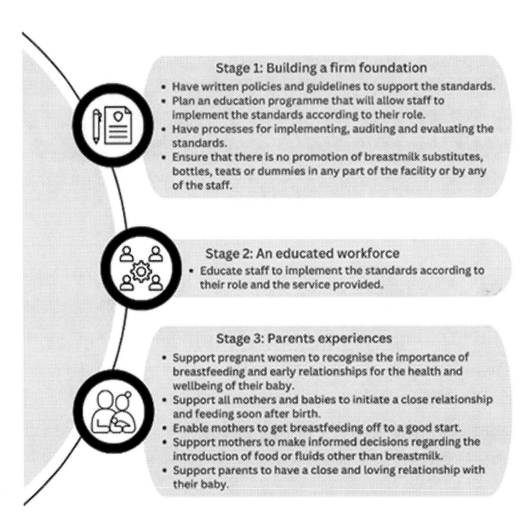

Stage 1: Building a firm foundation
- Have written policies and guidelines to support the standards.
- Plan an education programme that will allow staff to implement the standards according to their role.
- Have processes for implementing, auditing and evaluating the standards.
- Ensure that there is no promotion of breastmilk substitutes, bottles, teats or dummies in any part of the facility or by any of the staff.

Stage 2: An educated workforce
- Educate staff to implement the standards according to their role and the service provided.

Stage 3: Parents experiences
- Support pregnant women to recognise the importance of breastfeeding and early relationships for the health and wellbeing of their baby.
- Support all mothers and babies to initiate a close relationship and feeding soon after birth.
- Enable mothers to get breastfeeding off to a good start.
- Support mothers to make informed decisions regarding the introduction of food or fluids other than breastmilk.
- Support parents to have a close and loving relationship with their baby.

Figure 12.4 BFI maternity services standards.

Source: UNICEF UK. (2017).

provide a stringent framework based on evidence-based criteria, encompassing various sectors such as maternity, health visiting, neonatal care, children's hospitals, children's centres, and universities (Figures 12.4–12.6). The central aim of this program is to promote infant feeding practices and cultivate nurturing parent-infant relationships, ultimately enhancing the quality of care for nutrition, health and development. It operates through educational efforts and collaborative initiatives with healthcare professionals (UNICEF UK, 2019).

The importance of BFI is undeniable, given the imperative to promote and support breastfeeding. National initiatives and directives, such as the NHS long-term plan BFI standards (UNICEF UK, 2017) and NMC (2019), unequivocally endorse and support this cause. These authoritative documents underscore the value and significance of BFI in the healthcare sector.

Certificate of Commitment
- The Certificate of Commitment is the first award, given when the requirements for standards 1 and 3 are met.
- Standard 1:
- Make a written commitment to adhere to the Baby Friendly standards.
- Standard 3 The Code:
- Provide teaching without involvement, sponsorship or promotional materials from companies covered by the WHO International Code of Marketing of Breastmilk Substitutes (the Code).

Stage 1 Accreditation
- An assessment of the curriculum and supporting documents to ensure that all the learning outcomes are addressed.

Stage 2 - Full Accreditation
- Full accreditation involves an assessment of standard 2. This accreditation lasts for three years, after which a re-assessment of all standards is carried out.
- Standard 2 Knowledge & skills
- Ensure all students and staff are equipped with the knowledge and skills to implement the Baby Friendly learning outcomes in the relevant healthcare setting.
-

Figure 12.5 BFI university standards.

Source: UNICEF UK. (2018b).

BFI has gained recognition as a critical intervention for supporting both the duration and exclusivity of breastfeeding, as corroborated by a *Cochrane Review* (Trivedi, 2018). This reaffirms the significance of BFI in advancing breastfeeding practices. To ensure the enduring sustainability of BFI implementation, the Gold Achieving Sustainability (AS) Standards were introduced in 2018 (UNICEF UK, 2018b). These standards provide organisations with a structured approach to maintaining their commitment to BFI principles.

THE WHO CODE

In addition to the BFI, the WHO International Code of Marketing of Breastmilk Substitutes plays a significant role in shaping infant feeding practices globally (WHO,

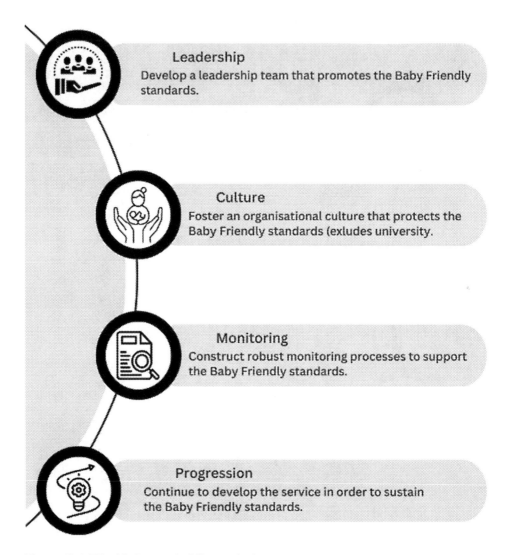

Figure 12.6 BFI achieving sustainability standards.

Source: UNICEF UK. (2018b).

1981). This code regulates the marketing and promotion of human milk substitutes, including infant formula, to protect and promote breastfeeding (Figure 12.7).

Breastfeeding duration and exclusivity are reduced when promotional materials from the CMF industry are shared. In 1981, the WHO initiated 'The Code' to limit the promotion of infant formula. Advertising of infant formula for infants under six months is prohibited in the UK, whereas advertisements for milks targeted at older babies are permitted. The advertisements indirectly encourage the use of infant formula, leading to the formation of misconceptions.

The formula milk industry advertises its products as a lifestyle choice, not a consequential decision for health and economics (Piwoz & Huffman, 2015). Accurate information and unbiased support for parents regarding infant milks is necessary.

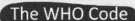

The WHO Code

1. **No promotion:** The WHO Code prohibits the advertising and promotion of CMF, ensuring that marketing practices do not undermine breastfeeding.
2. **No free samples:** healthcare facilities and professionals are not allowed to distribute free samples of CMF to pregnant women or new mothers.
3. **No gifts or sponsorships**: companies manufacturing CMF are prohibited from offering gifts or financial incentives to healthcare workers or facilities.
4. **Informational Labelling:** If CMF is available, abels must contain clear and accurate information about the benefits of breastfeeding and the risks of not breastfeeding.

Figure 12.7 WHO code.

Source: WHO (1981).

The infant formula industry seeks loopholes in regulations through the promotion of follow-on and toddler milks. Extending and strengthening legislation on human milk substitutes in the UK is crucial for protecting families from deceptive advertising (Brown et al., 2020).

21ST-CENTURY LOOPHOLES

Social media influencers, particularly micro-influencers, generate income by creating relatable content, connecting with followers, effectively establishing a presence in the digital marketing landscape (WHO, 2022). The prevalence of paid endorsements by influencers is increasing, as consumers now regard influencers with the same level of trust as their own family and friends (Swant, 2016). Adolescents idolise influencers and trust their endorsed brands, limiting critical evaluation of the advertisements (Lin et al., 2019). This raises concerns about how influencers shape future mothers' choices regarding infant feeding.

The utilisation of personalised social media content by formula companies often goes unnoticed as a form of advertising, enabling them to evade scrutiny from health authorities (WHO, 2022).

Monitoring becomes increasingly challenging because of the staggering volume, 229 million daily social media posts. The preservation of families is contingent upon the use of modern methodologies and the implementation of the Code. Considering the global concerns, the WHO recommends, governments implement and enforce legislation to prohibit the advertising and promotion of formula milk products.

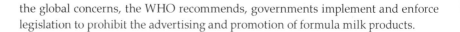

THE FUTURE OF INFANT FEEDING IN THE HEALTH PROMOTION CONTEXT

Prior to making policy changes and planning health promotion initiatives, it is crucial to comprehend and evaluate the non-modifiable and modifiable factors that influence infant feeding. The occurrence of breastfeeding challenges is not uncommon; however, their impact can be lessened. The pregnancy and birth experiences of women, along with the initiation and duration of breastfeeding, are positively influenced by dependable and lasting relationships with their social and professional caregivers, referred to as Continuity of Carer (Sandall et al., 2016). Partners, friends, family and broader societal norms have a direct impact on the success and positivity of infant feeding and early parenthood. Culturally sensitive, person-centred care pathways and behaviours from professionals or informal support are required to balance these influences. These should be supported by comprehensive and tailored education that aligns with current evidence, global and national strategies, and validated, evidence-based standards. Health promotion interventions need to remain mindful of potentially harmful discourses, driven usually by external aggressive marketing strategies, and to adopt an incremental goal setting approach to behaviour change.

Healthcare professionals of all backgrounds, particularly midwives who play a crucial role in perinatal physiology, must possess interprofessional education which is value-based and co-designed with service users. This ensures training aligns with the needs of women and families, and facilitates the provision of a consistent, safe, inclusive, and meaningful service for infant feeding. To promote forward-thinking public health strategies, it is crucial to integrate measures that strengthen workplace breastfeeding support and establish inclusive policies for parents to participate in their child's early years while still advancing professionally.

Incorporating emerging technologies and digital solutions cannot be disregarded within the framework of the digital natives' reality, as they enable greater adaptability and congruence with the future service users' requirements. New parents consistently express the need for greater personal and individual support, making in person, empathetic communication invaluable.

SUMMARY

- Biological Norm: Breastfeeding is the biological standard for infant nutrition.
- Support Over Slogans: Replace 'Breast is best' with unwavering, non-judgemental, and nuanced support for all mothers.
- Beyond Individual Choice: Recognise the complexities of breastfeeding that go beyond a mother's decision.
- Public Health Priority: Emphasise breastfeeding as crucial for public health, impacting individuals, families, society, and the planet.
- Policy and Education: Advocate for supportive policies, educational initiatives, community programs and workforce policies to encourage breastfeeding.

- Sustainable Future: Link breastfeeding to sustainable practices for improved health outcomes and environmental responsibility.
- Societal Environment: Foster societal conditions to normalise breastfeeding as a health-promoting and environmentally responsible choice.
- Informed Understanding: Deepen societal understanding of the benefits of breast-feeding for present and future generations.
- Role of the Midwife: Remain an advocate for infant feeding. Healthcare professionals, especially midwives, require interprofessional education and co-designed with service users to ensure alignment with the needs of women and families.

REFERENCES

Almohanna, A. A., Win, K. T., & Meedya, S. (2020). Effectiveness of internet-based electronic technology interventions on breastfeeding outcomes: Systematic review. *Journal of Medical Internet Research*, 22(5), e17361. https://doi.org/10.2196/17361

Alvarez-Pitti, J., de Blas, A., & Lurbe, E. (2020). Innovations in infant feeding: Future challenges and opportunities in obesity and cardiometabolic disease. *Nutrients*, 12(11), 1–22. https://doi.org/10.3390/nu12113508

Arshad, S. H., Holloway, J. W., Karmaus, W., Zhang, H., Ewart, S., Mansfield, L., Matthews, S., Hodgekiss, C., Roberts, G., & Kurukulaaratchy, R. (2018). Cohort profile: The isle of wight whole population birth cohort (IOWBC). *International Journal of Epidemiology*, 47(4), 1043–1044i. https://doi.org/10.1093/ije/dyy023

Azad, M. B., Nickel, N. C., Bode, L., Brockway, M., Brown, A., Chambers, C., Goldhammer, C., Hinde, K., McGuire, M., Munblit, D., Patel, A. L., Pérez-Escamilla, R., Rasmussen, K. M., Shenker, N., Young, B. E., & Zuccolo, L. (2020). Breastfeeding and the origins of health: Interdisciplinary perspectives and priorities. *Maternal and Child Nutrition*, 17(2), e13109. https://doi.org/10.1111/mcn.13109

Comparative proteomics of human and macaque milk reveals species-specific nutrition during postnataldevelopment. *Journal of Proteome Research*, 14(5), 2143–2157. https://doi.org/10.1021/pr501243m

Brown, A. (2018). The importance of supporting women who haven't been able to meet their breastfeeding goals. *Association of Breastfeeding Mothers (ABM) Journal.* Supporting women who haven't met their Breastfeeding goals – ABM

Brown, A. (2019). *Why Breastfeeding Grief and Trauma Matter.* London: Pinter & Martin.

Brown, A., Jones, S. W., & Evans, E. (2020). *Marketing of Infant Milk in the UK: What Do Parents See and Believe?* A report for First Steps Nutrition Trust: London.

Brown, A., & Shenker, N. (2021). Experiences of breastfeeding during COVID-19: Lessons for future practical and emotional support. *Maternal and Child Nutrition,* 17, e13088. https://doi.org/10.1111/mcn.13088

Byrom, A., Thomson, G., Dooris, M., & Dykes, F. (2021). UNICEF UK baby friendly initiative: Providing, receiving and leading infant feeding care in a hospital maternity setting – A critical ethnography. *Maternal & Child Nutrition,* 17(2), e13114. https://doi.org/10.1111/mcn.13114

Cadwell, K., Blair, A., Turner-Maffei, C., Gabel, M., & Brimdyr, K. (2020). Powdered baby formula sold in North America: Assessing the environmental impact. *Breastfeeding Medicine: the Official Journal of the Academy of Breastfeeding Medicine, 15*(10), 671–679. https://doi.org/10.1089/bfm.2020.0090

Cassidy, T. M., Dowling, S., Mahon, B. P., & Dykes, F. C. (2018). Exchanging breast-milk: Introduction. *Maternal & Child Nutrition, 14* (Suppl 6), e12748. https://doi.org/10.1111/mcn.12748

Çavdar, G., Papich, T., & Ryan, E. P. (2019). Microbiome, breastfeeding and public health policy in the United States: The case for dietary fiber. *Nutrition and Metabolic Insights, 12*. https://doi.org/10.1177/1178638819869597

Chang, Y.-S., Li, K. M., Li, K. Y., Beake, S., Lok, K. Y., & Bick, D. (2021). Relatively speaking? Partners' and family members' views and experiences of supporting breastfeeding: A systematic review of qualitative evidence. *Philosophical Transactions of the Royal Society B, 376*(1827). https://doi.org/10.1098/rstb.2020.0033

Christian, P., Smith, E., Lee, S., Vargas, A., Bremer, A., & Raiten, D. (2021). The need to study human milk as a biological system. *The American Journal of Clinical Nutrition, 113*(5), 1063–1072. https://doi.org/10.1093/ajcn/nqab075

Cook, E. J., Powell, F., Ali, N., Penn-Jones, C., Ochieng, B., & Randhawa, G. (2021). Improving support for breastfeeding mothers: A qualitative study on the experiences of breastfeeding among mothers who reside in a deprived and culturally diverse community. *International Journal for Equity in Health, 20*, 92. https://doi.org/10.1186/s12939-021-01419-0

Constantini, C., Joyce, A., & Britez, Y. (2021). Breastfeeding experiences during the COVID-19 lockdown in the United Kingdom: An exploratory study into maternal opinions and emotional states. *Journal of Human Lactation, 37*(4), 649–662. https://doi.org/10.1177/08903344211026565

Dagla, M., Mrvoljak-Theodoropoulou, I., Vogiatzoglou, M., Giamalidou, A., Tsolaridou, E., Mavrou, M., Dagla, C., & Antoniou, E. (2021). Association between breastfeeding duration and long-term midwifery-led support and psychosocial support: Outcomes from a Greek non-randomized controlled perinatal health intervention. *International Journal of Environmental Research and Public Health, 18*(4), 1988. https://doi.org/10.3390/ijerph18041988

Fantus, S. (2021). Experiences of gestational surrogacy for gay men in Canada. *Culture, Health & Sexuality, 23*(10), 1361–1374, https://doi.org/10.1080/13691058.2020.1784464

Fasano, A. (2018). Another reason to favor exclusive breastfeeding: Microbiome resilience. *Jornal de Pediatria, 94*(3), 224–225. https://doi.org/10.1016/j.jped.2017.10.002

Garratt, K. (2023). *Mental Health Policy and Services in England* (Research briefing CBP07547). London: House of Commons Library,.

Gianni, M. L., Bettinelli, M. E., Manfra, P., Sorrentino, G., Bezze, E., Plevani, L., Cavallaro, G., Raffaeli, G., Crippa, B. L., Colombo, L., et al. (2019). Breastfeeding difficulties and risk for early breastfeeding cessation. *Nutrients, Special Issue Human Milk and Lactation, 11*(10), 2266. https://doi.org/10.3390/nu11102266

Global Breastfeeding Collective. (2017). *Nurturing the Health and Wealth of Nations: The Investment Case for Breastfeeding.* UNICEF/WHO. https://www.who.int/publications/m/item/nurturing-the-health-and-wealth-of-nations-the-investment-case-for-breastfeeding

Global Breastfeeding Collective. (2022). *Global Breastfeeding Scorecard 2022: Protecting Breastfeeding through Further Investment and Policy Actions.* UNICEF/WHO, https://www.globalbreastfeedingcollective.org/media/1921/file

Gómez, L., Verd, S., de-la-Banda, G., Cardo, E., Servera, M., Filgueira, A., Ponce-Taylor, J., & Mule, M. (2021). Perinatal psychological interventions to promote breastfeeding: a narrative review. *International Breastfeeding Journal, 16*(8). https://doi.org/10.1186/s13006-020-00348-y

Grandahl, M., Stern, J., & Funkquist, E. L. (2020) Longer shared parental leave is associated with longer duration of breastfeeding: A cross-sectional study among Swedish mothers and their partners. *BMC Pediatrics, 20,* 159. https://doi.org/10.1186/s12887-020-02065-1

Jackson, L., De Pascalis, L., Harrold, J., & Fallon, V. (2021). Guilt, shame, and postpartum infant feeding outcomes: A systematic review. *Maternal & Child Nutrition, 17*(3), e13141. https://doi.org/10.1111/mcn.13141

Joffe, N., Webster, F., & Shenker, N. (2019). Support for breastfeeding is an environmental imperative. *BMJ, 367,* l5646. Support for breastfeeding is an environmental imperative - PubMed (nih.gov)

Krol, K. M., & Grossmann, T. (2018). Psychological effects of breastfeeding on children and mothers [Psychologische Effekte des Stillens auf Kinder und Mütter]. *Bundesgesundheitsblatt, Gesundheitsforschung, Gesundheitsschutz, 61*(8), 977–985. https://doi.org/10.1007/s00103-018-2769-0

Lau, C. Y. K., Lok, K. Y. W., & Tarrant, M. (2018). Breastfeeding duration and the theory of planned behavior and breastfeeding self-efficacy framework: A systematic review of observational studies. *Maternal and Child Health Journal, 22,* 327–342. https://doi.org/10.1007/s10995-018-2453-x

Lin, M., Vijayalakshmi, A., & Laczniak, R. (2019). Toward an understanding of parental views and actions on social media influencers targeted at adolescents: The roles of parents' social media use and empowerment. *Frontiers in Psychology; Frontiers in Psychology, 10,* 2664. https://doi.org/10.3389/fpsyg.2019.02664

McAndrew, F., Thompson, J., Fellows, L., Large, A., Speed, M., & Renfrew, M. (2012). *Infant Feeding Survey 2010.* London: Health and Social Care Information Centre.

McIntyre, L. M., Griffen, A. M., & BrintzenhofeSzoc, K. (2018). Breast is best . . . except when it's not. *Journal of Human Lactation, 34*(3). https://doi.org/10.1177/0890334418774011

Merritt, R., Vogel, M., Ladbury, P., & Johnson, S. (2019). A qualitative study to explore fathers' attitudes towards breastfeeding in South West England. *Primary Health Care Research & Development, 20,* E24. https://doi.org/10.1017/S1463423618000877

Mohd Hassan, S., Sulaiman, Z., & Tengku Ismail, T. A. (2021). Experiences of women who underwent induced lactation: A literature review. *Malaysian Family Physician: The Official Journal of the Academy of Family Physicians of Malaysia, 16*(1), 18–30. https://doi.org/10.51866/rv0997

Morse, H., & Brown, A. (2021). Accessing local support online: Mothers' experiences of local breastfeeding support Facebook groups. *Maternal & Child Nutrition, 17*(4), e13227. https://doi.org/10.1111/mcn.13227

Nursing and Midwifery Council. (2019). *Standards of Proficiency for Midwives.* London: NMC. standards-of-proficiency-for-midwives.pdf (nmc.org.uk)

Office for Health Improvement and Disparities. (2023). *Guidance: Infant Feeding Survey 2023.* https://www.gov.uk/guidance/infant-feeding-survey-2023

Oliver-Roig, A., Rico-Juan, J. R., Richart-Martínez, M., & Cabrero-García, J. (2022). Predicting exclusive breastfeeding in maternity wards using machine learning techniques. *Computer Methods and Programs in Biomedicine, 221,* 106837. https://doi.org/10.1016/j.cmpb.2022.106837

Pérez-Escamilla, R., Tomori, C., Hernández-Cordero, S., Baker, P., Barros, A. J. D., Bégin, F., Chapman, D. J., Grummer-Strawn, L., McCoy, D., Menon, P., Ribeiro Neves, P. A., Piwoz, E., Rollins, N., Victora, C. G., & Richter, L. (2023). Breastfeeding: Crucially important, but increasingly challenged in a market-driven world. *The Lancet (British Edition); Lancet, 401*(10375), 472–485. https://doi.org/10.1016/S0140–6736(22)01932-8

Piwoz, E. G., & Huffman, S. L. (2015). The impact of marketing of breast-milk substitutes on WHO-recommended breastfeeding practices. *Food and Nutrition Bulletin, 36*(4), 373–386. https://doi.org/10.1177/0379572115602174

Ryan, G., Callaghan, S., Rafferty, A., Murphy, J., Higgins, M., Barry, T., Mangina, E., Carroll, L., & McAuliffe, F. (2022). Virtual reality in midwifery education: A mixed methods study to assess learning and understanding. *Nurse Education Today, 119,* 105573. https://doi.org/10.1016/j.nedt.2022.105573

Reisman, T., & Goldstein, Z. (2018). Case report: Induced lactation in a transgender woman. *Transgender Health, 3*(1), 24–26. https://doi.org/10.1089/trgh.2017.0044

Roberts, D., Jackson, L., Davie, P., Zhao, C., Harrold Joanne A., Fallon, V., & Silverio, S. A. (2023). Exploring the reasons why mothers do not breastfeed, to inform and enable better support. *Frontiers in Global Women's Health, 4.* | https://doi.org/10.3389/fgwh.2023.1148719

Sandall, J., Soltani, H., Gates, S., Shennan, A., & Devane, D. (2016). Midwife-led continuity models versus other models of care for childbearing women. *The Cochrane Database of Systematic Reviews, 4*(4), CD004667. https://doi.org/10.1002/14651858.CD004667.pub5

Scottish Government, Children and Families Directorate. (2018). *Scottish Maternal and Infant Nutrition Survey 2017.* Edinburgh, UK: Scottish government. Healthcare quality and improvement directorate

Schnell, A. (2022). Successful co-lactation by a queer couple: A case study. *Journal of Human Lactation, 38*(4), 644–650. https://doi.org/10.1177/08903344221108733

Stanway, P., & Stanway, A. (1978). *Breast Is Best: A Commonsense Approach to Breastfeeding.* London: Pan Books.

Swant, M. (2016). Twitter says users now trust influencers nearly as much as their friends. *Adweek.* Retrieved 30 October 22, from https://www.adweek.com/performance-marketing/twitter-says-users-now-trust-influencers-nearly-much-their-friends-171367/

Tomori, C. (2023). Protecting, promoting and supporting breastfeeding in all policies: Reframing the narrative. *Frontiers in Public Health, 11.* https://doi.org/10.3389/fpubh.2023.1149384

Trivedi, D. (2018). Cochrane review summary: Support for healthy breastfeeding mothers with healthy term babies. *Primary Health Care Research & Development, 19*(6), 529–530. https://doi.org/10.1017/S1463423618000130

Tsutaya, T., & Mizushima, N. (2023). Evolutionary biological perspectives on current social issues of breastfeeding and weaning. *Yearbook Biological Anthropology, 181*(Suppl. 76), 81–93. https://doi.org/10.1002/ajpa.24710

Turner, S. E., Brockway, M., Azad, M. B., Grant, A., Tomfohr-Madsen, L., & Brown, A. (2023). Breastfeeding in the pandemic: A qualitative analysis of breastfeeding experiences among mothers from Canada and the United Kingdom. *Women and Birth*, *36*(4), e388–e396, https://doi.org/10.1016/j.wombi.2023.01.002

UNICEF UK. (2017). *Guide To the UNICEF UK Baby Friendly Initiative Standards*. UNICEF UK. Guide-to-the-Unicef-UK-Baby-Friendly-Initiative-Standards.pdf

UNICEF UK. (2018a) *Having Meaningful Conversations with Mothers: A Guide to Using the Baby Friendly Signature Sheets*. UNICEF Baby Friendly Initiative (BFI) UK. https://www.unicef.org.uk/babyfriendly/wp-content/uploads/sites/2/2018/10/Having-meaningful-conversations-with-mothers.pdf

UNICEF UK. (2018b). *Achieving Sustainability in Universities: Standards and Guidance*. UNICEF UK The Baby Friendly Initiative. https://www.unicef.org.uk/babyfriendly/wp-content/uploads/sites/2/2018/11/Achieving-Sustainability-in-Universities-Standards-and-Guidance-Unicef-UK-Baby-Friendly-Initiative.pdf

UNICEF UK. (2019). *UNICEF UK Baby Friendly Initiative Theory of Change*. UNICEF UK Baby Friendly Initiative. https://www.unicef.org.uk/babyfriendly/wp-content/uploads/sites/2/2019/04/Baby-Friendly-Initiative-Theory-of-Change.pdf

United Nations. (2015). *Every Woman, Every Child: Global Strategy for Women's Health, Child, and Adolescent (2016–2030)*. New York: United Nations. Available at: http://www.everywomaneverychild. org/wp-content/uploads/2017/10/EWEC_ Global StrategyUpdate_Full_EN_2017_web-1.pdf

United Nations. (2018) *Breastfeeding Is a Father's Responsibility*, https://www.un.org/en/academic-impact/breastfeeding-father%E2%80%99s-responsibility

United Nations General Assembly. (2015). *Transforming our world: the 2030 Agenda for Sustainable Development* (A/RES/70/1). Available at: https://www.refworld.org/docid/57b6e3e44.html

Victora, C. G., Bahl, R., Barros, A. J. D., França, G. V. A., Horton, S., Krasevec, J., Murch, S., Sankar, M., Jeeva, D. M., Walker, N., & Rollins, N. C. (2016). Breastfeeding in the 21st century: Epidemiology, mechanisms, and lifelong effect. *The Lancet (British Edition): Lancet*, *387*(10017), 475–490. https://doi.org/10.1016/S0140–6736(15)01024-7

Wedekind, S., & Shenker, N. (2021). Antiviral properties of human milk. *Microorganism*, *9*(4), 1–16. https://doi.org/10.3390/microorganisms9040715

World Health Organization. (1981). *International Code of Marketing of Breast-Milk Substitutes*. Available at: https://www.who.int/publications/i/item/9241541601

World Health Organization. (2003). *Global Strategy on Infant and Young Child Feeding*. Geneva: WHO. https://www.who.int/publications-detail-redirect/9241562218

World Health Organization. (2022). *Scope and Impact of Digital Marketing Strategies for Promoting Breast Milk Substitutes*, 9789240046085-eng.pdf (who.int)

Yang, H., Na, X., Zhang, Y., Xi, M., Yang, Y., Chen, R., & Zhao, A. (2023). Rates of breastfeeding or chestfeeding and influencing factors among transgender and gender-diverse parents: A cross sectional study. *eClinicalMedicine*, *57*, 101847. https://doi.org/10.1016/j.eclinm.2023.101847

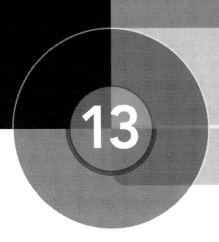

Perinatal Mental Health Promotion in Midwifery Practice

AMANDA FIRTH, IAN P S NOONAN, AND
CHARLOTTE ANNE KENYON

INTRODUCTION

This chapter will consider how midwives can promote the mental health of all people in their care. Women and birthing parents are acknowledged as the primary maternity service user, but perinatal mental health affects the whole family unit and therefore the wider potential impact of untreated perinatal mental illness is also explored. The term 'service user' is utilised here, referring collectively to all women and birthing parents using maternity services.

'Perinatal mental health' refers to the mental health of women and birthing parents during pregnancy and the first year postpartum (NICE, 2014). Statistics suggest that around 20% of the maternity population experience perinatal mental illness which includes conditions such as depression, anxiety disorders, eating disorders, addiction, psychosis, bipolar disorder and schizophrenia; with depression and anxiety being the most frequently diagnosed conditions (NICE, 2014).

Midwives, as leaders or coordinators of midwifery care, have a key role in assessing, promoting, and supporting the mental health of service users (NMC,

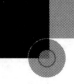

2019). This chapter will explore some of the barriers and facilitators that midwives experience when assessing and supporting women and birthing parents' perinatal mental health, suggesting ways that midwives can actively promote and support mental wellbeing.

WHY IS PERINATAL MENTAL HEALTH A KEY PUBLIC HEALTH CONCERN FOR MIDWIVES?

Untreated perinatal mental illness has interconnected issues which impact on both the individual and wider society. It is suggested that untreated perinatal mental illness in the UK has a long-term societal cost of around £8.1 billion per year, with almost three quarters of this figure attributed to the long-term impact on the child and family (Bauer et al., 2014). From a physical perspective, there is a correlation between maternal stress levels in pregnancy and increased rates of intrauterine growth restriction, premature birth and low birth weight (Misra et al., 2010; O'Hara et al., 2014). Additionally, the first 1,001 days of a child's life (from pregnancy to age 2) is a period of rapid brain development and an infant's interactions with people and the environment around them during this time forms the basis of future mental and emotional health (Department of Health and Social Care, 2021).

New parents with poor mental health are less likely interact with their infant and are more likely to isolate themselves from society, experience relationship breakdowns, become unemployed and have increased smoking or alcohol use (Slomian et al., 2019). Research suggests that infants and children of parents with perinatal mental illness are more likely to manifest behavioural problems, have lower educational achievement and experience mental illness themselves (Aktar et al., 2019). Midwives are in an optimal position to help address some of these potentially long-term health inequalities by ensuring that women and birthing parents receive effective support from maternity and perinatal mental health services as they transition to parenthood or expand their families.

CONSIDERING HOW TRANSITION TO PARENTHOOD MAY INFLUENCE MENTAL HEALTH

Pregnancy and transition to parenthood can increase a service user's vulnerability to perinatal mental health concerns. It is known that levels of formally diagnosed perinatal mental health conditions have increased in comparison to previous generations, perhaps partly due to increased societal discussion of mental health but also possibly attributed to women and birthing parents living in a fundamentally different society to that which their parents experienced (Howard & Khalifeh, 2020). One multi-generational research project suggests that perinatal depression is 51% more common in mothers from recent generations in contrast to their parent's generation (Pearson et al., 2018).

Becoming a parent is an intense and continuous learning curve which is best navigated with the support of a community, family and friends. Social isolation is a risk factor for conditions such as depression and anxiety, and may be increasing due to geographical mobility of service users in today's societies. Many service users no longer live close to their family, perhaps relocating due to job opportunities, reducing the amount of support available during that critical adjustment period (Solmeyer & Feinberg, 2011). Not all pregnancies are planned, and some relationships will breakdown during the perinatal period, which may have psychological, practical and financial implications, including emotional distress and grief, housing concerns, or worries about how the service user will be able to financially support a child. There is also a suggestion that social media may add to the societal pressures experienced by service users, which can have a negative impact on mental wellbeing (Pearson et al., 2018).

LEARNING ACTIVITY

Take time to speak with someone from a different generation to you. This might be a parent/ grandparent or someone else of a similar age. Ask them about their experiences of pregnancy and parenthood during that time.

- Who supported them through their pregnancy and transition to parenthood?
- What positively impacted on their experiences?
- What challenges did they experience and how did they overcome them?
- What was it like to be a parent in that generation?
- If appropriate to ask, how do they think this affected their mental health at the time?

Take time to reflect on which of those factors may be similar or different to the experiences of parents today.

DEFINING MENTAL HEALTH AND MENTAL ILLNESS

The World Health Organization (WHO) defines mental health as

a state of mental well-being that enables people to cope with the stresses of life, to realize their abilities, to learn well and work well, and to contribute towards their communities. Mental health is an integral component of health and well-being and is more than the absence of a mental disorder

(WHO, 2022, p. 8).

WHO (2022) states that mental health is dynamic rather than static, existing on a continuum. Some people with a diagnosed mental illness may perceive themselves to have high levels of mental wellbeing, and others may not have a formally diagnosed mental illness but may feel that their level of mental wellbeing is low.

These are important concepts to understand because midwives will care for service users with a range of needs including: existing mental illness, new onset of mental illness and symptoms of mental ill health which impact the service user's wellbeing but fall below the thresholds for treatment by formal healthcare services.

CONSIDERING MENTAL HEALTH FROM A SALUTOGENIC PERSPECTIVE

In healthcare professions, we are often prompted to consider health from the perspective of pathogenesis, the origin of disease. Yet for many women and birthing parents in our care, pregnancy and birth are not an illness. Some service users will have new or existing co-morbidities, such as gestational diabetes mellitis or hypertension, but may still view themselves as essentially healthy. Equally, some maternity service users may have existing well-controlled mental health conditions. Others will have exacerbations of existing conditions or a new onset of symptoms which negatively affect their health and wellbeing, requiring input from specialist perinatal mental health services.

Salutogenesis offers an alternative perspective on health, which has significant alignment with the WHO definition provided above. The theory of salutogenesis by Aaron Antonvosky (1979) is the opposite of pathogenesis and instead considers the origins of health and focusses on factors which promote or contribute to an individual's perception of good health.

LEARNING ACTIVITY

Antonovsky (1996) somewhat controversially proposed that people access 'disease care systems' rather than 'health care systems', meaning that healthcare focusses on the treatment of disease rather than the promotion of health.

1. How does this correspond with your experiences as a midwife working within a healthcare system?
2. How might this influence the perinatal mental health care offered to and received by maternity service users?
3. What health promotion responsibilities do you have in your role as a midwife?

Antonovsky proposed that an individual's perception of health constantly fluctuates on a continuum of 'ease' (total health) to dis-ease (see Figure 13.1).

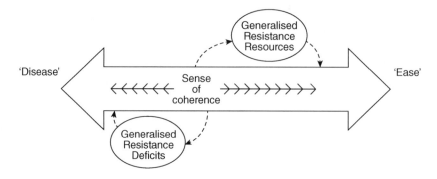

Figure 13.1 The Salutogenic model.

Source: Adapted from Antonovsky (1979).

He suggested that an individual's notion of health is determined by their ability to navigate stressors (the challenges in their life), proposing that although stressors may temporarily negatively impact health, they may also increase resilience to future stressors and therefore, increase perceptions of health and wellbeing in the future.

Antonovsky proposed that perceptions of health and wellbeing are influenced by an individual's 'sense of coherence'. Sense of coherence is defined as the ability to respond to a stressful situation, which is affected by the individual's *comprehensibility*, *manageability*, and *meaningfulness*. He suggested that to be able to respond appropriately to stressors, individuals need to be able to understand the environment they are within, have access to resources and coping strategies and have a life that is meaningful (see Figure 13.2).

Antonovsky believed that an individual's sense of coherence is influenced by the resources that they have available to help them cope with a stressor, naming these 'generalised resistance resources'. Generalised resistance resources are a subjective concept, with the importance of each variable dependent upon the individual. Figure 13.3 shows a non-exhaustive list including material resources such as financial security or accommodation, knowledge-based resources such as education and familiarity with societal systems (such as health care) and also access to social and cultural resources.

Antonovsky hypothesised that when a person has sufficient generalised resistance resources, this will strengthen their sense of coherence, therefore increasing their perception of health and wellbeing and moving them further along the continuum to 'ease' or total health. In contrast, when a person has a deficit of generalised resistance resources, this will decrease their sense of coherence and move their perception of health and wellbeing in the opposite direction, towards 'disease'.

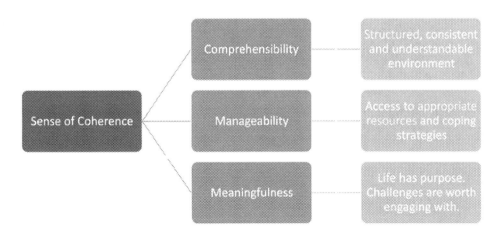

Figure 13.2 A sense of coherence.

Source: Adapted from Antonovsky (1979).

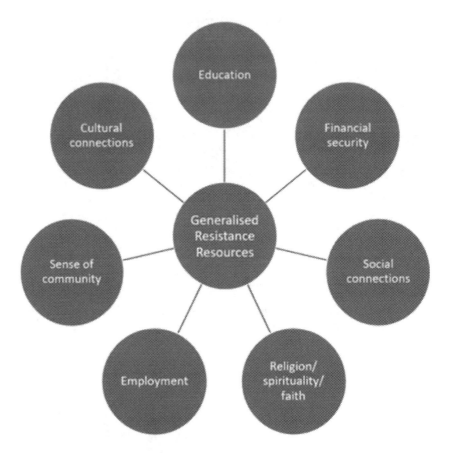

Figure 13.3 Generalised resistance resources.

Source: **Adapted from Antonovsky (1979).**

LEARNING ACTIVITY: APPLYING SALUTOGENIC THEORY TO A MIDWIFERY SCENARIO

You meet Sofia in a community midwife appointment. She is 28 weeks pregnant with her first baby and recently arrived from Ukraine where she worked as a teacher. Sofia is fleeing the war and she has travelled alone as her partner is completing military service. She hopes her parents will find a UK sponsor and will be able to join her before the baby is born. Sofia attends the appointment with an interpreter, she tells you that she feels well in herself, but visually she appears to be low in mood and tearful.

4. What factors may be affecting Sofia's sense of coherence? Think about this specifically in respect of her comprehensibility, manageability, and meaningfulness.
5. What can you do as a midwife help Sofia to increase her generalised resistance resources? List the different sources of support and signposting to other services that you could facilitate for Sofia.

See end of chapter for potential answers.

INDIVIDUAL CONSTRUCTS OF MENTAL HEALTH AND MENTAL ILLNESS

Although the beginning of this chapter offers a definition of mental health, it is important for midwives to recognise that personal constructs of mental health are filled with complexity and nuance. A midwife's own personal concept of mental health will likely differ from that of many of the service users that they care for. Service users may demonstrate different presentations of mental distress or describe their mental health in unfamiliar ways.

There are fundamental differences in how mental wellbeing is conceptualised across different cultures (Joshanloo, 2014). Joshanloo proposes that Western notions of mental wellbeing centre more on 'I' and individual concepts such as self-esteem and self-determination, whereas non-Western concepts of mental health are more likely to focus on collectivist principles such as relationships and family esteem or reputation.

Vocabulary used to describe mental health is socially constructed; defining morals and perspectives which are not universally applicable (Cromby, 2004). Language used by service users from racially diverse populations often demonstrate cultural differences in attitudes to mental health. One example is that narratives used by Black African, Caribbean, and Asian women sometimes refer to dishonour, religious stigma, and socially acceptable behaviour (Wittkowski et al., 2017). These perspectives may have a significant influence on service users' likelihood of disclosing symptoms to midwives and may affect their help-seeking behaviours (Edge & MacKian, 2010). Although UK perinatal mental health services portray a narrative of 'it's ok to not be ok', this may not correlate with all servicer user's beliefs about mental health. Being aware of this challenges the midwife to continually individualise their care, be sensitive in discussions on mental health and also acknowledge the need to develop continually evolving cultural competency.

TRAUMA-INFORMED CARE

It is important that midwives are aware that a service users' perinatal mental health may be influenced by past or present experiences of trauma. Trauma is a subjective concept. It is not the event or circumstances themselves, but the impact that this has on the psychological wellbeing of the individual. Two service users may experience a similar situation but manifest very different responses.

Trauma is defined as:

"an event, series of events, or set of circumstances that is experienced by an individual as physically or emotionally harmful or life threatening and that has lasting adverse effects on the individual's functioning and mental, physical, social, emotional or spiritual well-being." (SAMHSA, 2014, p. 7)

Although some maternity service users may commence their midwifery care aware of their previous trauma, for some service users, pregnancy or birth may unlock deeply buried past experiences. Examples include previous sexual abuse or sexual violence which may only be disclosed for the first-time during pregnancy.

Experiences of ongoing trauma may increase in pregnancy, such as domestic abuse, with the service user seeking help for the first-time during pregnancy (see Chapter 17 for more on violence against women and girls). For others, it may be the intrapartum period which initiates a trauma-response e.g. tokophobia (a fear of childbirth) or unresolved birth trauma from a previous birth experience (Law et al., 2021).

Trauma can affect anyone, but some people have a higher risk of experiencing trauma including service users from the following populations (Law et al., 2021):

- Migrants; particularly asylum seekers, refugees, and anyone who has experienced trafficking.
- Racially diverse groups.
- People experiencing homelessness/insecure housing.
- People living in poverty or destitution.
- People who live with physical or psychological health conditions, including addiction.

Of course, many service users may be part of more than one of these groups, therefore further increasing their risk of experiencing trauma. Although it is important to be aware of these increased risks, midwives must take care not to stereotype populations or groups. Instead, it is helpful to acknowledge the increased risk and have awareness of possible sources of trauma for some groups.

LEARNING ACTIVITY: BEING AWARE OF POSSIBLE SOURCES OF TRAUMA

Kadija is an asylum seeker from Eritrea, where she fled religious persecution. She arrived in the UK six weeks ago, is living in a hostel and has limited financial support from the government. Kadija doesn't want to talk much but discloses that she became pregnant during a long journey to the UK.

- Are there any factors in Kadija's short personal story which *may* indicate potential sources of trauma?
- How many of the groups listed above *might* Kadija feasibly be part of and how does this influence her risk of having experienced trauma?

Literature supports that midwives can feel overwhelmed by the trauma disclosed by women during perinatal mental health screening in the general maternity population (Bayrampour et al., 2018; Mollart et al., 2009) – see Chapter 15 for more on midwives' self-care). However, how healthcare practitioners respond to disclosure of trauma has a significant impact on the service user's future engagement with the maternity service and other healthcare provision (Law et al., 2021).

Law et al. (2021) outline four principles of trauma-informed care relevant to the perinatal period: compassion and recognition, communication and collaboration, consistency and continuity, and celebrating strengths and diversity. Table 13.1, adapted from Law et al.'s good practice guide, provides further information about how these may be demonstrated.

Table 13.1 Trauma informed good practice guide

Compassion and recognition	• Midwives need to be aware of sources of trauma, and the different impacts that these may have on service users. • When trauma is disclosed, midwives can show compassion by acknowledging and validating service users' experiences. • It is important that midwives ensure the service user feels believed and that they assess their immediate safety.
Communication and collaboration	• Communication with service users should be non-judgmental and sensitive. • Midwives can empower service users to feel able to collaborate with other healthcare professionals, ensuring that the service user feels in control of any referrals that are made.
Consistency and continuity	• Services need to work closely with each other, so that care pathways, referral processes and care provided does not add to the distress of the service user eg. needing to continually re-disclose the trauma to different providers. • The midwifery Continuity of Carer model would be especially valuable to service users with a history of trauma.
Celebrating strengths and diversity	• Midwives must also be aware that what is helpful for one service user, may be triggering for another. • They need to remain curious and to continually develop their cultural competency, acknowledging that factors such as religion and spirituality may influence service user's experiences and help-seeking behaviour. • Language barriers must be addressed so that service users have an equitable opportunity to discuss and receive support with trauma.

LEARNING ACTIVITY

You meet Beth at her booking appointment during her second pregnancy. When you ask about her previous obstetric history and birth she becomes visibly upset. Beth describes a full-term, category 1 caesarean section for prolonged fetal brady-cardia, which was completed under general anaesthetic. She remembers regaining consciousness on a recovery ward without her baby or partner. Beth tells you that she had tried to 'move on' from the experience but being pregnant again has led her to start replaying the memory over and over, unable to switch it off. Beth is fearful of birthing again but hasn't disclosed this to her partner or family. You are the first person that she has admitted her feelings to.

As a midwife how can you apply the principles of the good practice guide above to Beth's care? How will you demonstrate:

- Compassion and recognition?
- Communication and collaboration?
- Consistency and continuity?
- Celebrating strengths and diversity?

THE MIDWIFE'S ROLE IN SCREENING FOR COMMON PERINATAL MENTAL HEALTH CONDITIONS

Midwives should enquire about perinatal mental health at every maternity appointment, providing adequate time for service users to disclose any concerns (NICE, 2014). As part of universal midwifery care, midwives use validated screening tools to assess whether a service user would benefit from referral to other practitioners. The aim of this is to ensure that all service users are having their mental health assessed in an equitable way.

In the UK, perinatal mental health screening usually begins with the Whooley questions, a very short identification tool which asks two questions (see Table 13.2) (Whooley et al., 1997).

Where the answers to either of these questions is 'yes', the service user is asked if this is something that they would like help with. If the questions suggest that there may be perinatal mental illness, the midwife is encouraged to complete further screening and, where appropriate, refer to another healthcare professional or specialist perinatal mental health team for additional assessment and/or diagnosis (NICE, 2014). Further screening is often undertaken using the nine-item Patient Health Questionnaire (PHQ-9) or the Edinburgh Postnatal Depression Scale (EPDS), which is only used in the postnatal period (Cox et al., 1987; Spitzer et al., 1994). The Generalised Anxiety Disorder seven item questionnaire (GAD-7) may also be used when there are symptoms of anxiety (Spitzer et al., 2006).

There is an argument that mental health screening tools used in Western countries are biased towards Western symptoms of depression, and although they are validated for use in many different languages, they are not available in all languages needed (Tobin et al., 2015; Zubaran et al., 2010). There is also evidence that despite universal screening tools being used with women from racially diverse groups in the UK, there is less identification and subsequent management of symptoms in comparison to white British women (Prady et al., 2021). Prady et al.'s work demonstrates that health inequality is not restricted to language barriers, as identification was also reduced in racially diverse service users with no language concerns. Additionally, it is argued that depression screening tools are designed for self-completion, with the reliability and validity of the data decreasing when translated through an interpreter, who may struggle with cultural equivalence or vocabulary (Hayden et al., 2013). These are all important factors that midwives need to consider when undertaking mental health screening.

Table 13.2 The Whooley questions

Whooley questions
1. During the past month, have you been bothered by feeling down, depressed, and hopeless?
2. During the last month, have you been bothered by having little interest or pleasure in doing things?
If Yes to either or both of the above:
3. Would you like help with this?

Source: Whooley et al. (1997).

THE MIDWIFE'S ROLE IN PERINATAL MENTAL HEALTH PROMOTION FOR ALL

There remains a risk that mental health promotion is seen as something we only need to do for women who either have a mental illness or are at obvious risk of developing one during or after pregnancy. However, every interaction that a midwife has with a service user is an opportunity to either promote or demote mental health.

The ten elements of mental health promotion or demotion model considers these opportunities at a micro, meso, and macro level (MacDonald & O'Hara, 1998). The ten element model attempts to integrate the personal experience of mental health and illness, the impact on family and friends in addition to the causal factors of illness in an integrated bio-psycho-social approach.

- The micro level is primarily concerned with the relationship, interactions and interventions between the individual midwife and service user, their supporters, family and the immediate team.
- Meso-level interventions are those around the organisation of service delivery, inter-professional liaison and availability of services.
- Macro-level perspectives are concerned with maternal health care funding, priority within the NHS, social trends and issues like stigma that effect whole populations' views around mental health and mental illness (Figure 13.4).

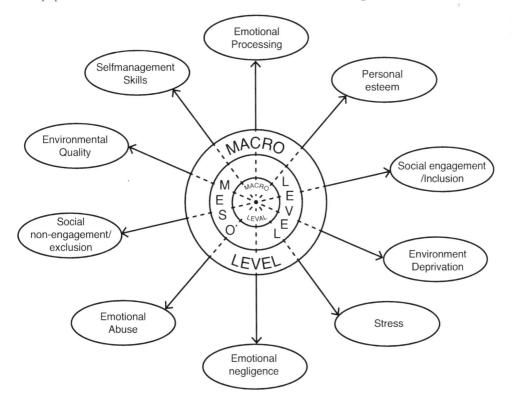

Figure 13.4 The ten elements of mental health promotion and demotion

Source: MacDonald and O'Hara (1998).

Midwives, in their role of promoting mental health for all service users, can particularly influence experiences at a micro and meso level of the MacDonald and O'Hara's model. At a micro level, a trusting relationship between the service user and midwife, where there is sufficient time within appointments for holistic assessment of wellbeing is important. It will provide space for authentic discussions about mental health and increase the likelihood that a service user will access and engage with any relevant support services, thereby promoting their mental health. Conversely, rushed appointments with unfamiliar midwives may decrease a service user's opportunity or desire to discuss their mental health, thereby acting as a demoting factor.

At a meso-level, midwives can promote mental wellbeing for all service users by ensuring that they are familiar with supporting agencies, referral mechanisms and by building collaborative relationships with the wider inter-disciplinary teams that are providing support and care. This will promote mental health by providing an experience where service users can more easily navigate the care pathways that have been provided for them. When midwives are unfamiliar of the support services available or have a fragmented inter-professional relationship with other service provision, women and birthing parents are more likely to become invisible or fall through gaps within the system.

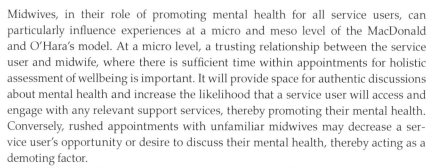

FURTHER EXPLORATION OF THE MIDWIFE'S ROLE IN ASSESSING AND SUPPORTING PERINATAL MENTAL HEALTH

Screening for symptoms of perinatal mental illness is a fundamental part of universal midwifery care, and there is an expectation that all registered midwives can proficiently assess and support women with their perinatal mental health; making referrals to the wider inter-disciplinary team and voluntary sector services as appropriate (NICE, 2014; NMC, 2019). However, the structure of service provision will be different depending on where the midwife works. In the UK there has been substantial investment in the development and improvement of specialist perinatal mental health services, but provision remains a post code lottery for many service users (Maternal Mental Health Alliance, 2022). In many areas, midwives and general practitioners will support service users with mental health symptoms classified as mild to moderate, with specialist perinatal mental health services leading on the care of service users with moderate to severe symptoms (Maternal Mental Health Alliance, 2022). The referral processes and services available may differ by geographical region and it is important that the midwife is familiar with the services and benchmarks for referral within the area that they work.

A recent report suggests that although service provision in the UK is rapidly improving, the midwifery workforce requires increased training in assessing and supporting women with perinatal mental health concerns (Bauer et al., 2022). This corresponds with narratives from midwives too, with some midwives reporting that they lack confidence and training in perinatal mental health screening; and others suggesting that midwives may find it difficult to discern whether a symptom such as fatigue, is a symptom of a perinatal health concern, or a physiological part of pregnancy (Coates & Foureur, 2019; Williams et al., 2016). A recent systemic review reports that health professionals frequently lack mental health literacy, which limits their ability to recognise and discuss symptoms of mental illness with service users (Branquinho et al., 2022). It is also argued that there is an increasing responsibility on midwives to support service users with mild to moderate symptoms, who do not meet the entry criteria for specialist services but relatively little guidance on how to do so effectively (Coates & Foureur, 2019).

Undoubtedly, in the UK and globally, many midwives work in maternity systems with evolving perinatal mental health services and differing levels of staff training. However, there is also the perspective that midwives are individually responsible for identifying and addressing gaps in their knowledge as indicated by the NMC revalidation requirements, which stipulate that midwives need to participate in continuing professional development in order to be able to provide safe, individualised and evidence-based care (NMC, 2018, 2021).

LEARNING ACTIVITY: SELF-ASSESSMENT OF PERINATAL MENTAL HEALTH LITERACY, INCLUDING THE ASSESSMENT AND SUPPORT OF SERVICE USERS IN YOUR CARE

Take some time to reflect on or find the answers the following:

- How would you rate your knowledge of common mental health conditions that service users may present with (e.g. anxiety and depression)?
- How confident do you feel in discussing mental health with service users?
- What perinatal mental health services are available in the region that you work?
- What is the criteria for referring someone into these services?
- Which perinatal mental health screening tools are used?
- How confident do you feel in using these tools?
- What areas of development do you have and what action will you take?

SUMMARY

- Perinatal mental health has an impact on the service user and the whole family unit.

- The impact on the child is particularly significant, with early support and intervention for the mother/birthing parent being a key method of minimising long-term inequalities.

- Transition to parenthood is a vulnerable period of time for women and birthing parents.

- It is helpful for midwives to consider mental health and wellbeing holistically, rather than diminishing it to just the absence of mental illness.

- Mental health and wellbeing are social constructs which may be influenced by many variables such as culture, religion, language, and social identity.

- Past or present trauma may influence service user's mental health and ability to engage with support.

- Screening for potential perinatal mental illness is a universal part of midwifery care, but it requires training and skills development to ensure that screening is used effectively.

- Midwives are responsible for promoting the mental health and wellbeing of all service users.

- Midwives can take positive action to ensure that they have the best available skills and knowledge to promote mental health and wellbeing for all women and birthing parents in their care.

Potential Answers for Sofia Case Study:

1. Sofia is adapting to living in a completely new and unfamiliar environment. These experiences will be affecting Sofia's sense of coherence. Her comprehensibility is challenged by needing to learn to navigate an environment which functions with unfamiliar processes e.g. UK health care system and welfare system. Her manageability is compromised as she is isolated from familiar resources and coping strategies. Sofia had a professional job in Ukraine but is not working in the UK and soon will be supporting a new baby with minimal family support. Sofia has meaningfulness and she is hopeful of being reunited with family, but the language barrier makes it much more difficult for her to ask for help adjusting to life in this new environment.

2. The midwife is perfectly placed to help Sofia increase her generalised resistance resources and could signpost or refer Sofia to activities such as local parents' groups, antenatal education, and English language classes. There may be a specific Ukrainian community group in the area to provide additional social support and cultural connection. The midwife could provide a continuity of carer model of midwifery to Sofia and ensure that each appointment has an interpreter present, so that Sofia can be encouraged to build a trusting relationship with the midwife and be able to discuss her physical and mental health comprehensively.

REFERENCES

Aktar, E., Qu, J., Lawrence, P. J., Tollenaar, M. S., Elzinga, B. M., & Bögels, S. M. (2019). Fetal and infant outcomes in the offspring of parents with perinatal mental disorders: Earliest influences. *Frontiers in Psychiatry, 10*, 391.

Antonovsky, A. (1979). *Health, stress, and coping.* San Francisco: Jossey-Bass.

Antonovsky, A. (1996). The salutogenic model as a theory to guide health promotion. *Health Promotion International, 11*(1), 11–18.

Bauer, A., Parsonage, M., Knapp, M., Iemmi, V., Adelaja, B., & Hogg, S. (2014). The costs of perinatal mental health problems. *Centre for Mental Health.* costsofperinatal.pdf (centreformentalhealth.org.uk)

Bauer, A., Tinelli, M., & Knapp, M. (2022). *The Economic Case for Increasing Access to Treatment for Women with Common Mental Health Problems During the Perinatal Period.* (14) (PDF) The economic case for increasing access to treatment for women with common mental health problems during the perinatal period (researchgate.net)

Bayrampour, H., Hapsari, A. P., & Pavlovic, J. (2018). Barriers to addressing perinatal mental health issues in midwifery settings. *Midwifery, 59*, 47–58.

Branquinho, M., Shakeel, N., Horsch, A., & Fonseca, A. (2022). Frontline health professionals' perinatal depression literacy: A systematic review. *Midwifery*, 103365. DOI: 10.1016/j.midw.2022.103365

Coates, D., & Foureur, M. (2019). The role and competence of midwives in supporting women with mental health concerns during the perinatal period: A scoping review. *Health & Social Care in the Community, 27*(4), e389–e405.

Cox, J. L., Holden, J. M., & Sagovsky, R. (1987). Detection of postnatal depression: Development of the 10-item Edinburgh Postnatal Depression Scale. *The British Journal of Psychiatry, 150*(6), 782–786.

Cromby, J. (2004). Depression: Embodying social inequality. *Journal of Critical Psychology, Counselling and Psychotherapy, 4*(3), 176–187.

Department of Health and Social Care. (2021). *The Best Start for Life: A Vision for the 1,001 Critical Days*. https://assets.publishing.service.gov.uk/media/605c5e61d3bf7f2f0d94183a/The_best_start_for_life_a_vision_for_the_1_001_critical_days.pdf

Edge, D., & MacKian, S. C. (2010). Ethnicity and mental health encounters in primary care: help-seeking and help-giving for perinatal depression among Black Caribbean women in the UK. *Ethnicity & Health, 15*(1), 93–111. https://doi.org/10.1080/13557850903418836

Hayden, M., Connelly, C. D., Baker-Ericzen, M. J., Hazen, A. L., & McCue Horwitz, S. (2013). Exploring perceptions and experiences of maternal depression in Latinas: A qualitative study. *Issues in Mental Health Nursing, 34*(3), 180–184.

Howard, L. M., & Khalifeh, H. (2020). Perinatal mental health: A review of progress and challenges. *World Psychiatry, 19*(3), 313–327.

Joshanloo, M. (2014). Eastern conceptualizations of happiness: Fundamental differences with western views. *Journal of Happiness Studies, 15*(2), 475–493. https://doi.org/10.1007/s10902-013-9431-1

Law, C., Wolfenden, L., Sperlich, M., & Taylor, J. (2021). *A Good Practice Guide to Support the Implementation of Trauma-Informed Care in the Perinatal Period.* NHS England and NHS Improvement.

MacDonald, G., & O'Hara, K. (1998). *Ten Elements of Mental Health, its Promotion and Demotion: Implications for Practice.* Society of Health Education and Health Promotion Specialists.

Maternal Mental Health Alliance. (2022). *A Sound Investment. Increasing Access to Treatment for Women with Common Maternal Mental Health Problems.* M. M. H. Alliance. a-sound-investment-report-centre-for-mental-health-2022-mmha.pdf (maternalmentalhealthalliance.org)

Misra, D., Strobino, D., & Trabert, B. (2010). Effects of social and psychosocial factors on risk of preterm birth in black women. *Paediatric and Perinatal Epidemiology, 24*(6), 546–554. https://doi.org/10.1111/j.1365-3016.2010.01148.x

Mollart, L., Newing, C., & Foureur, M. (2009). Midwives' emotional wellbeing: impact of conducting a structured antenatal psychosocial assessment (SAPSA). *Women and Birth, 22*(3), 82–88.

NICE. (2014). *Antenatal and Postnatal Mental Health: Clinical Management and Service Guidance.* Clinical guideline [CG192] (December 2014). Overview | Antenatal and postnatal mental health: clinical management and service guidance | Guidance | NICE

NMC. (2018). *The Code.* The Nursing and Midwifery Council. https://www.nmc.org.uk/globalassets/sitedocuments/nmc-publications/nmc-code.pdf

NMC. (2019). *Standards of Proficiency for Midwives.* https://www.nmc.org.uk/standards/standards-for-midwives/standards-of-proficiency-for-midwives/

NMC. (2021). *What Is Revalidation?* Nursing and Midwifery Council. https://www.nmc.org.uk/revalidation/overview/what-is-revalidation/

O'Hara, M. W., Wisner, K. L., & Asher, H. (2014). Best practice & research clinical obstetrics and gynaecology perinatal mental illness: De finition, description and aetiology. Best *Practice & Research Clinical Obstetrics & Gynaecology, 28,* 3–12. https://doi.org/10.1016/j.bpobgyn.2013.09.002

Pearson, R. M., Carnegie, R. E., Cree, C., Rollings, C., Rena-Jones, L., Evans, J., Stein, A., Tilling, K., Lewcock, M., & Lawlor, D. A. (2018). Prevalence of prenatal depression symptoms among 2 generations of pregnant mothers: The Avon longitudinal study of parents and children. *JAMA Network Open, 1*(3), e180725–e180725.

Prady, S. L., Endacott, C., Dickerson, J., Bywater, T. J., & Blower, S. L. (2021). Inequalities in the identification and management of common mental disorders in the perinatal period: An equity focused re-analysis of a systematic review. *PLoS ONE, 16*(3), e0248631.

SAMHSA. (2014). *SAMHSA's Concept of Trauma and Guidance for a Trauma-Informed Approach.* SAMHSA Administration. https://ncsacw.acf.hhs.gov/userfiles/files/SAMHSA_Trauma.pdf

Slomian, J., Honvo, G., Emonts, P., Reginster, J.-Y., & Bruyère, O. (2019). Consequences of maternal postpartum depression: A systematic review of maternal and infant outcomes. *Women's Health, 15,* 1745506519844044.

Solmeyer, A. R., & Feinberg, M. E. (2011). Mother and father adjustment during early parenthood: The roles of infant temperament and coparenting relationship quality. *Infant Behavior and Development, 34*(4), 504–514. https://doi.org/10.1016/j.infbeh.2011.07.006

Spitzer, R. L., Kroenke, K., Williams, J. B. W., & Löwe, B. (2006). A brief measure for assessing generalized anxiety disorder: The GAD-7. *Archives of Internal Medicine, 166*(10), 1092–1097.

Spitzer, R. L., Williams, J. B. W., Kroenke, K., Linzer, M., deGruy, F. V., Hahn, S. R., Brody, D., & Johnson, J. G. (1994). Utility of a new procedure for diagnosing mental disorders in primary care: the PRIME-MD 1000 study. *JAMA, 272*(22), 1749–1756.

Tobin, C., Napoli, P., Wood-Gauthier, M., & Di Napoli, P. (2015). Recognition of risk factors for postpartum depression in refugee and immigrant women: Are current screening practices adequate? *Journal of Immigrant and Minority Health, 17*(4), 1019–1024. https://doi.org/10.1007/s10903-014-0041-8

WHO. (2022). *World Mental Health Report: Transforming Mental Health for All.* WHO. https://iris.who.int/bitstream/handle/10665/356119/9789240049338-eng.pdf?sequence=1

Whooley, M. A., Avins, A. L., Miranda, J., & Browner, W. S. (1997). Case-finding instruments for depression: Two questions are as good as many. *Journal of General Internal Medicine, 12*(7), 439–445.

Williams, C. J., Turner, K. M., Burns, A., Evans, J., & Bennert, K. (2016). Midwives and women's views on using UK recommended depression case finding questions in antenatal care. *Midwifery, 35*, 39–46.

Wittkowski, A., Patel, S., & Fox, J. R. (2017). The experience of postnatal depression in immigrant mothers living in western countries: A meta-synthesis. *Clinical Psychology & Psychotherapy, 24*(2), 411–427. https://doi.org/10.1002/cpp.2010

Zubaran, C., Schumacher, M., Roxo, M. R., & Foresti, K. (2010). Screening tools for postpartum depression: Validity and cultural dimensions. *African Journal of Psychiatry, 13*(August), 357–365. https://doi.org/10.4314/ajpsy.v13i5.63101

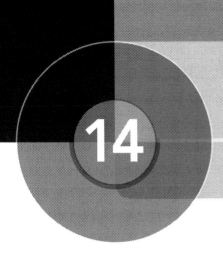

Maternal Suicide: A Key Public Health Issue for Midwifery Practice

14

ROSE BEAUMONT

INTRODUCTION

As explored in the previous chapter, perinatal mental health can affect up to 20% of expectant and new mothers and birthing parents (NHS England, NHS Improvement and National Collaborating Centre for Mental Health, 2018). Perinatal mental illness is linked to poorer maternal and neonatal outcomes and if left untreated can have a significant impact on long term outcomes for both the mother and wider family with an estimated cost to social and healthcare of £8.1 billion (NHS England, NHS Improvement and National Collaborating Centre for Mental Health, 2018). There are many different effects of mental health, but this chapter will aim to explore perinatal suicide, the leading cause of maternal death in the UK in the year following birth (MBRRACE, 2021, 2023). The 2018–2020 MBRRACE report (2023) shows that maternal death by suicide has tripled since the 2017–2019 MBRRACE report (MBRRACE, 2021) and 18% of all maternal deaths in the UK are attributed to suicide in this period. This chapter will also explore that this is not just a UK-wide problem, whilst global surveillance of suicide and perinatal mental health is poor, the evidence does suggest that globally maternal suicide accounts for approximately 20% of all global maternal deaths (Ghaedrahmati et al., 2017). Despite these statistics, there are no national or international public health initiatives aimed at reducing and preventing perinatal suicide. Research into perinatal suicide is in its infancy and minimal, and there is no published research about perinatal suicide prevention or evidence-based interventions to screen for suicidality. Moreover, the true burden of perinatal suicide is unknown, as it is a grossly underreported cause of maternal mortality due to issues with maternal mortality coding and stigma resulting in

DOI: 10.4324/9781003350071-14

many women not reporting mental health concerns due to fears of child removal, judgement and shame (MBRRACE, 2021). Despite the statistics both in the UK and globally, and evidence of rapidly rising rates of death by suicide in the UK and United States, perinatal suicide is a public health issue which remains largely unmet and urgently needs more focus. The midwife plays a key role in any future initiatives to screen for and prevent perinatal suicide.

BACKGROUND

There is a death globally from suicide in the general population, every 40 seconds. Global estimates expect death by suicide to increase by 50% by the year 2030 with pregnant or postpartum women representing a particularly vulnerable group due to the association of onset or relapse of psychiatric illness during this time (Orsolini et al., 2016).

Before exploring the issue of perinatal suicide, it is important to first explore suicide as a public health issue. With no specific policies targeting the issue of perinatal suicide, there is some aimed at prevention of suicide in the general population.

SUICIDE IN THE GENERAL POPULATION

Suicide is one of the leading causes of preventable deaths globally in the general population of those aged 15–49 (Our World in Data, 2019) with over 700,000 deaths per year and for every death by suicide, there are a further 20–30 suicidal attempts although the figure is believed to be much higher (Zalsman et al., 2016). Suicide is a serious global public health issue, and most are preventable with relatively low-cost evidence-based interventions and prevention strategies. Over the last 30 years, there have been some initial global suicide prevention efforts. These have provided steps towards improving knowledge and research, which has led to better understanding of the epidemiology of suicide (Goldsmith et al., 2002). This first-generation suicide research has led to the development of international and national policy on reducing suicide related deaths such as the development of Mental Health Action Plan 2013–2020 (World Health Assembly, 2013) and Preventing Suicide: A Global Imperative (WHO, 2014) and saw the inclusion of suicide reduction in the general population in the Sustainable Development Goals (SDGs) under 3.4.1 (United Nations, 2019) and WHO National suicide prevention strategies (WHO 2021). Whilst this is significant progress for suicide in the general population, there remains no global strategy to tackle maternal mental health and suicide (Table 14.1).

Table 14.1 Definitions of suicide and suicidality

Suicidal ideation: Thinking about dying by suicide, can be either active or passive
Active: Thinking about it and has a plan, the means, or the intent to attempt suicide
Passive: Thinking about it but does not have a plan, the means, or the intent. Passive suicidal ideation is more common in pregnancy and perinatal period than active suicidal ideation.
Suicidal attempt: Active attempt to end one's life by suicide
Suicidality: Someone is having suicidal ideation

PERINATAL SUICIDE

Death by suicide is the leading cause of maternal death in the UK in the first year following birth, and records illustrate it is on the rise particularly in women with multiple co-morbidities and social deprivation (MBRRACE, 2023). The 2019–2021 MBRRACE report indicates that rates of death by suicide tripled since the 2017–2019 MBRRACE report and wider global research suggests it is a leading cause of death in many other countries. There is an absence of quality data of suicide as a cause of maternal mortality globally, so the true burden is unknown, and it is an issue that gets little coverage. Countries with more vigorous maternal mortality surveillance systems to examine all causes of maternal deaths (the UK, Australia, the United States, Canada, the Nordic countries, and Sri Lanka) have all found suicide to be the leading cause of late maternal deaths and a significant cause of perinatal mortality (MBRRACE, 2023; Thornton et al., 2013; Koch & Geller, 2017; Bronson & Reviere, 2017; Agampodi et al., 2014, Vangen et al., 2017, Grigoriadis et al., 2017). Whilst there is limited data on maternal suicide in many other countries, data on suicide in the general population indicates 77% of all suicides occur in low- and middle-income countries, so it is likely a leading cause of maternal death across the globe (Khalifeh et al., 2016). Maternal suicide has far reaching implications on the family, and community.

LEARNING ACTIVITY

Before reading further, consider your learning from the previous chapter. Who do you consider might be more at risk of suicidal ideation or suicide in the perinatal period? Are you aware of any screening tools or pathways and policies to address maternal suicide in your area of practice?

UNDERREPORTING OF DEATH BY SUICIDE AS MATERNAL MORTALITY

Firstly, to understand the issue of maternal suicide, it is important to understand maternal mortality as well as the International Classification of Diseases (ICD). See Table 14.2 for the ICD classification.

The ICD is currently on its 11th revision and is revised to adapt to trends in disease and advancements in medical care and treatment. During the 10th revision, suicide during pregnancy, or within 42 days after either birth or termination of pregnancy, was re-classified as a direct cause of maternal death and any suicide between 43 days to 1 year following birth, was included as a late maternal death (WHO, 2012). Traditionally suicide and psychiatric death were not viewed as an obstetric cause but the change to definitions and inclusion criteria are reflective of growing research to support the brain-behaviour aetiology of the perinatal period and impact this can have on overall mental health (Mangla et al., 2019). Research into maternal mental health is relatively new; it is only in the last two decades that the link between brain-aetiology and behaviour and pregnancy has been understood. The lack of quality global data on maternal suicide (Agampodi et al., 2014; Humphrey, 2016) can also be attributed to the differences that exist

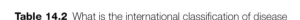

Table 14.2 What is the international classification of disease

The International Classification of Disease (ICD)

- allows the systematic recording, analysis, interpretation and comparison of mortality and morbidity data collected in different countries or regions and at different times;
- ensures semantic interoperability and reusability of recorded data for the different use cases beyond mere health statistics, including decision support, resource allocation, reimbursement, guidelines and more.
- during the 10th revision suicide during pregnancy, or within 42 days after either birth or termination of pregnancy, was re-classified as a direct cause of maternal death and any suicide between 43 days following to one year following birth, was included as a late maternal death (WHO, 2012).

Source: WHO (2023a).

in the classification and definition of maternal suicide in maternal death statistics (Knight et al., 2016). Maternal mortality is a key public health priority and is often viewed as an indicator of a country's health as lower rates are customarily associated with more advanced healthcare systems and medical progress (Mangla et al., 2019). Maternal mortality remains a significant source of preventable global premature death, with approximately 830 women dying from pregnancy-related causes every day (WHO, 2018). As a key indicator and focus of public health, there have been attempts to monitor and record maternal deaths in global and national maternal mortality statistics. Many national maternal mortality statistics do not include late maternal deaths and this impacts maternal suicide data as we know that most of these deaths occur after 42 days postpartum. There are often issues with pregnancy being added to death certificate particularly if beyond 42 days or if an early pregnancy loss such as miscarriage, termination or in cases of stillborn – yet we know these are risk factors for mental health.

Alterations to the global definition and inclusion criteria of maternal death (Mangla et al., 2019) have led to data variations as to how the death is coded on death certificates and national reporting databases, meaning many suicides are not reported accurately (Tabb et al., 2018). Although these recommendations have not been adopted by all countries and suicide is still considered to be grossly under-reported.

In addition, many women and birthing people do not seek support for perinatal mental health concerns meaning many are not diagnosed and psychiatric causes are not included on death certificates or databases (Mangla et al., 2019). It is also still deemed a coincidental death by numerous countries in their data reporting; this division of physical and mental health implies it is not a manifestation of biological conditions but a reflection of character or moral failure thus silencing women (Mangla et al., 2019). This we know has led to a gross underreporting of the true burden of maternal death by suicide. The focus of national and global health agenda is in tackling maternal mortality on the well-known and well researched causes such as haemorrhage and sepsis (Agampodi et al., 2014) despite research indicating perinatal suicide is a more common cause of maternal mortality and without the issue of underreporting taken into consideration. Whilst there has been a global reduction

Table 14.3 Definitions in relation to maternal mortality and death

Maternal death	The death of a women while pregnant or within 42 days of the end of the pregnancy* from any cause related to or aggravated by the pregnancy or its management, but not from accidental or incidental causes
Direct maternal death	resulting from obstetric complications of the pregnant state (pregnancy, labour and puerperium), from interventions, omissions, incorrect treatment or from a chain of events resulting from any of the above
Indirect maternal death	resulting from previous existing disease, or disease that developed during pregnancy and which was not the result of direct obstetric causes, but which was aggravated by the physiological effects of pregnancy
Late maternal death	occurring between 42 days and one year after the end of pregnancy* that are the result of direct or indirect maternal causes
Coincidental maternal death	from unrelated causes which happen to occur in pregnancy or the puerperium

*The end of pregnancy includes termination, miscarriage or birth and ectopic pregnancies.
Source: WHO (2018).

in maternal mortality, suicide rates remain unchanged since 2003 (Iacobucci, 2016) (Table 14.3).

STIGMA AND TABOO

It is well-documented that stigma and taboo of mental health and suicide leads to underreporting as well as inadequate and inaccurate cause of death data collection (WHO, 2018). Stigma, prejudice and taboo impact on how a person experience their mental illness and their use of mental health services and impact on reported rates (Oexle & Corrigan, 2018).

Stigma stops women seeking help instigated by the belief that they will be judged and demonised, and in some instances their children may be removed from their care, whilst social stigma makes women feel unable to speak out through fear of being stereotyped or outed by their community (Mangla et al., 2019; MBRRACE, 2021). Women regularly do not seek help during the perinatal period, some culturally do not consider themselves to have postnatal depression or identify with it and others fear the ramifications of admitting to struggle with motherhood, a universally understood and celebrated status (Mangla et al., 2019).

Different cultures have different perceptions of the aetiology of psychiatric illness and do not link mental and physical health but to attribute it to evil spirits, black magic, a taboo or the act of a "greater good" from immoral behaviour or karma (Gopalkrishnan, 2018). Diagnosis of psychiatric illness and reported rates of suicide are particularly likely to be lower in the countries such as India, where the act of suicide is punishable by law or in Islamic countries where self-harm and suicide is prohibited in the Qu'ran (Bhugra, 2010). This is important when considering the impact

Table 14.4 Cultural views on mental illness and suicide

Cultural impacts and views on mental illness and suicide
Beliefs link mental health with more traditional systems of medicine. The link between physical and mental health is not recognised but seen as an imbalance of energy.
Signs and symptoms of mental health illness are either not recognised or ignored. Alternative explanations are given such practical problems, a lack of sleep or support or given time it is something that will go away by itself.
Culturally seen as a failure as not fulfilling the position of women/mothers in society and is considered unacceptable
Illness and happiness are in God's hands and therefore not within the remit of the community to cure or manage it.
Mental illness is a sign of evil spirits and is not a medical condition'
Source: Adapted from Watson et al. (2019).

of globalisation and immigration and serving more diverse communities here in the UK. Furthermore, when considering the wider world views on mental health, the theory and practice of mental health has emerged from Western perceptions of health and health systems contradicting how other cultures view mental health (Gopalkrishnan, 2018). The ways in which different cultures express emotion, feel shame and have different resilience and coping mechanisms affects health-seeking behaviours and perceptions which can impact how mental health is viewed. Thus, the way mental health and suicide should be addressed should acknowledge cultural diversity.

When considering how different cultures may perceive mental health illness and intervention, it is also important to consider that much of the research is rooted in Western medicine where there is strong history of racism, particularly within psychiatry. This alienates many from seeking out support and will impact on how certain individuals may interact with perinatal mental health services. It is important we do not make presumptions about how a certain individual may view mental health due to their ethnicity, cultural or religious beliefs but also ensure that appropriate screening and referrals are made. Training in cultural competency is important for anyone working within perinatal mental health and an important consideration for midwives' carrying out screening for mental wellbeing (Marvin-Dowle et al., 2022) (Table 14.4).

There are many different factors which impact how mental health and suicidality may be viewed, cultural expectations, lack of awareness of mental health, community and cultural stigma and other beliefs mean that some women will not necessarily seek support or identify themselves as being unwell. Further, evidence shows that care is often fragmented, culturally insensitive and providers are dismissive particularly if a woman is from an ethnic minority (Watson et al., 2019).

PERINATAL SUICIDE RISK

Pregnancy presents a challenge for physical and mental health and women with a history of psychiatric disease or mood disorders are at a high risk of relapse or experiencing new onset severe mental illness (Vangen et al., 2017). Depression is the leading cause of suicide and globally fewer than 10% of individuals who experience depression receive effective treatments (WHO, 2014). It is well-established and researched that postpartum depression is a major risk factor for suicide with current global estimates of postnatal depression 16%–20% of all perinatal women (Lysell et al., 2018). However, research into the prevalence of common perinatal mental disorders in women in low- and middle-income countries found rates as high as 60% in India (Fisher et al., 2012). Meanwhile in high-income countries such as the United States, where the diagnosis of perinatal mental disorders is also on the rise, documented suicide rates in women have increased in every age group (Sengupta & Jantsen, 2019).

Whilst perinatal mental health disorders are not any more common than mental health disorders in non-pregnant women of childbearing age, women are two to three times more likely to experience depression and anxiety than men with the perinatal period presenting the greatest risk (Accortt & Wong, 2017), and illness tends to be more rapid in onset and more severe in symptoms. Women who die by suicide tend to use more violent and fatal means and these proportions remain unchanged over the 20 years of maternal mortality monitoring in the UK. Death rates by suicide in 2019–2021 were higher than deaths caused by sepsis and haemorrhage (MBRRACE, 2023) despite this there are no campaigns, minimal research, and no policies to specifically address maternal suicide (Chin et al., 2022). Women from ethnic minority groups have a higher incidence of mental health disorders are less likely to receive treatment and support for perinatal mental health and are disproportionately affected by perinatal suicide than white women (Watson et al., 2019) (Table 14.5).

[Suicide is more common in women with medical comorbidities or mental health diagnoses and mental health is more likely to be of rapid onset and deterioration (Mangla et al., 2019). Therefore, as pregnant women are now more likely to have medical comorbidities and mental health problems, prevention of maternal suicide represents an important obstacle to help reduce global and national health inequalities (Knight et al., 2018). Yet evidence is scarce to guide policy and initiatives for suicide prevention in perinatal women (Khalifeh et al., 2016). Much of the focus of the national and international policy, such as the SDG, aims in the reduction in maternal mortality to address causes of death such as haemorrhage, pre-eclampsia, and other complications. Even though maternal mortality statistics in the UK and many other countries globally indicates that work should be put into the implementation of support systems and mental health care for women during the childbirth continuum.

Table 14.5 Mode of death by suicide, UK and Ireland 2020 (MBRRACE, 2021)

Mode of death	Number of women (%) Total n = 25* women
Hanging	13 (52)
Overdose	4 (16)
Fall from height	4 (16)
Traffic/train	3 (12)
Lacerations	1 (4)

*For 3 women the mode of suicide could not be ascertained.
Source: MBRRACE (2021).

PANDAS is a charity dedicated to perinatal mental health. Approximately 20% of the calls to their helpline are from those feeling suicidal. There is some research which indicates pregnancy is a protective factor against perinatal suicide, but in the postpartum period, feelings of hopelessness, isolation and a belief that the child may be better off without them could be linked to the higher rates of suicide in the postnatal period. There are not always warning signs of suicide, but see Table 14.6 for some of the risk factors (PANDA Australia, 2023) identified for perinatal suicide. Statistically in the general population, those who die by suicide have seen a healthcare worker in the month prior to their death (WHO, 2023b).

Table 14.6 Risk factors for perinatal suicide

Risk factors for thoughts of suicide during the perinatal period include, but are not limited to:

- Severe or persistent or new symptoms of mental health distress
- Feelings of being a burden to others and/or feelings of despair and hopelessness
- Previous history of suicide thoughts and/or attempts.
- Personal experience of family member or friend who died by suicide
- History of mental health issues and/or substance use
- History of domestic abuse or violence (family or intimate partner)
- History of complex trauma
- People who are young
- People who are from LGBTQIAP+ communities
- Situational stressors (like housing, finances, unemployment, legal, immigration)
- Social isolation or limited social supports from partner, family, friends

Additional factors during the perinatal period that can increase the risk of suicidality

Pre-conception and during pregnancy

- Experience of fertility issues or perinatal loss
- Experience of miscarriage or abortion or abortion for fetal abnormality
- Unplanned and/or unwanted pregnancy
- Impact of a diagnosis of hyperemesis gravidarum- physical, mental, and social
- High-risk pregnancies -physical, mental, or social complexity

Post-birth

- Diagnosis of postnatal depression, bipolar disorder and/or postnatal psychosis
- Traumatic birthing experience
- Premature birth, NNICU/SCBU admission or baby is unwell
- Becoming a parent of multiple babies
- Bonding and attachment issues
- Trying to manage sleep deprivation, mental health changes, feeding and sleep/settle difficulties-especially in the early weeks-leaving the person feeling overwhelmed
- Hopes/expectations of parenthood vs. the reality of parenthood leading to feelings of loss and even grief
- Self-esteem issues: feeling inadequate, or a failure as a parent or feeling trapped or ashamed or guilty of their thoughts in terms of their baby and themselves as a parent.

Source: PANDA Australia (2023).

Case Study

Olenka is G3P0 currently 38 weeks pregnant following IVF with a donor egg. She moved to UK at 29 weeks pregnant due to her husband's work. They are currently in temporary accommodation and searching for permanent housing. She had antenatal care in Germany and booked in the UK at 31 weeks. She reports no medical history but reports a history of generalised anxiety disorder which has been historically medicated and has had some counselling in past. She attends her 38-week appointment with her community midwife and reports feeling very low and hopeless, she has had some suicidal thoughts (Table 14.7).

Consider the following:

- What her risk factors are for perinatal suicide?
- Does she have any protective factors?
- What would be a suitable care plan?

SCREENING FOR PERINATAL SUICIDE AND THE ROLE OF THE MIDWIFE

The position of the midwife is unique and provides holistic care of pregnant and postnatal woman including their physical, mental and emotional health. The Perinatal Mental Health pathways were published in 2018 and included universal screening for mental health wellbeing and encouraged a focus on person-centred, compassionate and respectful care (NICE, 2021). A key part of the pathways is to increase timely access to specialist perinatal mental health services – yet since their implementation suicide rates have risen in the UK. It is important that research to understand this trend is undertaken when we are at a time when investment

Table 14.7 Protective factors against perinatal suicide

- Having people around that a woman can talk to, who listen without judgment and with compassion- simple but can decrease the risk of suicide.
- During pregnancy and early months of parenting having and developing a strong support network made up of family, friends, other new parents, or peer support groups.
- Accessing and gaining support from health professionals – Midwives, GPs, Health Visitors
- Accepting offers of help and support- especially important during the transition from work and social life to becoming a parent- which can feel lonely and overwhelming at times.
- Recognise that relationships can and will shift with the partner, with the family and with friends especially if they are not parents. Recognising it is important to talk it through with them and gain support including professional support such as partnership counselling.

Source: Adapted from PANDA Australia (2023).

Table 14.8 Screening tools for mental wellbeing (NICE, 2021)

The Whooley questions:
- During the past month, have you often been bothered by feeling down, depressed, or hopeless?
- During the past month, have you often been bothered by having little interest or pleasure in doing things?

Two-item generalised anxiety disorder scale (GAD-2)
- Over the last 2 weeks, how often have you been bothered by feeling nervous, anxious or on edge?
- Over the last 2 weeks, how often have you been bothered by not being able to stop or control worrying?

Source: NICE (2021).

to perinatal services is being made, why it is not sufficient. One theory that if the screening tools used for perinatal mental wellbeing (see Table 14.8) are inadequate, and a lack of a suicidality scale or screening tool. Howard et al. (2018) observed that many midwives and women see the questions asked to screen for mental well-being as a tick box exercise and are less routinely asked than other health questions, especially in those from racially diverse communities – a major issue considering they are more likely to suffer a maternal death. Therefore, as Midwives, we must consider the importance of regularly screening for mental health for all clients and especially those more at risk and from racially diverse communities. Further research into near-miss suicide in pregnancy (Easter et al., 2019) also shows that the escalation of care in near-miss events is often influenced by professionals understanding on perinatal mental illness – further highlighting a need for better pathways, research, and education for those working with the perinatal population.

LEARNING ACTIVITY

Consider the risk factors for suicidality and the screening tools recommended by NICE (2021) to assess maternal mental health (Whooley and GAD-2)
- Are these good tools to assess suicidal ideation?
- Do we screen adequately for the risks?

IMPACT OF MATERNAL SUICIDE

The suicide of a parent has significant developmental and psychological effects on children (O'Brien et al., 2015). The link between familial suicide is well-established (Brent & Melham, 2008) and other impacts include (Reid et al., 2022)

- Loss of primary care giver
- Separation and abandonment issues
- Increased risk of bipolar disorder
- Increased risk of death by suicide themselves
- Poorer motor skills and language development

The impact of perinatal suicide creates issues which lie at the core of public health aims to reduce inequality, improve health, and tackle poverty. As the leading cause of maternal death in the UK, it is important that this public health issue receives research and national policy and initiatives.

CONCLUSION

- Perinatal suicide is a leading cause of maternal death both in the UK and globally and is increasing.
- This area of perinatal health needs better research and policies to specifically address it and promote how to prevent/lessen the risk.
- It is a public health need that is unmet, and midwives and health visitors are ideally placed to screen for suicidality so should be included in any research and development of pathways to address this issue.
- It has far-reaching effects on those left behind and puts the child/children at an increased risk of suicide themselves.

REFERENCES

Accortt, E.E., and Wong, M.S. (2017) It is time for routine screening for peri-natal mood and anxiety disorders in obstetrics and gynaecology. *Obstetric and Gynaecological Survey.* 72(9), 553–563. https://doi.org./10.1097/OGX.0000000000000477.

Agampodi, S., Wickramage, K., Agampodi, T., Thennakoon, U., Jayathilaka, N., Karunarathna, D., and Alagiyawanna, S., (2014) Maternal mortality revisited: The application of the new ICD-MM classification system in reference to maternal deaths in Sri Lanka. *Reproductive Health Journal.* 11(1), 17. https://doi.org/10.1186/1742–4755-11–17.

Bhugra, D., (2010). Commentary: Religion, religious attitudes and suicide. *International Journal of Epidemiology.* 39(6), 1496–1498.

Brent, D. A., and Melhem, N. (2008). Familial transmission of suicidal behavior. *The Psychiatric Clinics of North America.* 31(2), 157–177.

Bronson, J., and Reviere, R. (2017) Pregnancy-associated deaths in Virginia due to homicides, suicides and accidental overdoses compared with natural causes. *Violence Against Women.* 23(13), 1620–1637.

Chin, K., Wendt, A., Bennett, I.M., and Bhat, A. (2022) Suicide and maternal mortality. *Current Psychiatric Reports.* 24(4), 239–275. https://doi.org/10.1007/s11920-022-01334-3

Easter, A., Howard, L.M., and Sandall, J. (2019) Recognition and response to life-threatening situations among women with perinatal mental illness: A qualitative study. *BMJ Open.* https://doi.org/10.1136/bmjopen-2018-025872

Fisher, J., Cabral de Mello, M., Patel, V., Rahman, A., Tran, T., Holton, S., and Holmes, W. (2012) Prevalence and determinants of common perinatal mental disorders in women in low- and lower- middle-income countries: A systematic review. *Bulletin of the World Health Organisation.* 90(2), 139–149.

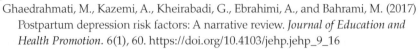

Ghaedrahmati, M., Kazemi, A., Kheirabadi, G., Ebrahimi, A., and Bahrami, M. (2017) Postpartum depression risk factors: A narrative review. *Journal of Education and Health Promotion.* 6(1), 60. https://doi.org/10.4103/jehp.jehp_9_16

Goldsmith, S.K., Pellmar, T.C., Kleinman, A.M., and Bunney, W.E. (2002) Chapter 8: Programs for reducing suicide. In: *Reducing Suicide.* Washington: National Academies Press, pp 273–330.

Gopalkrishnan, N. (2018) Cultural diversity and mental health: Considerations for policy and practice. *Frontiers in Public Health.* 6(179). https://doi.org/10.3389/fpubh.2018.00179

Grigoriadis, S., Wilton, A.S., Kurdyak, P.A., Rhodes, A.E., VonderPorten, E.H., Levitt, A., Cheung, A., and Vigod, S.N. (2017) Perinatal suicide in Ontario, Canada: A 15-year population-based study. *Canadian Medical Association Journal.* 189(34), E1085–E1092. https://doi.org/10.1503/cmaj.170088

Howard, L.M., Ryan, E.G., Trevillion, K., Anderson, F., Bick, D., Bye, A., Byford, S., O'Connor, S., Sands, P., Demilew, J., Milgrom, J., and Pickles, A. (2018) Accuracy of the Whooley questions and the Edinburgh postnatal depression scale in identifying depression and other mental disorders in early pregnancy. *British Journal of Psychiatry.* 212(1), 50–56. https://doi.org/10.1192/bjp.2017.9.

Humphrey, M.D. (2016) Maternal mortality trends in Australia. *The Medical Journal of Australia.* 205(8), 244–346. https://doi.org/10.5694/mja16.00906

Iacobucci, G. (2016) Maternal deaths from suicide must be tackled, say experts. *British Medical Journal.* 355, i6585. Available [online] https://doi.org/10.1136/bmj.i6585

Khalifeh, H., Hunt, I.M., Appleby, L., Howard, L.M. (2016) Suicide in perinatal and non-perinatal women in contact with psychiatric services: 15 year findings from a UK national inquiry. *The Lancet Psychiatry.* 3(3), 233–242. https://doi.org/10.1016/S2215-0366(16)00003-1

Knight, M., Nair, M., Br)ocklehurst, P., Kenyon, S., Neilson, J., Shakespeare, J., Tuffnell, D., Kurinczuk, J. J., and MMBRACE-UK collaboration. (2016) Examining the impact of introducing ICD-MM on observed trends in maternal mortality rates in the UK 2003–13. *BMC Pregnancy and Childbirth.* 16, 178.

Koch, A.R. and Geller, S.E. (2017) Addressing maternal deaths due to violence: The Illinois experience. *American Journal of Obstetrics & Gynecology.* Nov;217(5):556. e1-556.e6. doi: 10.1016/j.ajog.2017.08.005. Epub 2017 Aug 24. PMID: 28844823.

Lysell, H., Dahlin, M., Viktorin, A., Ljungberg, E., D'Onofrio, B.M., Dickman, P., and Runeson, B. (2018) Maternal suicide – Register based study of all suicides occurring after delivery in Sweden 1974–2009. *PLoS One.* 13(1). https://doi.org/10.13771/journal.pone.019-133

Mangla, K., Hoffman, M.C., Trumpff, C., O'Grady, S., and Monk, C. (2019) Maternal self-harm deaths: An unrecognized and preventable outcome. *American Journal of Obstetrics and Gynecology.* 221(4), 295–303. https://doi.org/10.1016/j.ajog.2019.02.056

Marvin-Dowle, K., Oshaghi, G., Fair, F., Ratcliffe, J., and Soltani, H. (2022) Training on cultural competency for perinatal mental health peer supporters. *British Journal of Midwifery.* 30(12), 668–676.

MBRRACE-UK. (2021) *Saving Lives, Improving Mothers' Care – CORE Report Lessons Learned to Inform Maternity Care from the UK and Ireland Confidential Enquiries into Maternal Deaths and Morbidity 2017–19.* Oxford: National Perinatal Epidemiology Unit, University of Oxford.

MBRRACE-UK. (2023) *Saving Lives, Improving Mothers' Care State of the Nation Surveillance Report: Surveillance Findings from the UK Confidential Enquiries into Maternal Deaths 2019–21*. Oxford: National Perinatal Epidemiology Unit, University of Oxford.

National Institute for Health and Care Excellence. (2021) Antenatal and postnatal mental health: *Clinical guideline CG192*. (nice.org.uk)

NHS England, NHS Improvement, National Collaborating Centre for Mental Health (2018) *The Perinatal Mental Health Care Pathways*. NHS England: London.

O'Brien, K.H., Salas-Wright, C.P., Vaughn, M.G., and LeCloux. M. (2015) Childhood exposure to parental suicide attempt and risk for substance use disorders. *Addictive Behaviours*. 46, 70–76.

Oexle. N., and Corrigan. P.W. (2018) Understanding mental illness stigma toward persons with multiple stigmatized conditions: Implications of intersectionality theory. *Psychiatric Services*. 69, 587–589.

Orsolini, L., Valchera, A., Vecchiotti, R., Tomasetti, C., Iasevoli, F., Fornaro, M., De Berardis, D., Perna. G., Pompili. M., & Bellantuono, C. (2016) Suicide during perinatal period: epidemiology, risk factors, and clinical correlates. *Frontiers in Psychiatry*. 12(7) https://doi.org/10.3389/fpsyt.2016.00138

Our World in Data. (2019) *Suicide*. Available [online] https://ourworldindata.org/suicide

PANDA Australia. (2023) *Perinatal Suicide: Signs, Safety and Support Options*. Available [online] https://panda.org.au/articles/perinatal-suicide-signs-safety-and-support-options/

Reid, H., Pratt, D., Edge, D., and Wittkowski, A. (2022) Maternal suicide ideation and behaviour during pregnancy and the first postpartum year: A systematic review of psychological and psychosocial risk factors. *Frontiers in Psychiatry*. 24, 13. https://doi.org/10.3389/fpsyt.2022.765118.

Sengupta, B., and Jantzen, R., (2019) Incidence of female suicide in New York City: How important are socioeconomic factors? *Social Psychiatry and psychiatric epidemiology*. 54, 89–98.

Tabb KM, Huang H, Valdovinos M, Toor R, Ostler T, Vanderwater E, Wang Y, Menezes PR, Faisal-Cury A. Intimate Partner Violence Is Associated with Suicidality Among Low-Income Postpartum Women. J Womens Health (Larchmt). 2018 Feb;27(2):171-178. doi: 10.1089/jwh.2016.6077. Epub 2017 May 24. PMID: 28537476.

Thornton C, Schmied V, Dennis CL, Barnett B, Dahlen HG. Maternal deaths in NSW (2000-2006) from nonmedical causes (suicide and trauma) in the first year following birth. Biomed Res Int. 2013;2013:623743. doi: 10.1155/2013/623743. Epub 2013 Aug 19. PMID: 24024205; PMCID: PMC3760299..

United Nations. (2019) *The Sustainable Development Goals Report 2019*. Available [online] — SDG Indicators (un.org)

Vangen, S., Bødker, B., Ellingsen, L., Salrvedt, S., Gissler, M., Geirsson, R.T., Nyfløt, L.T., (2017) Maternal deaths in the Nordic countries. *Acta Obstetricia et Gynecologica Scandinavica*. 96, 1112–1119.

Watson, H., Harrop, D., Walton, E., Young, A., & Soltani, H., (2019) A systematic review of ethnic minority women's experiences of perinatal mental health conditions and services in Europe. *PLoS One*. https://doi.org/10.1371/journal.pone.0210587

World Health Assembly Resolution. (2013) *Comprehensive Mental Health Action Plan 2013–2020*. Available [online] http://apps.who.int/gb/ebwha/pdf_files/WHA66/A66_R8-en.pdf?ua=1

World Health Organisation (WHO). (2012) *The WHO Application of ICD-10 to Deaths During Pregnancy, Childbirth and the Puerperium: ICD MM*. Available [online] https://iris.who.int/bitstream/handle/10665/70929/9789241548458_eng.pdf?sequence=1&isAllowed=y

WHO. (2014) *Preventing Suicide: A Global Imperative*. Available [online] https://www.who.int/publications/i/item/9789241564779

WHO. (2018) *Maternal Mortality*. Available [online] https://www.who.int/news-room/fact-sheets/detail/maternal-mortality

WHO. (2021) *Suicide Worldwide in 2019*. Available [online] 9789240026643-eng.pdf (who.int)

WHO. (2023a) *International Statistical Classification of Diseases and Related Health Problems. ICD-11*. [online] Available at https://www.who.int/standards/classifications/classification-of-diseases

WHO. (2023b) *Preventing Suicide* [infographic]. https://www.who.int/images/default-source/departments/mentalhealth/suicide/suicide_prevention_health_workers.jpg?sfvrsn=5dcfa797_3

Zalsman, G., Hawton, K., Wasserman, D., van Heeringen, K., Arensman, E., Sarchiapone, M., Carli, V., Hoschl, C., Barzilay, R., Balazs, J., Purebl, G., Kahn, J.P., Saiz, P.A., Bursztein Lipiscas, C., Bobes, J., Cozman, D., Hegerl, U., and Zohar, J. (2016) Suicide prevention strategies revisited: 10-year systematic review. *The Lancet Psychiatry*. 3(7), 646–659.

FURTHER RESOURCES – FOR BOOK WEBSITE:

UN General Assembly. (2015) *Transforming Our World: The 2030 Agenda for Sustainable Development*. Available [online] at: www.refworld.org/docid/57b6e3e44.html

United Nations World Population Review. (2023). *Suicide Rate by Country 2023*. Available [online] at: http://worldpopulationreview.com/countries/suicide-rate-by-country/

WHO. (2008) *Improving Maternal Health. Millennium Development Goal 5*. Available [online] Millennium Development Goals (MDGs) (who.int)

WHO. (2011) *Intimate Partner Violence During Pregnancy Information Sheet*. Available [online] at: WHO_RHR_11.35_eng.pdf

WHO. (2015) *Thinking Healthy: A Manual for Psychological Management for Perinatal Depression*. Available [online] at: https://www.who.int/mental_health/maternal-child/thinking_healthy/en/

WHO. (2023) *World Health Statistics Data Visualisation Dashboard. SDG Target 3.4: NonCommunicable Diseases and Mental Health – Suicide*. [online] Available at: http://apps.who.int/gho/data/node.sdg.3-4-viz-2?lang=en

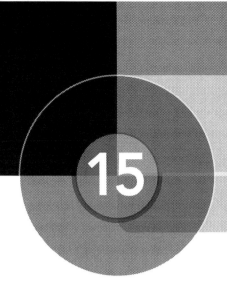

Midwives' Self-Care and Resilience

15

RUTH SANDERS AND KELDA FOLLIARD

INTRODUCTION

The professional practice of midwifery is known and understood across the literature to be emotionally demanding for the individuals working within maternity care systems (Hunter 2004; Hunter & Warren, 2014). Midwives spend a large proportion of their time discussing public health and training and informing people about issues related to the communities they serve (Crabbe & Hemingway, 2014). However, as members of these communities, there is also a need for self-reflection and awareness of their own position and needs. This means ensuring that midwives can both respond to these public health messages and remain healthy and resilient in their own lives.

The challenging landscape of midwifery work globally is well-documented (United Nations Population Fund, International Confederation of Midwives & World Health Organization, 2021). In the UK, the midwifery profession is acutely aware of the pressure to provide safe services, as highlighted in a growing number of reports into maternity services where care failings have been evident (Independent Review Group, 2022). Literature about the poor psychosocial health of the midwifery workforce population is not new (Hunter, 2004), and there continues to be high-profile discussion of dissatisfaction with pay and conditions, and shortages of maternity staff. An increasingly concerning picture of retention issues and worries around how to sustain the midwifery workforce has emerged (Cramer & Hunter, 2018). A steep decrease in the number of pre-registration midwifery applicants, coupled with an increase in the numbers of midwives leaving the profession, indicates clear potential

DOI: 10.4324/9781003350071-15

for an unstable midwifery workforce. Against this backdrop, the need to identify ways in which midwives can sustain their health and wellbeing is undeniable.

An awareness of these issues has underpinned some work around midwives' wellbeing, notably the Royal College of Midwives (RCM) Caring for You campaign, the International Confederation of Midwives Advocacy Toolkit (ICM, 2022), and the work of Professional Midwifery Advocates (PMAs) (Capito et al., 2022). The NHS Health and Wellbeing Framework (NHS, 2021) aims to provide organisations with guidance around supporting the wellbeing of their workforce. A criticism of occupational health and workplace wellbeing initiatives has been the lack of a whole system approach to provision, which is needed for their success (British Medical Association [BMA], 2018; Brand et al., 2017). Not only are individual midwives threatened by a lack of investment in their wellbeing and workplace or organisational dysfunction, equally at risk is the integrity of the midwifery profession and the health of the women, birthing people, and families it serves (Pezaro et al., 2015).

This chapter discusses the concept of resilience, and the environmental and cultural factors that challenge midwives' capacity for self-care. Personal internal mechanisms for self-care are introduced, alongside practical suggestions for midwives wishing to build their own means of maintaining their wellbeing despite the multiple professional challenges that exist.

THE CONCEPT OF RESILIENCE

REFLECTIVE ACTIVITY

- When you think about resilience, what does this mean for you and your own practice?
- What would a list of personal and professional attributes which you consider demonstrate aspects of resilience look like?
- What might the potential challenges in creating a resilient environment be, for your clinical environment?

Midwifery practice is challenging and much of the day-to-day work includes professional decision-making which can cause ideological conflict for midwives. This arises when midwives attempt to care for women and birthing people within a complex environment of competing demands, all of which though rewarding can profoundly affect midwives' ability to practice effectively (Hunter & Warren, 2013; Tant, 2020).

The notion of resilience in midwifery practice has shifted over time, initially being understood as a positive characteristic and defined as the ability to "bounce back" (Aburn et al., 2016), a way of positively adapting to changing environments and being able to "withstand or recover quicky from difficulty" (Oxford English Dictionary, 2023). These definitions assume that resilient people will simply return to the state prior to the difficulty encountered without further discussion of the cause and effect that working environments, systems, and practices can have upon the individual.

More recently resilience as a concept has come under scrutiny within the midwifery profession as something of a slogan used to describe whether an individual is able to consistently cope in a high pressured and dynamically changing environment (Hunter & Warren, 2022). This is echoed in discussions across wider health care communities of practice and social media conversations and places the onus on the individual to change rather than scrutiny of unhealthy working cultures which may be at the root of the problem. Traynor (2018) argues that the current understanding of resilience supports the present 'status quo' which can leave practitioners feeling personally responsible for systemic failures.

Discussion of resilience as predominantly related to individual practitioners, rather than the wider institution, places the emphasis on an individual's ability to cope in the face of adversity rather a system lacking structures to promote a healthy workplace and facilitate the work of midwifery caring. This can cause moral injury, with midwives unable to provide the care they strive for despite working to support service users to their best ability. Midwifery participants from Cull et al.'s (2020) study demonstrate this in a powerful quote:

> The feeling of failure when you've physically exhausted yourself and couldn't possibly do any more is demoralising. Above everything, not giving women and babies the care, they deserve is the worst aspect (MW 316).

> *(Cull et al., 2020: 552)*

This feeling of failing the population that midwives serve is common in this study, with midwives reporting a lack of control about working patterns, sporadic collegial support and untenable work pressures adding to a fear about increased risk of making mistakes and the inability to do their jobs to the full scope of their ability culminating in the experiencing of moral injury.

THE CONTEXT OF MIDWIFERY PRACTICE

Midwifery involves a high level of emotional work, due to the intensity of providing interpersonal support during a time of huge transition and challenge, encompassing joy, pain and loss for women, birthing people, and families (Rayment, 2015). Furthermore, Barker (2011) notes that the emotional work of midwives impacts the quality of relationship with the clients they support. Meaningful emotional investment is inherent in midwifery work, and challenges are felt from the beginning of the practitioner's journey, prior to registration. Eaves and Payne (2019) examined the relationship between resilience, stress, burnout, and intention to leave the profession among 150 student midwives in the UK. The study showed that higher levels of stress were more likely to lead to disengagement, and high stress and low resilience predicted the intention to leave midwifery. Resilience did not moderate the effects of stress, but was a factor in reducing intention to quit, suggesting that commitment and dedication may play a role alongside resilience in mediating the negative effects of workplace stress.

Pezaro et al. (2018) found that midwives' levels of stress were visible to the people in their care, with women reporting that midwives often appeared rushed, out of control, with several participants observing midwives' emotional distress.

Participants reported that the mothers themselves aligned these workforce issues to a lack of compassion for workers, poor working practice behaviours, leading to midwives becoming demoralised, ultimately culminating in a poor or diminished standard of care. This lack of workplace support for midwives was perceived as problematic for mothers, with them being potentially placed in a 'burdensome' role, not wanting to ask for help in case this adds to the midwife's stress at being asked to perform yet another task. Compassion becomes lost between colleagues and towards clients in this climate, and participants suggested that midwives may even turn to service users for support, eroding the trust they had in their care provider to meet the needs of them as a new family (Pezaro et al., 2018). This emphasises that when the midwifery workforce is suffering, this is directly impacting the population they are seeking to support, adding guilt, stress and frustration to an already-fractious workforce.

Recognising the importance of understanding the experience of student midwives, Williams and Hadley (2022) tested a measure of resilience in a cohort of undergraduate learners and were able to establish determinants of resilience, which included satisfaction, confidence and the value of reflection. In common with Eaves and Payne (2019), the authors noted the role of perseverance as a personal attribute in motivating students to continue in the profession. The development of resilience is not a linear process and for student midwives there may be points during their programme of study when this is challenged; this is a valuable finding for educators considering how best to support students (Williams & Hadley, 2022).

On registration, midwives have described entering environments of hierarchy and complex power dynamics, where practice is mismatched with their philosophical perceptions of midwifery, leading to personal distress and professional dissatisfaction (Griffiths et al., 2019). Registered midwives' perceptions of the concept of burnout have been explored, showing excessive workload as the root cause, manifesting in stress and exhaustion alongside reduced capacity for motivation, empathy, and coping (Doherty & O'Brien, 2022a). These findings support those of Sidhu et al. (2020), whose global review of midwifery burnout highlighted workload, alongside exposure to traumatic events, as a key factor. The authors also noted that midwives with fewer years post-qualification experience were at greatest risk of burnout. There can be a dissonance between expectations formed during training programmes and the reality of preceptorship; greater support and recognition of the challenges of entering this new environment could assist staff retention.

There is an association between staff with poor self-care and suboptimal wellbeing who are suffering from burnout and heightened self-reported clinical and medication errors (Cramer & Hunter, 2019; Hall et al., 2016). Cramer and Hunter (2018) provided a detailed examination of modifiable and non-modifiable risk factors and the relationships between these for midwives' emotional wellbeing, noting variables including low staffing, high workload, colleague support, lack of continuity of carer, challenging clinical situations and low clinical autonomy. Personal risk from not being able to cope can arise from reliance on unhealthy coping mechanisms, including the use of alcohol and illicit substances (Pezaro et al., 2020).

In the face of such occupational stresses, methods that facilitate coping and maintenance of wellbeing are key. A group of Australian midwives interviewed by McDonald et al. (2016) described the ways in which they embedded resilience in their workplace, with themes including support networks, personal characteristics, and the ability to organise work for personal resilience emerging. The authors highlighted midwives' access to self-efficacy and coping strategies, with resilience at the core, as enablers for midwives to manage workplace adversity.

REFLECTIVE ACTIVITY

- Consider how resilience is discussed in your place of work?
- How is self-care promoted in your working environment?
- Are you aware of support structures within your workplace?
- Do you access these, or would you if you felt the need?
- How might you access support?

COLLEGIAL WORKING

Improving workplace culture was cited as the primary mechanism for reducing burnout among midwives by Doherty and O'Brien (2022b). Midwives interviewed highlighted several environmental and cultural elements which would contribute positively to improved wellbeing. These included building professional working relationships, support and acknowledgement from team members, regular collegial debriefing, having access to a quiet space and the opportunity for clinical rotation. One participant highlighted the value of Schwartz rounds as a positive tool for processing emotional aspects of care in a supportive environment. Schwartz rounds are forums for healthcare staff to undertake a group debrief focusing on the emotional and psychological elements of a clinical situation or theme and have been shown in a range of clinical settings to improve wellbeing and teamwork (Doherty, 2021). The implementation of Schwartz rounds in an Irish maternity hospital were evaluated positively (Cullen, 2021), including when adapted to blended and virtual formats during the COVID pandemic (Doherty, 2021).

Thumm and Flynn (2018) synthesised the attributes of a successful midwifery practice climate and noted that relationships between clinicians are key, highlighting that collaborative practice is consistent with core midwifery values. The essential components of collaboration included respect and trust, shared global vision and effective communication. Therefore, cultural practice that supports these components will improve job satisfaction and protect the wellbeing of midwives and the wider team, building a psychologically safe working environment. Nash (2021) describes the use of the A-equip model and role of the Professional Midwifery Advocate (PMA) in supporting midwives' wellbeing (NHSE, 2017) and how poor teamwork contributes to midwives' stress and a culture of blame. The authors emphasise the importance of civility and how Restorative Clinical Supervision can support personal reflection and insight, enhancing teamwork.

A key element of the role of the PMA is one of leadership, and the type of leadership modelled within an organisation is essential to driving improvements in culture. Compassionate leadership, where collegial relationships are nurtured in a respectful and empathic way, causes individuals to feel cared for and positively impacts on wellbeing (West, 2021). A compassionate leadership approach is essential for organisations to address issues of inclusivity within the workplace (Ross et al., 2020). Positive leadership does not only apply to senior clinicians; the

Future Midwife standards highlight leadership skills as an essential component of midwifery from the point of registration (NMC, 2019).

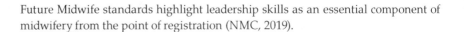

PRACTICE POINT

- What influences your choices about discussing resilience with colleagues?
- What are the enablers and barriers to discussing resilience with colleagues?

ENVIRONMENTAL AND CULTURAL FACTORS

The COVID-19 pandemic shone a light on the aspects of working in healthcare where resilience is most challenged. A Polish study exploring nurses and midwives' intention to leave the profession during the pandemic, highlighted the relationship between occupational stress and resilience with job satisfaction and intention to leave. Occupational stress and job dissatisfaction were associated with high intention to leave in 25% of participants (Piotrowski et al., 2022). However, the issues facing maternity services in the UK predate the pandemic. Piotrowski et al.'s findings are confirmed by a study conducted by Hunter et al., on behalf of the Royal College of Midwives (2018), which found higher levels of stress, depression, and burnout than the general population with two thirds of the respondents having considered leaving the profession in the previous six-month period. This chronic understaffing and the response to critique creating in maternity units a tendency to defensiveness driving authoritarian culture and this undermining the autonomy, flexibility, and competence of staff (Downe, 2022). Downe argues, it is this environment which contributes to burnout.

Different midwifery models of care can impact how midwives feel about their practice within the framework of maternity care. Midwifery practice exists within a hierarchical system, and although autonomous as practitioners in their own profession, there can be challenges in working practices such as the fragmentation of care, moving frequently between different working environments such as community and hospital-based settings and movement between in-hospital areas (Crowther et al., 2016).

Wider maternity provision can create organisational challenges for midwives due to the changeable nature of the multidisciplinary team. Obstetrics and midwifery have different philosophical outlooks which can create potential professional conflicts (Mharapara et al., 2023). The hierarchy in most healthcare settings means that medics are often situated at the top of the decision-making structure, leaving midwives potentially limited in their ability to facilitate choice for others, with diminished control and autonomy in their working environments (Ebert, 2020). Ebert (2020) argues that to remain safe practitioners, midwives need to align themselves with institutional expectations and a specific management style often emphasising a problem-solving and task-focused approach to care. This can impact midwifery autonomy and value for the midwifery role in the wider team, with midwives' desire to conform to the underlying institutional structures being in opposition to the needs of the service users.

While some environmental factors require significant national effort from policymakers and service leaders to address, there are cultural factors which can be improved through grassroots initiatives which focus on trauma-informed working and civility. Bullying has been recognised as a cultural facet of maternity services and can be experienced by student and registered midwives alike (Capper et al., 2021; Catling et al., 2017). In recognition of the importance of civility and kindness to supporting the wellbeing of clinicians in maternity services, Health Education England commissioned the Capital Midwife programme to develop a civility toolkit (Health Education England [HEE], 2021). The toolkit encourages midwives to promote civil behaviour and speaking up among colleagues and to champion self-care. Principles underpinning trauma-informed care for service users, safety, trust, choice, collaboration, empowerment and cultural consideration are equally recognised as important for staff in the workplace, and in England the Office for Health Improvement and Disparities (OHID) published a working definition of trauma-informed practice aimed at service users and staff (OHID, 2022).

The 'Job Demands-Resources' theory (Bakker & Demerouti, 2017) can be used to analyse how the work environment affects wellbeing and performance. This model proposes that there are two separate strands at play across organisations. The demands of midwifery practice, including work-related pressures, exhaustion, and complex client situations, erode individual's ability to manage and reduce perceptions of health and wellbeing (see Figure 15.1). Job resources assist in self-development of employees in the presence of social support systems such as restorative supervision and the work of PMAs, Schwartz rounds, autonomy for their professional status, and the ability practice to their full ability (Demerouti & Bakker, 2022). This, in turn, affects levels of job satisfaction which could in turn, impact midwives' resilience.

PERSONAL INTERNAL MECHANISMS

Scaling up midwifery is a global priority and yet the sustainability of the profession is threatened by levels of burnout and attrition (Sidhu et al., 2020). Globally levels of burnout amongst midwives are high (Creedy et al., 2017; Hunter et al., 2019) and increasing compared to other health professions such as nursing, with rates reported between 15% and 55% of midwifery professionals (Henrickson et al., 2016; Hunter et al., 2018). Burnout is defined as a state of vital or chronic exhaustion (Doherty & O'Brien, 2022a; WHO, 2016) within the WHO's International Classification of Diseases (ICD-10), discussed across the literature as a chronic state also featuring low levels of personal accomplishment, feelings of depersonalisation, a loss of motivation and symptoms of distress (Pezaro et al., 2016; Sidhu et al., 2020).

There are associations between burnout and post-traumatic stress disorder (PTSD), and with a third of midwives experiencing work-related stress, depression, and anxiety (Smith, 2021), coping strategies to assist with daily stresses of midwifery practice are necessary for a functioning profession. Resilience is tied to sustainability of the future midwifery workforce, and identity, connection, and protection have been found to be important features for student midwives' coping mechanisms (Maddock & Oates, 2022). Clohessy et al.'s concept analysis (2019) found that self-efficacy, social support and optimism all contribute developing resilience in student midwives, and these need to be fostered in educational institutions and then carried forwards into the future workplace.

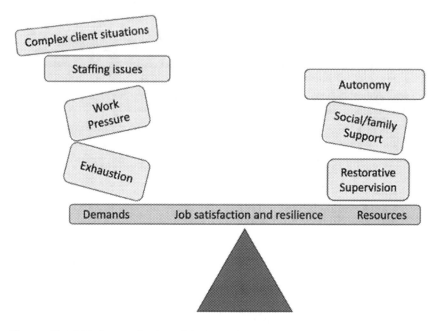

Figure 15.1 Midwifery application of job demands-resources theory.

There are clear links between the cumulative nature of witnessing traumatic childbirth and signs of distress, which can result in a decline in empathy. This decline in empathy and associated compassion fatigue is directly linked to patient experience, with investigations such as the Francis Report (2013) reporting poor patient experience including an increase in medical errors, infection, and mortality rates (Hall et al, 2016). Due to the empathetic relationships which midwives form with women and birthing people, midwives are more at risk of the emotional trauma of caring, including vicarious traumatisation or secondary trauma (Pezaro et al, 2016) associated in witnessing traumatic childbirth events (Davies & Coldridge, 2015). Experiencing vicarious trauma is increasingly recognised as a concern among midwives, including symptoms of detachments, depersonalisation, anxiety, grief, confusion, withdrawal, and flashbacks (Pezaro et al., 2016), none of which are conducive to safe and effective patient midwife relationships or personal wellbeing. Ängeby et al. (2022) found that self-criticism among midwives working on labour ward was associated with greater levels of compassion fatigue and so self-examination is necessary to ensure that these feelings can be reframed positively by identifying successful dimensions within caring episodes.

MODEL FOR SELF-CARE: A SHARED LANDSCAPE FOR MIDWIFERY RESILIENCE

To achieve a sustainable and flourishing midwifery workforce, the onus cannot be on the individual alone. Instead, organisations need to take responsibility for the culture of resilience using a system wide approach and enabling individual midwives to nurture and nourish their profession and themselves, in turn impacting the families they serve. We must acknowledge that midwives as a part of their everyday work are placed in situations of stress, overwhelm and heightened emotion, some of which can be positive as well as negative. We must consider the ability of midwives to thrive, and achieve psychological equilibrium, a type of midwifery homeostasis, within the context, organisations and systems of their work.

A scoping review by Sist et al. (2022) identified that the three constructs for self-care among nurses and midwives are mindfulness, compassion, and resilience, all necessary for practitioners to care effectively. There are numerous personal, environmental and cultural aspects of midwifery practice which can support or threaten the individual's capacity for wellbeing.

Use this example as a guide to complete your own list of internal personal factors in your work life.

These elements are all likely to be present to a varying degree within a midwife's work, and the work of maintaining a balance between competing positive and negative influences on wellbeing is ongoing. Visualising these component parts and this act of balancing may help midwives to understand how to make the adjustments needed to ensure the scales do not tip in favour of threats to resilience. Conceptualising this in terms of internal and external factors helps midwives to understand which aspects are within their control and which are not. Table 15.1 shows this balance in terms of internal mechanisms, and Table 15.2 illustrates external factors.

Table 15.1 Summary of internal personal factors – balancing what supports resilience and what threatens it

Internal personal factors (personal characteristics, circumstances and behaviours)	
Supports:	*Threatens:*
Self-reflection and awareness	Vicarious traumatisation
Self-efficacy	Self-criticism
Personal accomplishment	Burnout
Social support	Compassion fatigue
Optimism	Personal responsibility for system failures
Competence	Unhealthy coping mechanisms – use of
Identity	Alcohol and illicit substances
Connection	
Protection	

Use this box to complete your own list of internal personal factors in your work life.

Internal personal factors (personal characteristics, circumstances, and behaviours)	
Supports:	*Threatens:*

Table 15.2 Summary of external factors – balancing what supports resilience and what threatens it

External factors: organisational/systems/cultural considerations	
Supports:	*Threatens:*
Opportunity for clinical rotation	Bullying
Support	Poor teamwork
Acknowledgement	Culture of blame
Debriefing	Critique of profession
Access to a quiet space	Demanding client situations
Flexibility	Dissatisfaction with pay and conditions
Restorative supervision	Shortages of maternity staff
Positive relationships between clinicians	Lack of a whole system approach to
Collaborative practice	provision
Trauma-informed working	Competing demands
Civility	Moral distress & injury
Colleague support	High workload
Visionary leadership	Lack of continuity of carer
	Challenging clinical situations
	Low clinical autonomy

Can you complete a list of external factors which impact your wellbeing at work?

External factors: organisational/systems/cultural considerations	
Supports:	*Threatens:*

LEARNING ACTIVITY

- Using Table 15.1 as a guide to complete your own list of internal personal factors in your work life.
- Using Table 15.2 as a guide complete a list of external factors which impact your wellbeing at work.

TOWARDS A STATE OF SALUTOGENESIS: THE STRESS BUCKET

Just as there are factors which can add to levels of overwhelm and stress, there are elements of midwifery work which can add to a sense of wellbeing and positive states of health.

The stress bucket analogy (Brabban & Turkington, 2002) can be used to enable individuals to consider how to maintain a balance of life factors to positively support overall wellbeing. The analogy accepts that there are stressors inevitably encountered by individuals but encourages individuals to reflect on how the stress bucket can be prevented from overflowing – to think about the helpful and unhelpful elements in life and maintain equilibrium. A tap at the bottom of the bucket allows stressors to flow out of the bucket, and the operation of the tap is facilitated by the existence of helpful coping mechanisms.

REFLECTIVE ACTIVITY

- Draw a stress bucket for yourself and place in it all the things that may be causing your stress in your work?
- Make a list of helpful coping mechanisms – the things that will help you to turn the tap on the bucket and allow the stress to flow out.
- You may find it helpful to think of your professional needs as a framework to consider what is in the bucket, and what may be required to prevent it from overflowing.

There are many aspects of midwifery practice which can impact whether self-care occurs while midwives provide safe, holistic support for individuals and communities. Environmental, cultural, and organisational elements can challenge midwives to the point where they experience burnout, or even feel unable to continue in the profession.

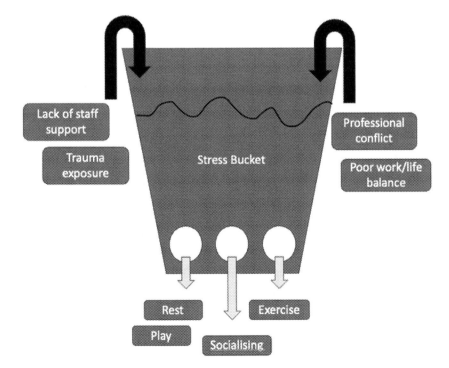

Figure 15.2 The stress bucket.

Despite this, midwives continue to find joy and inspiration in their work, fuelled by things they have found which nourish their midwifery practice. Consider the following:

- Is it possible to look at your work from a position of salutogenesis, rather than focusing on what may be problematic?
- Look to the aspects that bring you joy and see if there are techniques and strategies to help you grow.
- Are there individuals in your workplace who can nurture you and provide you with hope for your own practice and that of our profession?
- Think back to those moments which moved you to become a midwife in the first place.
- What inspired and uplifted you to become a midwife?
- If our capacity as midwives to provide self-care to ourselves is challenged, what can we ensure that we pack in our clinic bag to maintain ourselves

SUMMARY

- Environmental, cultural, and organisational elements can challenge midwives to the point where they experience burnout, or even feel unable to continue in the profession.
- Much of the very special emotion our work elicits is related to seeing people overcome the challenge that pregnancy, labour, and birth can present.
- It is in these moments that individuals look to us, as midwives, to provide strength, power, support and facilitation to overcome what can feel like an experience of great adversity.
- Midwifery self-care is a necessity but relies on a psychologically safe working environment where kindness, empathy and affirming practice experiences are accessible and easily available universally to colleagues as well as clients (Smith, 2021).
- We can, with support, focus, and self-compassion harness that strength we provide and turn it inwards, holding ourselves and our colleagues, in gentle yet empowering hands in such turbulent professional times.

REFERENCES

Aburn, G., Gott, M., & Hoarn, K (2016) What is resilience? An integrative review of the empirical literature. *Journal of Advanced Nursing.* 72(5), 980–1000. https://doi.org/10.1111/jan.12888.

Ängeby, K., Rubertsson, C., Hildingsson, I., & Edqvist, M. (2022) Self-compassion and professional quality of life among midwives and nurse assistants: A cross-sectional study. *European Journal of Midwifery.* 6(July), 1–11. https://doi.org/10.18332/ejm/149520.

Bakker, A. B., & Demerouti, E. (2017) Job demands-resources theory: Taking stock and looking forward. *Journal of Occupational Health Psychology.* 22, 273–285. https://doi.org/10.1037/ocp0000056

Barker, S. (2011). *Midwives Emotional care of Women becoming Mothers.* Newcastle upon Tyne: Cambridge Scholars Publishing.

BMA. (2018). *Supporting Health and Wellbeing at Work*. Available at: https://www.bma.org.uk/media/2076/bma-supporting-health-and-wellbeing-at-work-oct-2018.pdf

Brabban, A., & Turkington, D. (2002) The search for meaning: Detecting congruence between life events, underlying schema and psychotic symptoms. In Morrison, A. P. (Ed.), *A Casebook for Cognitive Therapy for Psychosis*. New York: Brunner-Routledge

Brand, S. L., Thompson Coon, J., Fleming, L. E., Carroll, L., Bethel, A., & Wyatt, K. (2017). Whole-system approaches to improving the health and wellbeing of healthcare workers: A systematic review. *PloS One*. 12(12), e0188418.

Capito, C., Keegan, C., Lachanudis, L., Tyler, J., & McKellow, C. (2022) Professional midwifery advocates: Delivering restorative clinical supervision. *Nursing Times* [online]. 118(2), 26–28.

Capper, T., Muurlink, O., & Williamson, M. (2021). Social culture and the bullying of midwifery students while on clinical placement: A qualitative descriptive exploration. *Nurse Education in Practice*. 52, 103045. https://doi-org.uea.idm.oclc.org/10.1016/j.nepr.2021.103045

Catling, C.J., Reid, F., & Hunter, B. (2017).. *Women and Birth*. 30(2), 137–145.

Clohessy, N., McKellar, L., & Fleet, J. (2019). Bounce back –bounce forward: Midwifery students experience of resilience. *Nurse Education in Practice*. 37, 22–28.

Crabbe, K., & Hemingway, A. (2014). Public health and wellbeing: A matter for the midwife? *British Journal of Midwifery*. 22, 9.

Cramer, E., & Hunter, B. (2018). Relationships between working conditions and emotional wellbeing in midwives. *Women and Birth*. 32, 531–532.

Creedy, D.K., Sidebotham, M., Gamble, J., Pallant, J., & Fenwick, J. (2017). Prevalence of burnout, depression, anxiety and stress in Australian midwives: A cross sectional survey. *BMC Pregnancy & Childbirth*. 17 (13).

Crowther, S., Hunter, B., McAra-Couper, J., Warren, L., Gilkison, A., Hunter, M., Fielder, A., & Kirkham, M. (2016) Sustainability and resilience in midwifery: A discussion paper. *Midwifery*. 40, 40–48.

Cull, J., Hunter, B., Henley, J., Fenwick, J., & Sidebotham, M. (2020). "Overwhelmed and out of my depth": Responses from early career midwives in the United Kingdom to the Work, Health and Emotional Lives of Midwives study. *Women and Birth*. 33(6), e589–e557. https://doi.org/10.1016/j.wombi.2020.01.003

Cullen S. Implementing Schwartz Rounds in an Irish maternity hospital. Ir J Med Sci. 2021 Feb;190(1):205-208. doi: 10.1007/s11845-020-02268-6. Epub 2020 Jun 2. PMID: 32488464.

Davies, S.D., & Coldridge, L. (2015). 'No Man's Land': An exploration of the traumatic experiences of student midwives in practice. Midwifery, 31(9), 858–864.

Demerouti, E., & Bakker, A. (2022). Job-demands resources theory in times of crises: New propositions. *Organizational Psychology Review*. 13(3), 1–28. https://journals.sagepub.com/doi/10.1177/20413866221135022

Doherty, J. (2021). Using blended and virtual scwartz center rounds to support maternity staff in Ireland during the COVID-19 pandemic. *Journal of Nursing Practice*. 5, 1.

Doherty, J., & O'Brien, D. (2022a). A participatory action research study exploring midwives' understandings of the concept of burnout in Ireland. *Midwifery*. 35, e163–e171.

Doherty, J., & O'Brien, D. (2022b). Reducing midwife burnout at organisational level – Midwives need time, space and a positive workplace culture. *Women and Birth.* 35(6), e563–e572. https://doi.org/10.1016/j.wombi.2022.02.003

Downe, S. (2022). Maternity services are in crisis – Here's how to fix them. *The New Statesman.* https://www.newstatesman.com/spotlight/healthcare/2022/12/maternity-services-crisis-staffing-fix [Accessed 02 April 23]

Eaves, J.L., & Payne, N. (2019) Resilience, stress and burnout in student midwives. *Nurse Education Today,* 79,: 188–193. https://doi.org/10.1016/j.nedt.2019.05.012.

Ebert, L. (2020). Midwifery decision-making. Feeling safe to support women's choice in the maternity care environment. In Jefford, E., & Jomeen, J. (Ed.), *Empowering Decision –Making in Midwifery a Global Perspective.* Abingdon, OXON: Routledge.

Francis, R. (2013). *Report of the mid Staffordshire NHS Foundation Trust public inquiry executive summary.* London: The Stationery Office.

Griffiths, M., Fenwick, J., Carter, A.G., Sidebotham, M., & Gamble, J. (2019). Midwives transition to practice: Expectations and experiences. *Nurse Education in Practice.* 41, 102641. https://doi.org/10.1016/j.nepr.2019.102641

Hall, L.H., Johnson, J., Watt, I., Tsipa, A., O'Connor, D.B. (2016). Healthcare staff wellbeing, burnout, and patient safety: A systematic review. *PLoS One.* 11(7), e0159015. https://doi.org/10.1371/journal.pone.0159015

HEE. (2021). *Growing Our Culture of Kindness: Civility Toolkit.* https://www.hee.nhs.uk/sites/default/files/documents/CM%20civility%20toolkit%20March%2022.pdf [Accessed 02 April 23]

Henrickson, L., & Lukasse, M. (2016). Burnout among Norwegian midwives and the contribution of personal and work-related factors: A cross sectional study. *Sexual & Reproductive Healthcare.* 9, 42–47.

Hunter, B. (2004). Conflicting ideologies as a source of emotion work in midwifery. *Midwifery.* 20, 261–272.

Hunter, B., Fenwick, J., Sidebotham, M., & Henley, J. (2019) Midwives in the United Kingdom: Levels of burnout, depression, anxiety and stress and associated predictors. *Midwifery.* 79, 102526.

Hunter, B., Henley, J., Fenwick, J., Sidebotham, M., & Pallant, J. (2018). *Work Health and Emotional Lives of Midwives in the United Kingdom: The UK WHELM Study.* https://www.rcm.org.uk/media/2924/work-health-and-emotional-lives-of-midwives-in-the-united-kingdom-the-uk-whelm-study.pdf

Hunter, B., & Warren, L. (2013). *Investigating Resilience in Midwifery: Final Report.* Cardiff: Cardiff University.

Hunter, B., &Warren, L. (2014). Midwives' experiences of workplace resilience. *Midwifery,* 30(8), 926–934. https://doi.org/10.1016/j.midw.2014.03.010.

Hunter, B., & Warren, L. (2022). Revisiting resilience. *The Practising Midwife.* 25(5), 08–13.

ICM. (2022). *ICM Advocacy Toolkit for Midwives.* https://www.internationalmidwives.org/assets/files/advocacy-files/2021/10/11103-icm_midwivesadvocacytoolkit.pdf [Accessed 11 December 2023]

Independent Review Group. (2022). *Ockenden Report.* London: Independent Review Group.

Maddock, A., & Oates, J. (2022) Connections, rituals and identities: Healthcare students' descriptions of objects that represent resilience. *Journal of Mental Health Training, Education & Practice.* 17(3), 274–287. https://doi.org/10.1108/JMHTEP-05-2021-0053.

Mharapara, T., Clemons, J., Greenslade-Yeats, J., Ewertowska, T., Awhina Staniland, N., & Ravenswood, K. (2023) Toward a contextualized understanding of well-being in the midwifery profession: An integrative review. *Journal of Professions and Organization.* 9(3), 8–363. https://doi.org/10.1093/jpo/joac017

Mcdonald, G., Jackson, D., Vickers, M.H., & Wilkes, L. (2016) Surviving workplace adversity: a qualitative study of nurses and midwives and their strategies to increase personal resilience. *Journal of Nursing Management.* 24(1),: 123–131. https://doi.org/10.1111/jonm.12293

Nash, K. (2021). Improving the culture of care. *British Journal of Midwifery.* 29(9), 486–488.

NHSE. (2017). *A-EQUIP A Model of Clinical Midwifery Supervision.* https://www.england.nhs.uk/wp-content/uploads/2017/04/a-equip-midwifery-supervision-model.pdf. [Accessed 13 October 2023]

NHS. (2021) *NHS Health and Wellbeing Framework.* Available at: https://www.england.nhs.uk/publication/nhs-health-and-wellbeing-framework/#heading-1

NMC. (2019). *Standards of Proficiency for Midwives.* standards-of-proficiency-for-midwives.pdf (nmc.org.uk) [Accessed 11 December 2023]

OHID. (2022). *Working Definition of Trauma-Informed Practice.* London: Office for Health Improvement and Disparities.

Oxford English Dictionary. (2023). Resilience. In *Oxford English Dictionary.* Oxford: Oxford University Press.

Pezaro S, Clyne W, Turner A, Fulton EA, Gerada C. 'Midwives Overboard!' Inside their hearts are breaking, their makeup may be flaking but their smile still stays on. Women Birth. 2016 Jun;29(3):e59-66. doi: 10.1016/j.wombi.2015.10.006. Epub 2015 Oct 27. PMID: 26522961.

Pezaro, S., Patterson, J., Moncrieff, G., & Ghai, I. (2020). A systematic integrative review of the literature on midwives and student midwives engaged in problematic substance use. *Midwifery.* 89, 102785. https://doi.org/10.1016/j.midw.2020.102785

Pezaro, S., Pearce, G., & Bailey, E. (2018). Childbearing women's experiences of midwives' workplace distress: Patient and public involvement. *British Journal of Midwifery.* 26(10), 659–669. https://doi.org/10.12968/bjom.2018.26.10.659

Pezaro, S., Clyne, W., Turner, A., Fulton, E.A., & Gerada, C. (2015). 'Midwives overboard!' Inside their hearts are breaking, their makeup may be flaking but their smile still stays on. *Women and Birth.* 29, e59–e66.

Piotrowski A, Sygit-Kowalkowska E, Boe O, Rawat S. Resilience, Occupational Stress, Job Satisfaction, and Intention to Leave the Organization among Nurses and Midwives during the COVID-19 Pandemic. Int J Environ Res Public Health. 2022 Jun 2;19(11):6826. doi: 10.3390/ijerph19116826. PMID: 35682410; PMCID: PMC9180178.

Rayment, J. (2015). Emotional labour: How midwives manage emotion at work. *The Practising Midwife.* 18(3), 9–11.

Ross, S., Jabal, J., Chauhan, K., Maguire, D., Randhawa, M., & Dahir, S. (2020). *Workforce Race Inequalities and Inclusion in NHS Providers.* London: The Kings Fund.

Sidhu R, Su B, Shapiro KR, Stoll K. Prevalence of and factors associated with burnout in midwifery: A scoping review. Eur J Midwifery. 2020 Feb 11;4:4. doi: 10.18332/ejm/115983. PMID: 33537606; PMCID: PMC7839164.

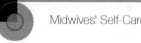

Sist, L., Savadori, S., Grandi, A., Martoni, M., Baiocchi, E., Lombardo, C., & Colombo, L. (2022). Self-care for nurses and midwives: Findings from a scoping review. *Healthcare (Basel).* 7(10).

Smith, J., (2021). *Nurturing Maternity Staff.* London: Pinter & Martin.

Tant, M., (2020). Resilience and midwives: Whose responsibility is it anyway? *The Practising Midwife* 23(5).

Thumm, E.B., & Flynn, L. (2018). The five attribute of a supporting midwifery practice climate: A review of the literature. *Journal of Midwifery and Women's Health.* 63(1), 90–103.

Traynor, M. (2018). What's wrong with resilience? *Journal of Research in Nursing.* 23(1), 5–8.

United Nations Population Fund, International Confederation of Midwives, World Health Organization. (2021). *State of the World's Midwifery 2021.* New York: United Nations Population Fund. [Accessed 08/ August 23]

West, M.A. (2021). *Compassionate Leadership: Sustaining Wisdom, Humanity and Presence in Health and Social Care.* United Kingdom: The Swirling Leaf Press.

World Health Organisation. (2016). WHO Classification of Diseases ICD-10. https://icd.who.int/browse10/2016/en#/Z73.0

Williams, J., & Hadley, J., (2022). An exploration of the development of resilience in student midwives. *BJM.* 30(4), 202–207.

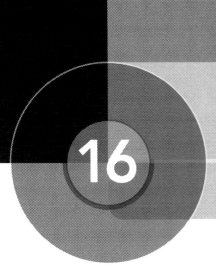

Sexual Health Promotion in Midwifery Practice

SARAH KIPPS

16

INTRODUCTION

Pregnancy and childbirth are a special period in a woman and birthing person's life and involve significant physical, hormonal, psychological, social, and cultural change. It is imperative that a holistic approach is undertaken, and midwives recognise that sexual health is an essential part of comprehensive health care. Positive sexual health outcomes are important to individuals and are recognised by the government as a major public health issue. Some achievements in the general sexual health targets have been noted, namely a decline in teenage pregnancy and an increase in universal HIV testing in other clinical areas (DoH 2013a). But there are still major challenges – there were 447,694 sexually transmitted infection diagnoses across the population in England in 2018 (UK Health Security Agency 2019), up to 45% of pregnancies and one-third of births were unplanned or associated with feelings of ambivalence (Public Health England [PHE] 2018) and in 2018, an estimated 7,500 people were living with undiagnosed HIV and two in five were diagnosed at a late stage (PHE 2019).

Midwives are in an ideal position to improve sexual health having unique access to the private sphere of a woman and her family's life and can use targeted measures to address sexual health issues and promote positive sexual health outcomes. However, in midwifery practice, promoting sexual health is more than likely than others to be omitted. (McCance & Cameron 2014, Walker & Davis 2014). This can be for a variety of reasons:

- midwives feeling unskilled and unprepared to tackle the issue.
- the fear of uncovering something that the midwife cannot deal with.

- the perceived idea that new mothers are not interested in contraception and sexual health matters post birth.
- the idealisation of the new mother as a non-sexual being.

(Fennell & Grant 2019, Åling et al. 2021)

The chapter will discuss the midwife's role during the journey through pregnancy to motherhood and examine how midwives can facilitate positive sexual health promotion throughout this time. This is not without its challenges, but sexual health promotion is an integral part of a midwife's role, and delivering this ensures the sexual wellbeing of the women who are being cared for, as well as their partners and families (ICM 2019).

WHAT IS SEXUAL HEALTH?

Sexual health is a multi-faceted concept that is not just narrowly defined by issues such as sexually transmitted infections (STIs), pregnancy and contraception but includes positive, respectful, pleasurable, and safe sexual relationships free of coercion, discrimination, and violence (WHO 2023). Physical sexual health does not just imply the absence of disease but being enabled to make positive health choices and access to services when needed. Sexual health can be altered during pregnancy and after childbirth, optimal sexual health outcomes can vary according to the differing needs of individual women and their partners. For some, it will be resuming sexual intercourse, for some feeling comfortable in a postnatal body and for others expressing love to their partner in a non-sexual but tender way. The midwife's role in facilitating sexual health is therefore varied and includes anticipating sexual health problems, informing about changes in physical and psychological states that can impact on sexual health, promoting positive sexual health choices and having the ability to recognise and refer on to other agencies if specialist intervention is needed. The role of the midwife in sexual health, most importantly, is recognising that sexual health is an integral part of holistic care and to omit this means that women's and birthing people's health needs are not being wholly met.

THE MIDWIFE'S ROLE IN SEXUAL HEALTH PROMOTION

The role of midwives in public health and sexual health promotion is enshrined in professional organisation competencies recognising that midwives, due to their close relationship with women during the maternity episode, are in a unique position to give this information and advice. The Nursing and Midwifery council in 2019 issued 'Standards of proficiency for midwives' highlighting the standards that a qualified midwife needs to attain. "The standards of proficiency in this document specify the knowledge, understanding and skills that midwives must demonstrate at the point of qualification, when caring for women across the maternity journey…across all care settings" (NMC 2019, p. 3). The standards are divided into six domains. The domains inter-relate and build on each other and reflect what is expected of a new midwife to know, understand and be capable of doing safely and proficiently. Within these domains the role of midwives in promoting and delivering sexual and contraceptive care is recognised. Domain 1 asks the midwives to understand and promote women's sexual and reproductive rights. In Domain 3, midwives must give information and access to resources and services for women regarding reproductive health and contraception. In Domain 6, midwives are asked to conduct person centred conversations which must include "sexual and reproductive health, pre-conception, contraception, unintended pregnancy, abortion and STI's" (NMC 2019) (Figure 16.1).

Further emphasis on the midwife's role in sexual health was highlighted in the priority for sexual health improvements by the Department of Health and Social Care (DoH 2013b), including reducing unwanted or unintended pregnancy after

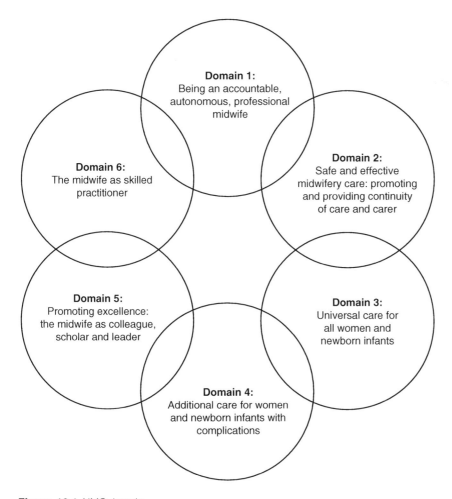

Figure 16.1 NMC domain.

childbirth and screening for and identifying infection in antenatal screening programmes for HIV, Hepatitis B, and syphilis.

Several studies have indicated that although sexual health promotion is viewed positively by midwives, it is not given as much attention as other subjects when caring for pregnant and postnatal women (McCance & Cameron 2014; Walker & Davis 2014). Research from adult and mental health nursing also shows that sexual health is not given a priority and highlighted some reasons why there can be resistance to addressing the sexual health needs of patients (Fennell & Grant 2019, Åling et al. 2021). These can all be applied to midwives.

- Embarrassment
- Lack of knowledge/time
- Not enough education and training
- Ageism
- Personal convictions
- Fear of offending
- Not knowing how to broach the subject.

APPROACHING SEXUAL ISSUES IN PRACTICE

There has been extensive work into how to overcome these barriers and initiate sexual health discussion. One of the first encounters the midwife will have with the woman is at the initial booking interview. This is a time when a comprehensive sexual health assessment can be undertaken.

NICE (2021a) emphasises that the environment in which antenatal appointments take place should enable people to discuss sensitive issues – this means somewhere private and quiet where there will be no interruptions. There are many issues to discuss at this first appointment and the midwife may well feel that there is so much to cover that sexual health is not a priority. However, it is important to remember that this is the first meeting the pregnant person has with the midwife and may have unmet needs and questions. They need to feel listened to in a safe environment where any concerns or fears can be explored. As part of the booking all are encouraged to screen for HIV, syphilis, and Hepatitis B to avoid any vertical transmission to the unborn child (PHE 2021). Having these routine tests can encourage them to disclose any other sensitive issues and queries about the need for other tests e.g., chlamydia. PHE do not recommend routine chlamydia testing for pregnant women, but screening should be considered for women who have had a chlamydia contact, women who are reporting symptoms (e.g., dysuria, abnormal discharge, pelvic pain) or women under 25 where the prevalence of this bacterial infection is high. In young women aged 15–24 accessing the Chlamydia screening programme, there were 68,882 chlamydia diagnoses, an increase of 21.8% compared to 2021 (Gov.uk 2023). Self-swabs, for chlamydia and gonorrhoea, can be performed in private by the woman while producing a urine sample (Table 16.1).

Pregnant women carry the same STI risk from unprotected sexual intercourse as any other women. The ramifications of undiagnosed STI in a pregnant woman can be very serious, resulting in significant morbidity for the unborn child as well as the woman herself (Gerwen et al. 2022). Mother to baby transmission of STIs can result in stillbirth, neonatal death, congenital deformities, low birth weight and prematurity and sepsis (WHO 2023). If a woman discloses signs or symptoms of an STI e.g., unusual discharge, pain, lesions, or ulcerations on the vulva, a prompt appointment with a Genito-Urinary Medicine (GUM) clinic is recommended.

It is important to remember that many pregnant women have fears and worries that they feel are exclusive to them – questions that are universally phrased can help the woman to feel that her worries are shared e.g., "many women are worried about being sexually active during pregnancy, do you have any concerns?"

It can be useful to use a recognised framework to guide sexual health assessment. Originally developed by Annon in 1976,, the PLISSIT model was enhanced by

Table 16.1 Key skills for sexual history taking

Environment	Sensitivity, privacy, and confidentiality should be always shown. Consider the environment. Is it private? Can the client be overheard? **Active listening skills** should be employed, avoiding distractions such as looking at the computer screen.	Privacy and Confidentiality enable the client to feel comfortable to disclose personal information. (BASHH 2019)
Introduction	Give a friendly introduction and eye contact – if culturally appropriate.	This helps set the scene and aid comfort and confidence (BASHH 2019)
Questions	Use 'universal' questions-questions which are explicitly asked of all patients. Use 'bridging' questions, which link general lifestyle questions to sexual history questions. Use 'Open-ended' questions and 'closed' questions	This may help when introducing sensitive questions. **Closed questions** are useful for gaining practical information such as demographics. **Open questions** help the client express thoughts and feelings and give a sense of these thoughts being validated. If just Closed questions are used this tends to limit the range of responses and make the woman feel not listened to (RCN 2015)

(Continued)

Table 16.1 *(Continued)* Key skills for sexual history taking

Incorporating diversity	Do not assume a heteronormative model. Use expressions such as partner and do not assume heterosexual relationships.	This ensures an inclusive approach is maintained. (RCN 2016)
	Clarify how the patient identifies regarding sexuality and gender.	Understanding the difference between sex which is assigned at birth and gender which is related to a person's identity is imperative to understanding the patient presenting themselves for care and treatment.
	Establish the **preferred pronoun** the patient would like to use and how they would prefer to be addressed.	Midwives should understand that gender identity is not necessarily fixed and can be fluid over time. (RCN 2015) – see Chapter 6 Health Promotion considerations for clients from the LGBTQ+ community.

Table 16.2 Ex-PLISSITT model

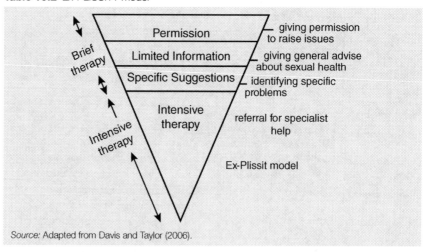

Source: Adapted from Davis and Taylor (2006).

Davis and Taylor (2006) and renamed the Ex-PLISSIT model with permission giving at each stage. The model has different levels of intervention, and the therapy is provided by a third party. The midwife's role in this is to have the knowledge of the model and know where to refer to know, for psychosexual counselling and to have the resources to do so (Table 16.2).

Make a list of sexual health issues women may wish to discuss with you as a midwife.

Think of how you will approach and respond to these issues and what resources you will use for assistance.

Do you know the local sexual health services e.g., GUM, contraception, abortion, Female genital mutilation (FGM), rape, and sexual assault, psychosexual in your area and do you have a referral pathway to these services in place?

SEXUAL HEALTH ISSUES DURING PREGNANCY AND BEYOND

SEXUAL ACTIVITY IN PREGNANCY

Women may have worries about their sexual health during pregnancy and beyond, and during midwife appointments if perceived as a safe environment to verbalise thoughts and feelings, these worries may be expressed. The transition to parenthood is a time of immense transformation for both women and men. The area of intimacy and the sexual functioning of new parents is one of the most affected by this transformation and the most vulnerable (Drozdowsky et al. 2019).

Many factors can lead to this change during pregnancy. These include physical changes, hormonal changes, psychological changes, fears and myths and cultural beliefs about sexual activity during pregnancy. Evidence shows that sexual function declines during pregnancy specifically during the third trimester. This reduction does not resolve immediately post-birth but persist during the first three to six months postpartum before steadily recovering (Drozdowsky et al. 2019, Johnson 2011, Pauleta et al. 2010, Korzeniewski et al. 2019). Johnson (2011) argues that rather than pathologising these changes, they should be viewed and presented as a normal sequence of events that gradually recovers over time.

Physical and hormonal factors which reduce sexual activity can include fatigue, nausea, back pain and infections, for example, urinary tract infections, candidiasis and vulvar varicose veins. In the third trimester, the sheer weight of the pregnancy and pressure on the bladder and other organs can cause a decrease in sexual frequency and desire, masturbation and oral sex also tend to decline during late pregnancy (see Table 16.3). If sexual intercourse is desired, adjustments may have to be made to coital positioning (Johnson 2011).

Psychological changes can also affect sexual desire and activity. Pregnancy involves a period of transition; as with all transition, there can be anxiety as well as happiness. Feeling of ambivalence about the pregnancy, changes in body shape and worries about changes to a relationship can all affect sexual desire. There also exist fears and myths about sexual intercourse during pregnancy and, of course, there are some conditions, which are contraindications to sexual intercourse (Johnson 2011) (See Table 16.4). However, outside of these contraindications, sexual intercourse is safe and acceptable and should be encouraged for women who desire sexual intercourse within their relationship.

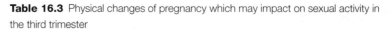

Table 16.3 Physical changes of pregnancy which may impact on sexual activity in the third trimester

Deep engagement of fetal head
Stress urinary incontinence
Haemorrhoids
Weight of partner on uterus
Subluxation of pubic symphysis and sacroiliac joints
Vaginal discomfort/dyspareunia
Pelvic and vaginal vasocongestion

Source: From Johnson (2011).

Table 16.4 Contraindications to sexual intercourse during pregnancy

Absolute contraindications
Unexplained vaginal bleeding
Placenta previa
Preterm premature dilation of the cervix
Preterm premature rupture of the membranes
Relative contraindications
History of premature delivery
Multiple gestation

Source: From Johnson (2011).

SEXUAL ACTIVITY IN THE POSTPARTUM PERIOD

Many women experience physical sexual health issues after birth and older research into postpartum sexual activity concentrated very much on these aspects of sexual dysfunction such as dyspareunia, lack of lubrication and lack of libido (O'Malley et al. 2021). More recent research has incorporated broader aspects of sexual functioning postpartum, acknowledging that women can face psychological, body, hormonal, relationship and sociocultural changes. These can all affect sexual functioning and desire (Serrano Drozdowskyj 2020).

Concentrating on purely physical aspects of sexual health as expressed through penetrative sexual intercourse postpartum raises a number of issues. It ignores different ways of expressing sexuality such as kissing, mutual masturbation and experiencing closeness. It also promotes a heteronormative model with no mention of same sex sexuality. Many of the studies also use resumption of penetrative intercourse as a measure of positive sexual health. This ignores an important psychosocial component in that women may feel under pressure to commence sexual intercourse despite genital pain. (McBride 2017). O'Malley et al. (2021) argue that observing these other aspects of postpartum sexual health does not detract from the evidence that many do experience physical sexual health issues after birth but using only physical dysfunction as a measurement is problematic. The authors suggest adopting a more holistic approach that encompasses emotional and social factors which can assist midwives to counsel and support women during the possible change to their sexual health after birth and to develop strategies to help them.

Factors that impact on sexual function post birth include:

- Fatigue-sleep quality
- Identity and role adjustment – becoming a mother.
- Difficult birth and trauma
- Change in romantic relationship.
- Decreased lubrication and increased vaginal dryness, especially among those breastfeeding.
- Fear of wakening the baby, especially if the baby sleeps in the mother's bedroom.
- Not hearing if the baby cries
- Decreased sense of attractiveness

(McBride et al. 2017).

There is mixed evidence about the mode of delivery and its effect upon sexual health postpartum (McBride et al. 2017). Mode of delivery and perineal trauma, including episiotomy, perineal tears and lacerations, can all impact sexual function (McBride et al. 2017). Gutzeit et al. (2020) in their study showed that while sexual function does decline during pregnancy and beyond, severe perineal trauma and lactation have the most serious negative effect on sexual function in the postpartum period. Korzeniewski et al. (2019) concur with this finding and found women who experience the most severe problems such as pain and dyspareunia were more likely to have suffered perineal trauma at birth. The severity of pain varied depending on the degree of perineal trauma, severe pain more commonly being reported following a second-degree trauma compared to a first-degree trauma or an intact perineum.

Dyspareunia was shown in some studies to persist up to six months in women who had experienced an instrumental vaginal birth. An increased delay in resumption of sexual intercourse plus perineal pain, and self-reported perception of sexual health/sexual problems was found in women who underwent instrumental vaginal birth as opposed to those who had a spontaneous vaginal delivery or caesarean section (Hicks et al. 2004).

PRACTICE POINTS

PHYSIOLOGICAL AND HORMONAL EFFECTS OF BREASTFEEDING ON SEXUAL ACTIVITY

- Low oestrogen levels can result in decreased vaginal lubrication and atrophy of the vaginal epithelium; so during sexual activity, there can be little or no vaginal secretions. This can lead to reduced physical arousal and painful intercourse.
- Increased prolactin levels can impact sex hormone levels which may have an influence on sexual desire, sexual arousal, and orgasm.
- When a woman is lactating, she may have a milk ejection reflex when she experiences orgasm. She may also find her breast a source of discomfort during lovemaking if they are overly full or leaking milk.
- New mothers may struggle with their role as a new mother and their role as a sexual being, and this may cause a clash between her breasts performing a biological function and the sexual connotation of her breasts (O'Malley et al. 2021).

- With a drive to increase breastfeeding rates and prolong duration, it is important that women are informed of the changes that may affect their sexual health and the fact that these changes are normal physiological events.
- Practical advice includes use of vaginal lubricants, oestrogen pessaries and open discussion with partners that can help breastfeeding women feel reassured about their sexual health

Woolhouse et al. (2012) found in their study of women's experiences of sex and intimacy after childbirth that a drop in libido was found to cause feelings of guilt and failure despite it being a very common phenomenon. The authors believe that women have internalised the socially constructed message that mothers can 'be it all', and when faced with the realities of motherhood, feelings of guilt and inadequacy are somewhat inevitable.

Midwives can play an important role in recognising these issues around intimate relationships during pregnancy and beyond and tackling them head on. Johnson (2011) argues for targeted counselling for women on the impact of pregnancy, childbirth, and the post-partum period on their sexual health. This should be performed throughout the antenatal period and reinforced by all members of the team. However, Korzeniewski et al. (2019) found that sexual functioning changes or problems were rarely explored by Health Care Professionals and there was a general lack of focus on all aspects of sexual intimacy postnatally. The authors review continued to add weight to previous findings that women receive little information and advice post-natally, regarding sexual functioning changes, or problems they may encounter during this period, discussions centred on contraception or timing to resume intercourse, with many women describing they wanted to ask something, but felt they could not.

Quilliam (2010) concurs that the first challenge is to bring the issue into the consulting room in a way that clients can engage with. This may not be as simple as it sounds – both sides may be embarrassed, uninformed, and unresourced. Midwives need to normalise the issue by being relaxed, friendly, armed with phrases such as "People often ask me whether it's OK to have sex..." or "In case you're wondering, your love life can carry on until..." and be prepared to wait out client hesitation.

O'Malley and Smith (2013a) feel it is important to consider discussions about sexual health, including changes in sexual health patterns, during the antenatal period and in antenatal classes. This normalises the subject and leads to facilitating open, honest discussion between practitioners, women, and their partners. O'Malley and Smith (2013b) believe the postnatal six-week check is an excellent opportunity to discuss sexual wellbeing for the majority of women. This can range from advice around specific issues such as recommending lubrication for vaginal dryness and using sexual positions that allow for more shallow penetration or give women more control over penetration, referring for more in-depth sexual health counselling for those who identify with more ongoing sexual health concerns. However, for some women, this will be too late and the check-up may not occur at the six week mark with many current GP services. Resuming sexual activity, postpartum is not a spontaneous act, women and birthing people considered their mode of birth, presence of perineal trauma and their physical and emotional recovery (O'Malley et al. 2021). Having the support of a midwife or health care professional in this consideration is invaluable. If midwives can promote sexual health in every encounter with women from the antenatal period to the post-partum period, there is more of a chance that women will feel that this is an important part of their overall health care and feel empowered to discuss these issues at the six-week check.

PROMOTING POSITIVE BODY IMAGE

Pregnancy is a time when women face substantial changes to their body shape and weight in a short period of time. Changes in body shape and body image can have a dramatic effect on sexual and intimate relationships. Postpartum body image can be impacted by scars, changed abdomen shape, enlarged breasts, stretch marks and change in body weight (O'Malley et al. 2021). In 2010, the Government Equalities Office report 'Two for the Price of One' acknowledged the pressure that women feel during and after pregnancy to achieve a perfect body. This is not helped by media pictures of celebrities achieving a 'perfect body' after delivery (Hopper & Aubrey 2015). There seems to be a cultural assumption that a mother's job is to present herself as if nothing life changing or body changing has happened (Orbach & Rubin 2014). Some women found that their post-partum bodies left them feeling unat-tractive and self-conscious. A woman's body image consists of her attitudes and self-perceptions about her appearance, which have developed from biological, psy-chological and sociocultural influences. Experiencing a sense of bodily acceptance is critical to healthy sexual functioning. Women who reported feeling more negative about their bodies post-partum had lower levels of desire and arousal; increased avoidance; and decreased pleasure, orgasm, and sexual satisfaction (Drozdowsky et al. 2019).

In most Western countries, socially constructed ideals about how a woman's body should look include being thin and having shapely breasts, but a woman's body does not fulfil these social requirements during the perinatal period (or at any time) and this can lead to a deterioration in a woman's view of her body image.

However, this is by no means universal, and some celebrate their sense of empowerment and respect for their bodies following childbirth. Many women have posted pictures of their post-partum bodies at '#takebackpostpartum' celebrating the power of their bodies in giving new life.

Orbach and Rubin (2014), while recognising the heavy workload that midwives face, recommend that they incorporate body image into their consultations and create positive body image models by advertising model diversity in pictures used around the clinical area ensuring there are pictures of happy, healthy women of all different shapes and sizes. The guidance also encourages health professionals to be mindful of the language used. around body size and shape and expectations post-partum. Women and their body image needs to be discussed sensitively regarding the physi-cal, psychological, and emotional changes in the post-natal period. This support when provided during pregnancy and beyond this can make a significant difference to body image satisfaction.

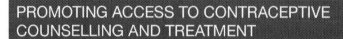

PROMOTING ACCESS TO CONTRACEPTIVE COUNSELLING AND TREATMENT

Rapid, repeat pregnancies are associated with worse outcomes for mother and child. Short inter-pregnancy intervals (IPI) of less than 12 months have been linked to increased risk of preterm birth, low birth weight, small for gestational age and increases in maternal morbidity and mortality (Thwaites et al. 2019). Currently, the World Health Organization (Marston et al. 2007) recommends a 24-month IPI after childbirth (WHO) (Table 16.5).

During pregnancy, high levels of sex steroid hormones suppress pituitary gonadotrophins. Within 30 days of delivery, placental sex steroid levels decrease, and gonadotrophins increase, thus stimulating the activity of the ovaries. The earliest date of ovulation in non-breastfeeding women is thought to be Day 28 and menstruation may return by Week 6. As sperm can live up to seven days in the genital tract, there is a potential risk of pregnancy from Day 21 after birth, and contraception needs to be started from then on. In women who exclusively breastfeed, suckling disrupts the frequency and amplitude of gonadotrophin pulses, and, despite ovarian follicular activity, ovulation is suppressed. Ovulation returns when the frequency and duration of suckling episodes decrease (Faculty of Sexual and Reproductive Health [FSRH] 2020).

NICE guidelines advise that methods of contraception should be discussed within the first week of giving birth (NICE 2006). This role usually falls to the midwife and undertaken when the mother is discharged from postnatal care. The FSRH, however, recommend that women should be given the opportunity to discuss contraception at all stages of antenatal, intrapartum and postpartum care (FSRH 2020). Walker et al. (2021) in a study of midwife's views on discussing contraception felt that this discussion should happen all along the pregnancy journey with the antenatal period being the time to 'plant the seed' leading to a more extended discussion later with women having time to make decisions about contraception postnatally. The FSRH agree that advice about contraception after childbirth may be better discussed antenatally, especially since many methods can be provided at the time of delivery e.g. intrauterine contraception (IUC) or during the hospital stay e.g. sub dermal implant. Prior to giving birth, women may have more time to think through their options than immediately after giving birth when the requirements of caring for a baby and recovering from delivery may take priority over contraceptive decision-making (FSRH 2020).

The FSRH also recommend that maternity service providers should ensure that women post-partum have access to the full range of effective contraceptive methods

Table 16.5 Percentage of adverse outcomes during pregnancy and birth at 6 months and 18 months

Morbidity risk	At 6/12 (%)	At 18/12 (%)
Maternal morbidity	0.62	0.26
Fetal and infant outcome risks	2.0	1.4
Spontaneous pre-term delivery (148,544 pregnancies)	5.3	3.2

Source: Schummers et al. (2018).

and that these should be available immediately after childbirth. The emphasis should be on the most effective methods with long-acting reversible contraception (LARC) promoted due to its superior efficacy, lack of user failure and the fact that it does not impact on breast feeding. To support this service the FSRH have introduced a new FSRH qualification in 2017 open to doctors, nurses and midwives for sub-dermal implant insertion only, without the requirement to achieve a competency in removals as well (www.fsrh.org).

There is also support from the FSRH for an increase in fitting post-partum Intra Uterine contraception (PPIUC). Immediate postpartum IUC insertion (within 48 hours of childbirth) has shown to be safe, convenient, cost effective and associated with high continuation rates (FSRH 2023). The insertion can take place as soon as the placenta is delivered at caesarean section or up to 48 hours after vaginal birth. A routine check-up is recommended four to six weeks post insertion where the threads may need to be trimmed due to the involution of the uterus leaving long threads in the vagina (FSRH 2023). However, in contrast to the sub-dermal implant, there are no current national UK training schemes for the fitting of intrauterine methods postnatally and relatively few experienced trainers (Cooper et al. 2018).

Despite the support for immediate post-natal contraception from the FSRH, this is not routinely or universally available in UK NHS maternity hospitals. At present only a small minority of midwives are trained to fit contraceptive implants or prescribe contraceptive methods, and appear restricted to those caring for those groups seen to be vulnerable e.g. teenagers or those with mental health problems (Thwaites et al. 2019, Walker et al. 2021, Thwaites et al 2019).

Walker et al. (2021) in their study of midwives' views on giving postnatal contraceptive advice and administering treatment find that although midwives are very supportive of this activity and feel it fits into the 'continuity of care' model which is practiced in the UK, they do express worries about the reality of performing these tasks with other demands made on the midwives workload. Lack of training as a barrier to provision was cited in many studies as well as time pressures, low prioritisation of this training and disputes over funding (McCance & Cameron 2014, Walker et al. 2021). One study showed that midwives viewed their role in discussing contraception as a minor one, and due to lack of privacy, time and knowledge would rather signpost women to their general practitioner at the six-week check (McCance & Cameron 2014).

The issue with waiting to discuss contraception until the six-week check is the risk that new mothers could become pregnant again before contraception is commenced or women who have not recommenced sexual intercourse feel alienated from the discussion and miss the opportunity to engage with a health care professional at this time. They also need to find the time with competing demands of a newborn to engage with a service to discuss and commence contraception. Walker et al. (2021) in their study of midwives found that they understood the need to make an appointment with a doctor after six weeks was a hazardous discontinuity of care which could result in an unintended pregnancy.

Studies of women themselves find support and interest in midwives supplying contraception and expressed the view this was convenient and highly acceptable (Walker et al. 2014). When a service is supported such as the APPLES study (Access to Postpartum LARC in Edinburgh South) which offered routine ante natal contraception counselling and post-natal provision of chosen method with training provided for midwives, both midwives and new mothers expressed satisfaction (Cameron et al. 2017).

Thwaites et al. (2017) found that opportunities for post-natal counselling were missed and there remained confusion about the safety of breastfeeding with contraception. This was despite daily breastfeeding sessions taking place on the ward. As more women are encouraged to breastfeed, it is important that consistent, accurate advice about breastfeeding, the effectiveness of this in protecting against pregnancy and the options for contraception that are safe during breastfeeding are discussed.

Exclusive breastfeeding can work as an effective contraceptive, but only if strict criterion is met about frequency of feeds. This is known as lactational amenorrhoea method (LAM) (Table 16.6).

PRACTICE POINTS

Important information points to be given about postnatal contraception ideally throughout their pregnancy journey but at the latest in the immediate postnatal period before discharge:

- The choice of contraceptive method should be initiated by Day 21 after childbirth.
- Although contraception is not required in the first 21 days after childbirth most methods can be initiated immediately except for the combined hormonal contraceptive (CHC) method.
- Emergency contraception is indicated for women who have had unprotected sexual intercourse from 21 days after childbirth but not before this.
- Women who are not breastfeeding and are without additional risk factors for Venous thromboembolism (VTE) should wait until 21 days after childbirth before initiating a CHC method (Jackson 2011).
- Women who are breastfeeding should wait until six weeks after childbirth before initiating a CHC method. These women should be informed that there is currently limited evidence regarding the effects of CHC use on breastfeeding.
- Women should be advised that additional contraceptive precautions (e.g. barrier method/abstinence) are required if hormonal contraception is started 21 days or more after childbirth. Additional contraceptive precaution is not required if contraception is initiated immediately or within 21 days after childbirth.
- Intra-uterine contraception can be safely inserted immediately after birth (within 10 minutes of delivery of the placenta) or within the first 48 hours after uncomplicated caesarean section or vaginal birth. After 48 hours, insertion should be delayed until 28 days after childbirth.
- Progestogen only implant can be safely started at any time after childbirth including immediately after delivery
- Progestogen only injectable can be started at any time after childbirth, including immediately after delivery.
- Progestogen only pill can be started at any time after childbirth, including immediately after delivery.
- Male and female condoms can be safely used by women after childbirth. Women choosing to use a diaphragm should be advised to wait at least six weeks after childbirth before having it fitted because the size of diaphragm required may change as the uterus returns to normal size.

FSRH (2020)

Table 16.6 LAM

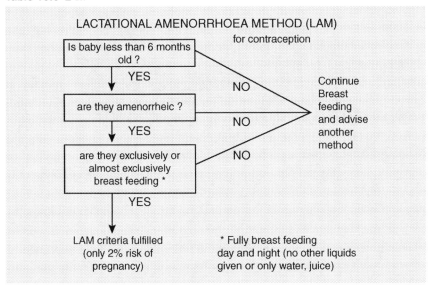

LACTATIONAL AMENORRHOEA METHOD (LAM)
for contraception

Is baby less than 6 months old ? — YES → are they amenorrheic ? — YES → are they exclusively or almost exclusively breast feeding * — YES → LAM criteria fulfilled (only 2% risk of pregnancy)

NO / NO / NO → Continue Breast feeding and advise another method

* Fully breast feeding day and night (no other liquids given or only water, juice)

There are a range of contraceptives that are safe to use immediately post-partum while breastfeeding, including progestogen-only methods: pills, implants, intra-uterine copper devices and intrauterine system, for example, Mirena, Women who are breastfeeding should be informed that the available evidence indicates that progestogen-only methods of contraception have no adverse effects on lactation, infant growth or development (FSRH 2020).

Contraception choice is also affected by individual preferences, cultural beliefs and attitudes, personal and family health issues, and whether the woman is return-ing to work. Giving the woman an opportunity to explore all the options, her own individual preferences and her suitability for the different methods takes time and knowledge. It may be that the midwife does not have the time to explore all the options fully, but it is imperative that women are given some access to contraceptive advice even if it is signposting to websites, local clinics or providing up to date lit-erature on the subject (Support For Women | SHEWISE | United Kingdom). Results from a survey in Wales showed 84% of women were interested in receiving contra-ception prior to discharge with the majority wanting LARC. The recommendation was to provide a patient-centred postnatal contraception service within the mater-nity service. This certainly was the case in the past with a contraceptive nurse visit-ing the postnatal ward on a regular basis (Oliver et al. 2015).

There seems to be very little consensus about the best time to discuss contra-ception for the pregnant or new mother. Normalising the subject and including it at every stage along the journey through pregnancy to the postnatal period would cover the differing needs of all women and is the approach recommended by the FSRH (2020). However, studies into midwives' skills and expertise in the subject do point out that an investment in ongoing skills training in the subject is essen-tial as well as giving midwives the time and space to perform this essential role (McCance & Cameron 2014; Walker & Davis 2014).

SUMMARY

- Sexual health is a broad concept and implies being able to make positive health choices and being able to access services when needed.
- The role of the midwife in sexual health promotion is to recognise that sexual health is an integral part of overall health, and its omission would mean that holistic care is not being offered.
- Sexual health can be altered during pregnancy and childbirth in a variety of ways – physical, emotional, and psychological.
- The role of midwives in public health and sexual health promotion is enshrined in professional organisation competencies and government directives.

Sexual health promotion and sexual health discussion should be an integral part of the pregnancy journey and beyond.

- Sexual health should be discussed in an environment which is private and quiet, and midwives should use their communication skills to facilitate a frank and honest discussion which enables the pregnant woman to disclose any fears and worries she may have.
- Pregnant and postnatal women may have concerns surrounding sexual activity in pregnancy and beyond, issues with body image and questions about postnatal contraception.
- Challenges to sexual health promotion can be overcome by training and giving midwives time and space to perform this role.

REFERENCES

Åling, M., Lindgren, A., Löfall, H., & Okenwa-Emegwa, L. (2021). A scoping review to identify barriers and enabling factors for nurse–patient discussions on sexuality and sexual health. *Nursing Reports, 11*(2), 253–266. https://doi.org/10.3390/nursrep11020025

BASHH (British Association of Sexual Health and HIV). (2019). *UK National Guideline for Consultations Requiring Sexual History Taking.* http://www.bashh.org/BASHH/Guidelines/Guidelines/BASHH/Guidelines/Guidelines.aspx

Cameron, S., Craig, A., Sim, J., Gallimore, A., Cowan, S., Dundas, K., Heller, R., Milne, D., & Lakha, F. (2017). Feasibility and acceptability of introducing routine antenatal contraceptive counselling and provision of contraception after delivery: The APPLES pilot evaluation. *BJOG: An International Journal of Obstetrics & Gynaecology, 124*(13), 2009–2015 https://doi.org/10.1111/1471-0528.14674

Cooper, M., Boydell, N., Heller, R., & Cameron, S. (2018). Community sexual health providers' views on immediate postpartum provision of intrauterine contraception. *BMJ Sex Reproductive Health, 44*, 7–102. https://doi.org/10.1136/bmjsrh-2017-101905

Davis, S., & Taylor, B. (2006). Using the extended PLISSIT model to address sexual healthcare needs. *Nursing Standard, 21*(11), 35–40. https://doi.org/10.7748/ns2006.11.21.11.35.c6382

DoH. (2013a). *A Framework for Sexual Health Improvement in England.* London: DoH.

DoH. (2013b). *Nursing and Midwifery contribution to Public Health.* London: DoH

Serrano Drozdowskyj E, Gimeno Castro E, Trigo López E, Bárcenas Taland I, Chiclana Actis C. Factors Influencing Couples' Sexuality in the Puerperium: A Systematic Review. Sex Med Rev. 2020 Jan;8(1):38-47. doi: 10.1016/j.sxmr.2019.07.002. Epub 2019 Aug 22. PMID: 31447412.

Fennell, R., & Grant, B. (2019). Discussing sexuality in health care: A systematic review. *Journal of Clinical Nursing, 28*(17–18), 3065–3076.

FSRH. (2020). *Clinical Guidance. Contraception after Pregnancy.* London: FSRH.

FSRH guideline (March 2023) intrauterine contraception. (2023). *BMJ Sexual & Reproductive Health, 49*(Suppl 1), 1–142.

Gerwen, O. T., Muzny, C. A., & Marrazzo, J. M. (2022). Sexually transmitted infections and female reproductive health. *Nature Microbiology, 7*(8), 1116–1126. https://doi.org/10.1038/s41564-022-01177-x

Gov.UK. (2023). *Sexually Transmitted Infections and Screening for Chlamydia In England: 2022 Report.* London UK: Health Security agency.

Gutzeit, O., Levy. G., & Lowenstein, L. (2020). Postpartum sexual function: Risk factors for postpartum sexual dysfunction. *Sexual Medicine, 8*(1), 8–13. https://doi.org/10.1016/j.esxm.2019.10.005

Hicks, T. L., Goodall, S. F., Quattrone, E. M., & Lydon-Rochelle, M. T. (2004). Postpartum sexual functioning and method of delivery: Summary of the evidence. *Journal of Midwifery & Women's Health, 49*(5), 430–436. https://doi.org/10.1016/j.jmwh.2004.04.007

Hopper, K., & Aubrey, J. (2015). Bodies after babies: The impact of depictions of recently post-partum celebrities on non-pregnant women's body image. *Sex Roles, 74*, 24–34.

ICM. (2019). *Essential Competencies for Midwifery Practice* (Essential Competencies for Midwifery Practice | International Confederation of Midwives (international-almidwives.org)) (accessed 10 August 2023).

Jackson, E. (2011). Controversies in postpartum contraception: When is it safe to start oral contraceptives after childbirth? *Thrombosis Research, 127*, S35–S39. https://doi.org/10.1016/s0049-3848(11)70010-x

Johnson, C. E. (2011). Sexual health during pregnancy and the postpartum (CME). *The Journal of Sexual Medicine, 8*(5), 1267–1284. https://doi.org/10.1111/j.1743-6109.2011.02223.x

Korzeniewski, R., Kiemle, G., & Slade, P. (2019). Mothers' experiences of sex and sexual intimacy in the first postnatal year: A systematic review. *Sexual and Relationship Therapy, 36*(2–3), 219–237. https://doi.org/10.1080/14681994.2019.1671969

Marston, C., Conde-Agudelo, A., World Health Organization, Department of Making Pregnancy Safer, & World Health Organization, Reproductive Health and Research. (2007). *Report of a WHO Technical Consultation on Birth spacing, Geneva, Switzerland, 13–15 June 2005.*

McBride, H. L., & Kwee, J. L. (2017). Sex after baby: Women's sexual function in the postpartum period. *Current Sexual Health Reports, 9*(3), 142–149. https://doi.org/10.1007/s11930-017-0116-3

McCance, K., & Cameron, S. (2014). Midwives' experiences and views of giving postpartum contraceptive advice and providing long-acting reversible contraception: A qualitative study. *Journal of Family Planning and Reproductive Health Care*, *40*(3), 177–183. https://doi.org/10.1136/jfprhc-2013-100770

NICE (National Institute for Clinical Excellence). (2021a). *NICE Guideline NG21 Antenatal Care*. London: NICE.

NICE (National Institute for Clinical Excellence). (2021b). *NICE Guideline NG194 Post natal care*. London: NICE.

NMC (Nursing and Midwifery Council). (2019). *Standards of Proficiency for Midwives*. http://www.nmc-org.uk

Oliver, M., Erasmus, H., & Al Dabbagh, R. (2015). Are women interested in receiving contraception in the immediate post natal period? *Poster Presentation at the Annual Scientific Meeting*. London: FSRH.

O'Malley, D., Higgins, A., & Smith, V. (2021). Exploring the complexities of postpartum sexual health. *Current Sexual Health Reports*, *13*(4), 128–135. https://doi.org/10.1007/s11930-021-00315-6

O'Malley, D., & Smith, V. (2013a). Altered sexual health after childbirth: Part 1. *The Practising Midwife*, *16*, 30–32.

O'Malley, D., & Smith, V. (2013b). Altered sexual health after childbirth: Part 2. *The Practising Midwife*, *16*, 27–29.

Orbach, S., & Rubin, H. (2014). *Two for the Price of One: The Impact of Body Image During Pregnancy and After Birth*. London: Government Equalities Office Gov. UK.

Pauleta, J. R., Pereira, N. M., & Graça, L. M. (2010). Sexuality during pregnancy. *The Journal of Sexual Medicine*, *7*(1), 136–142. https://doi.org/10.1111/j.1743-6109.2009.01538.x

Public Health England. (2018). *Health Matters: Reproductive Health and Pregnancy Planning*. London: PHE.

Public Health England. (2019). *Towards Zero HIV Transmission by 2030*. London: PHE.

Public Health England. (2021). *Infectious Diseases in Pregnancy Screening (IDPS) Care Pathway*. London: PHE.

Quilliam, S. (2010). Sex during pregnancy: Yes, yes, yes! *Journal of Family Planning and Reproductive Health Care*, *36*(2), 97–98. https://doi.org/10.1783/147118910791069448

RCN. (2015). *Sexual Health Competencies an Integrated Career and Competence Framework for Sexual and Reproductive Health Nursing Across the UK*. RCN: London.RCN. (2016). *Faircare for Trans Patients: A RCN Guide for Nursing and Health Care Professionals*. RCN: London.

Schummers, L., Hutcheon, J. A., Hernandez-Diaz, S., Williams, P. L., Hacker, M. R., VanderWeele, T. J., & Norman, W. V. (2018). Association of short interpregnancy interval with pregnancy outcomes according to maternal age. *JAMA Internal Medicine*, *178*(12), 1661. https://doi.org/10.1001/jamainternmed.2018.4696

Thwaites, A., Tran, A. B., & Mann, S. (2019). Women's and healthcare professionals' views on immediate postnatal contraception provision: A literature review. *BMJ Sexual & Reproductive Health*, *45*(2), 88–94. https://doi.org/10.1136/bmjsrh-2018-200231

UK Health Security Agency. (2019). *Health Matters: Preventing STI's.* https://ukhsa.
blog.gov.uk

Walker, S. H., & Davis, G. (2014). Knowledge and reported confidence of final year
midwifery students regarding giving advice on contraception and sexual health.
Midwifery, 30(5), e169–e176. https://doi.org/10.1016/j.midw.2014.02.002

Walker SH, Hooks C, Blake D. The views of postnatal women and midwives on
midwives providing contraceptive advice and methods: a mixed method con-
current study. BMC Pregnancy Childbirth. 2021 Jun 2;21(1):411. doi: 10.1186/
s12884-021-03895-2. PMID: 34078302; PMCID: PMC8170056

World Health Organization. (2023). *Sexual Health.* [online] www.who.int. Available
at: https://www.who.int/health-topics/sexual-health#tab=tab_2 [Accessed 18
September 2023].

Woolhouse, H., McDonald, E., & Brown, S. (2012). Women's experiences of sex
and intimacy after childbirth: Making the adjustment to motherhood. *Journal of
Psychosomatic Obstetrics & Gynecology, 33*(4), 185–190. https://doi.org/10.3109/
0167482x.2012.720314

Contraceptive choices after you've had a baby – Contraception – Sexwise. www.
sexwise.org.uk (accessed 20 September 2023). Contraceptive Choices After You've
Had Your Baby (fpa.org.uk)

Education & Training – Faculty of Sexual and Reproductive Healthcare (fsrh.org). www.
fsrh.org.uk (accessed 21 July 2023). Education & Training | FSRH

Violence against Women and Girls

17

HANNAH RAYMENT-JONES AND
ELSA MONTGOMERY

INTRODUCTION

Violence against women and girls is the most widespread form of abuse worldwide and crosses cultural and economic boundaries. It is a fundamental breach of human rights that is recognised as a significant public health problem, with serious consequences on physical, mental, sexual and reproductive health (Garcia-Moreno et al., 2006). Reducing this violence and its associated health impacts has been prioritised by the UK government's Women's Health Strategy (Department of Health & Social Care, 2022). The World Health Organization (WHO, 2021) estimates that about one in three women worldwide have experienced either physical and/or sexual intimate partner violence (IPV) or non-partner sexual violence in their lifetime. This violence takes on many different forms, including physical, psychological and sexual abuse; intimate partner (or domestic) violence; female genital mutilation; child marriage and forced marriage; sex trafficking; and 'honour-based' violence. Most of this violence is thought to be perpetrated by a current or former spouse/partner or family member.

DOI: 10.4324/9781003350071-17

The adverse physical and mental health outcomes that women and girls experience because of abuse leads to an increased use of health care resources. Midwives frequently and often unknowingly encounter women who are experiencing or are affected by violence. Maternity services can provide women a safe environment where they can confidentially disclose experiences of violence and receive a supportive response. They can also be a place of distress where women who have experienced abuse can encounter a lack of control and re-traumatisation. Therefore, it is imperative that those working in maternity services understand this complex issue to care for women and girls appropriately and strengthen support networks for their future. This chapter focuses on IPV and childhood sexual abuse (CSA) and provides an overview of epidemiology, the impact on women and girls, particularly around the time of pregnancy and birth, and the role of maternity services and the midwife.

INTIMATE PARTNER VIOLENCE: AN OVERVIEW AND EPIDEMIOLOGY

The most common type of violence against women is IPV, otherwise known as domestic violence or abuse, which refers to any behaviour within an intimate relationship (including intimate partners and family members) that causes physical, psychological or sexual harm to those in the relationship. Family members are defined as immediate relatives, whether directly related, in-laws or stepfamily (United Nations, 2023). IPV is manifested by physical, sexual or emotional abusive acts as well as controlling behaviours. Table 17.1 depicts some types of IPV (Heise & Garcia-Moreno, 2002). It occurs in all settings and among all socioeconomic, religious, and cultural groups, but there are specific areas of concern for those from specific ethnic groups such as (commonly termed) 'honour-based violence', female genital mutilation, and forced marriage. The overwhelming global burden of IPV is borne by women (Sardinha et al., 2022).

Although people irrespective of gender experience IPV, both cis and trans women are considerably more likely to experience repeated and severe forms of violence (Garthe et al., 2018; Sardinha et al., 2022). Globally, approximately 38% of all murders of women are committed by their intimate partners, compared to 6% of

Table 17.1 Forms and examples of intimate partner violence

Forms of violence	Examples
Physical	Slapping, hitting, biting, kicking, beating, choking
Sexual	Forced sexual intercourse and others forms of sexual coercion
Emotional (psychological)	Insults, belittling, constant humiliation, intimidation, tricking, threats of harm, threats to take away children
Control	Isolation from family and friends, monitoring movements, restricting access to financial resources, employment, education, or medical care

Source: Adapted from Heise and Garcia Moreno (2002).

men murdered by their intimate partner (WHO, 2021). Adolescent girls and young women, women belonging to ethnic minorities, transwomen and women with disabilities or those who are unemployed are at a disproportionate risk (Sardinha & Catalán, 2018).

A growing number of population-based surveys have attempted to measure prevalence, most notably the WHO multi-country study on women's health and domestic violence, which collected data on IPV from more than 24,000 women in ten countries, representing diverse cultural, geographical and urban/rural settings (Garcia-Moreno et al., 2006). Figure 17.1 shows the prevalence of lifetime physical violence by an intimate partner according to severity of violence for ever-partnered women, by site.

In the UK, recent figures from the Crime Survey for England and Wales (Elkin, 2022) reported that 7% of women aged 16 years and over experienced IPV, equating to an estimated 1.7 million women. It estimates that approximately one in five adults had experienced some form of IPV since the age of 16, and that this number has steadily risen in the past few decades. This increase could be due to increased victim reporting. The Crown Prosecution Service (CPS) domestic abuse-related charging rate in England and Wales also increased for the first time in four years to 72.7% in 2022 (Elkin, 2022).

The data on reported incidents of IPV merely show the tip of the iceberg. This is due to myriad of reasons leading to victims of IPV being less likely than victims of other violence to report their experiences. This reluctance to report incidents may be because of the belief that it is not a matter for police involvement, fear of being reported to social care or the home office in cases of irregular migration, 'victim blaming', a significant fear of reprisal from the perpetrator, or fear of not being believed, or that the risks of disclosure are perceived to outweigh the benefits (Decker et al., 2019).

There are high-level global and national commitments to reduce violence against women and girls, with a consistent focus on IPV. The UN's Sustainable Development Goals (SDGs) have placed an emphasis on eliminating all forms of violence against women and girls (SDG target 5.2) as a pathway to achieving SDG 5: 'Achieve gender equality and empower all women and girls' (WHO, 2021). Many national governments, including the UK, have laws that explicitly criminalise IPV, but there remains legal inconsistency across the globe.

PREVALENCE OF INTIMATE PARTNER VIOLENCE IN PREGNANCY

Estimating the prevalence of IPV in pregnancy is difficult; significant variations in estimates across the globe are often due to different definitions of IPV and how many disclosures are reported and/or recorded. To establish a baseline prevalence, the WHO commissioned a large, multinational study across 15 countries into the prevalence of physical violence reported in pregnancy, which was found to be between 1% and 15%. Between 20% and 50% of these women reported direct trauma to the abdomen, and over 90% of the perpetrators were the biological fathers of the fetus (Ellsberg et al., 2008). A more recent systematic review collated worldwide literature

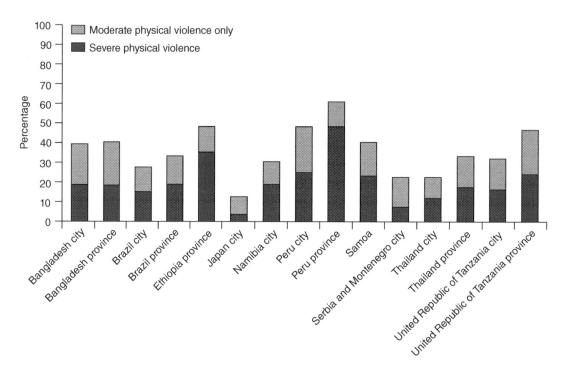

Figure 17.1 Prevalence of IPV by severity across sites.

Source: Garcia-Moreno et al. (2006).

from over 50 countries, on prevalence rates of different types of IPV in pregnancy, finding one-quarter of pregnant women or mothers exposed to IPV on average and wide variation between countries (Román-Gálvez et al., 2021). When combining countries, it found that that, on average, one in ten mothers were exposed to physical IPV, 1 in 5 to psychological IPV and 1 in 20 to sexual IPV. The differences between countries showed that IPV rates were the highest in Africa (except for psychological IPV which was higher in North America) and lowest in Europe. In the East of Africa and Southeast of Asia, the rates are twice or more as high as the rest. These estimates should be viewed with caution given the low-quality nature of the studies included; however, an analysis of the WHO Global Database on Prevalence of Violence Against Women of over 2 million women found similar estimates; 27% of ever-partnered women aged 15–49 years were estimated to have experienced IPV in their lifetime. They found that violence starts early with 24%–26% of women aged 15–24 years having already experienced IPV at least once since the age of 15. Again, regional variation was found, with low-income countries reporting higher IPV compared with high-income countries.

To add to the complexity, some contexts report a higher prevalence of IPV during pregnancy than before or after the pregnancy, and others a smaller prevalence during pregnancy. This may be due to cultural variations, and/or fear of disclosure during pregnancy due to safeguarding practices or immigration control (Rayment-Jones et al., 2019). That said, various enquiries into maternal deaths have identified IPV as a major factor leading to death in the perinatal period (Campbell et al., 2021).

The studies above all found higher prevalence of IPV in countries that are affected by conflict. This demonstrates the importance of considering the different social, economic, and political circumstances that are associated with IPV and how these can limit women's ability to leave abusive relationships, such as financial insecurity, gender inequitable norms, high amounts of societal stigma, discriminatory family and immigration law and inadequate support services (Sardinha & Catalán, 2018; Sardinha et al., 2022).

It is crucial to reflect on how COVID-19 restrictions and 'lockdowns' exacerbated the rates and severity of IPV, impeding victims' ability to disclose, seek help or leave abusive relationships. Again, a socioeconomic divide became apparent; economic independence is a critical factor in the prevention of IPV. For many women who experience IPV, the financial entanglement with an abusive partner is too convoluted to sever without an alternative source of economic support. The pandemic caused significant job losses, particularly among racially diverse communities, migrants and those without higher education. In addition, public health restrictions put in place to combat the spread of COVID-19, including travel restrictions, reduced access to healthcare, safe spaces and IPV support including emergency housing and shelters exacerbating the experiences of IPV (Evans et al., 2020).

THE IMPACT OF INTIMATE PARTNER VIOLENCE

IPV can have devastating and long-lasting effects on the victims and their families' health and quality of life. A U.S. analysis of the economic cost of IPV estimated that health care costs were 42% higher for women experiencing IPV (McLean & Gonzalez Bocinski, 2017).

The associated health consequences are varied and women suffering IPV obviously do not all have the same set of symptoms or experiences. Although victims of IPV are frequently visiting health care services, they generally do not present with obvious trauma or specific symptoms (Coker et al., 2000). This phenomenon is thought to be because of long-term negative health consequences for victims, even after abuse has ended, manifesting as poor health status, poor quality of life and high use of health services (Bonomi et al., 2009). However, there is a wealth of evidence showing that bruising is one of the most common injuries sustained by women through IPV, followed by a multitude of physical and mental health problems listed in Table 17.2.

The adverse consequences of IPV on children must also be considered when caring for families experiencing abuse and developing interventions to reduce its prevalence. Up to 60% of children directly witness IPV and are used in threats or as a spy, with repercussions such as removal from the family due to safeguarding concerns or living in a refuge with their mother. Children exposed to IPV have a higher risk of physical, emotional, behavioural, and educational problems that persist into adulthood (Pinheiro, 2006).

Table 17.2 Physical and mental health problems associated with intimate partner violence

Physical health risks	Stress-related/ functional disorders	Mental health risks
Bruises and welts	Headaches/migraine	Depression
Lacerations and abrasions, abdominal or thoracic injuries	Irritable bowel syndrome	Anxiety
Fractures/broken bones and teeth	Gastrointestinal symptoms	Phobias
Sight and hearing damage	Fibromyalgia	Suicide
Head injury	Dysmenorrhoea	Alcohol and drug abuse
Attempted strangulation	Dyspareunia	Eating and sleep disorders
Back and neck injury/ chronic pain	Various chronic pain syndromes	Physical inactivity
Arthritis	Exacerbation of asthma	Poor self-esteem
Sexually transmitted infections	Angina and chest pain	Post-traumatic stress disorder
Smear abnormalities	Bladder and kidney infections Stomach ulcers	Smoking self-harm unsafe sexual behaviour cancer worries

INTIMATE PARTNER VIOLENCE AND PREGNANCY

The nature of violence can alter during pregnancy, with physical violence aimed directly at the woman's abdomen having a direct effect on the mother and the fetus (Bullock et al., 2006). Women who experience violence in pregnancy have an almost 40% higher risk of morbidity, leading to antenatal admission, such as hypertension, premature rupture of membranes and anaemia (Aizer, 2011). Table 17.3 shows physical and psychological health outcomes found directly and indirectly related to IPV in pregnancy. We also need to consider that negative maternal behaviours, insufficient nutrition, poor access and engagement with maternity care, and increased stress levels associated with IPV can all contribute to poor perinatal outcomes (Pires de Almeida et al., 2013; Sardinha et al., 2022).

At its extreme, IPV in pregnancy causes death to the mother and the unborn. The most recent review into maternal deaths in the UK between 2019 and 2021 (Knight et al., 2023) found that 12% of the women who died during or up to a year after pregnancy were at severe and multiple disadvantaged. The main elements of multiple disadvantages were a mental health diagnosis, substance use and domestic abuse. The report highlighted that information about domestic abuse was missing from 30% of the records of all women who died. Multiple adversity, including mental health, substance abuse, migrant, or asylum seeker status and non-English speaking, was a major theme amongst the women who were murdered, which may have made disclosing IPV even more difficult. The avoidable deaths of these women emphasise the need for complex and nuanced care. The report recommends that healthcare providers working with pregnant women ask about IPV in a kind,

Table 17.3 Health outcomes associated with intimate partner violence in pregnancy

Physical	Psychological
Hypertension	Depression
Premature rupture of membranes	Anxiety
Preterm labour and birth	Pressured into pregnancy and/or abortion
Fetal distress	Negative attitudes towards pregnancy
Anaemia	Poor relationship with the unborn
Low birth weight	Less likely to breastfeed
Miscarriage	Decreased confidence in ability to parent
Oedema	Childhood behavioural problems
Vomiting and dehydration	
Urinary and renal tract infections	
Weight loss during pregnancy	
Operative delivery	
Placental abruption, antepartum haemorrhage	
Placenta previa	
Rupture of the uterus, liver or spleen	
Maternal, fetal and neonatal death	

sensitive way at the earliest opportunity i.e., at the booking appointment and when they are alone allowing for a private one to one discussion.

IDENTIFYING INTIMATE PARTNER VIOLENCE IN PRACTICE

The most effective way to identify IPV is by directly asking women; in fact, research has shown that survivors want to be asked (Chang et al., 2005). Routine enquiry not only identifies women at risk of a plethora of adverse health outcomes but raises awareness, reduces stigma, and demonstrates an intolerance of violence against women. However, some midwives are reluctant to embrace enquiry into IPV because they lack the confidence, knowledge and system support to do so, or feel unable to respond with effective advice and support in the event of a disclosure (Hegarty et al., 2020).

Many organisations aiming to prevent IPV recognise that healthcare providers should be trained to understand the relationship between IPV and women's poor health and respond appropriately. The WHO (2012) identified the importance of maternity services in the identification of violence due to the multiple entry points throughout the antenatal period. Women may not disclose on the first occasion they are asked; therefore, it is important to bear in mind the need to make routine enquiries on a number of occasions and prioritise continuity of care (Barron, 2014; Rayment-Jones, 2023a). Midwives are in a unique position to offer support and safe referral; however, this is often hampered by the poor coordination of services, inadequate knowledge and by midwives own experiences, beliefs, and attitudes concerning IPV and who is at risk (Hegarty et al., 2020). It must be remembered that health professionals, too, can be victims of abuse and that IPV occurs across all social classes and within all ethnic groups.

The NICE (2010) guidelines for women with complex social factors highlighted five key issues for midwives enquiring about and women disclosing violence:

1. Fear of the potential involvement of social services and child custody.
2. Anxiety that their partner will find out they have disclosed the abuse.
3. Insufficient time for health care professionals to deal with the issue appropriately.
4. Insufficient support and training for health care professionals in asking about domestic abuse.
5. Perception of domestic abuse as a taboo subject that should not be discussed.

Recommendations continue to focus on the practicalities of routine enquiry including: compulsory education for undergraduate curricula and continued professional development for midwives and include a structure for referral to appropriate support and follow-up; this may increase midwives confidence and likelihood to enquire.

If appropriate, women should be asked about IPV in pregnancy during social history taking at booking or at another opportune point during their antenatal care. The MBRRACE report (Knight et al., 2021) recommended women should be seen alone at least once during the antenatal period to facilitate disclosure. This can be difficult for women who are experiencing abuse as controlling partners often accompany them. This scenario can be seen as a warning sign to health professionals, and innovative schemes to identify and direct help towards women in this situation have been set up in Trusts across the UK. These include IPV information in toilets, placing a small sticker on their urine pot to alert staff and the provision of information disguised as a bar code number on their notes for the 24 Hour National Domestic Violence Helpline run by Women's Aid and Refuge. The Helpline is free, staffed 24 hours a day by fully trained female helpline workers and all calls are completely confidential. There is a wealth of literature and useful resources for midwives to support these conversations.

If, during an appointment, it is deemed safe to proceed, a midwife can broach the subject using direct but open-ended questions. The qualitative study by Chang et al. (2005) identified women want the person asking the question to give a reason for doing so to reduce suspicions and minimise stigma. This reason could be given in the form of discussing routine screening due to the known increased incidence of IPV in pregnancy. Women also want a safe and supportive environment, and to be given information around access to support regardless of whether they disclose IPV or not. Once it is deemed safe to proceed, a midwife can broach the subject using the following direct but open-ended questions and responses (Hegarty et al., 2008) (Table 17.4):

Figure 17.2 below shows the Duluth 'Power and Control' training model (Pence & Paymar, 1993), which was developed by survivors of IPV to illustrate the many different abusive behaviours of perpetrators. It can be used as a tool to open up discussions on relationships and understand who might be at risk and why through consideration of different forms of abuse. It is stressed, however, that IPV remains common in all demographic groups. Cook and Bewley (2008) emphasise that there is no 'typical' victim, and it is unhelpful, and even stigmatising, to focus attention on one single population, just as it is important not to assume that any individual is at 'low risk'.

Table 17.4 Direct and open ended questions & responses

Questions	Responses
How are things at home?	Everybody deserves to feel safe at home.
Who lives at home with you?	You don't deserve to be hit or hurt. It is not your fault.
Are there any problems at home? Tell me about your relationship.	I am concerned about your safety and wellbeing.
Does anyone ever try to control what you do?	You are not alone, and help is available.
Is there somebody that you are frightened of or who hurts you?	Abuse is common and happens in all kinds of relationships. It tends to continue.

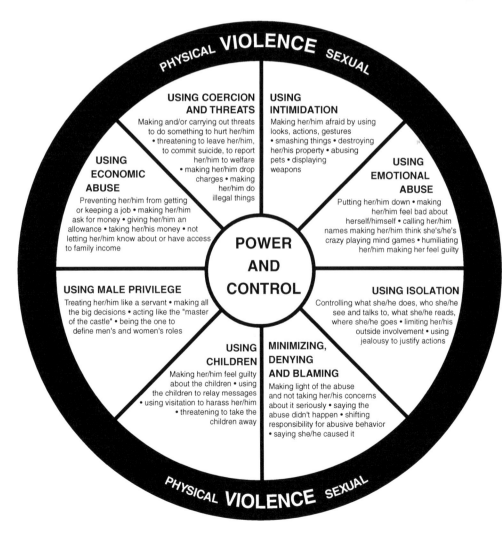

Figure 17.2 The Duluth Power and Control Wheel training model.

Source: Developed by Domestic Abuse Intervention Project, Duluth, MN, https://www.theduluthmodel.org/.

REFERRAL AND SUPPORT: THE MIDWIFE'S ROLE

The lack of a coherent and consistent process for reporting abuse can be discouraging for people seeking help through the healthcare and legal systems. Certain populations, such as minoritised ethnic groups who have long faced oppression and brutality by police, migrants and those with social care involvement may be reluctant to involve the police when IPV escalates (Rayment-Jones et al., 2019; Evans et al., 2020). It is imperative that processes are not only in place to identify and effectively communicate with those experiencing IPV, but also pathways for safe and meaningful support when a disclosure is made. If a midwife suspects IPV or a woman discloses, the midwife must act quickly and appropriately by assessing risk and providing information. This should be carried out in a non-judgemental and sensitive manner, ensuring that the woman is fully informed and involved in the decision-making process (Sohal & Johnson, 2014). It is crucial that any action taken does not in any way increase the danger the woman is facing. Barron (2014) suggests the following seven actions that could be taken to ensure safety, but it should be noted that this guidance is specific to the UK context:

1. For assessing immediate danger, the following questions may be helpful:
   a   Is your partner here with you?
   b. Where are the children?
   c. Is it safe for you to return home today?
   d. Do you have any immediate concerns?
   e. Do you have a place of safety?
   f. If you feel a woman is at immediate risk, do any of the following:
       i.   Contact independent intimate partner or domestic violence advisor and safeguarding leads.
       ii. Police: 999.
       iii. Contact a friend/family member not known to the perpetrator.
       iv. Contact Refuge (0808 2000 247) for emergency accommodation.
2. Give her time to talk about her experience, listen to her and show you believe her.

3. Give her contact numbers and information about how to protect herself and her children. The aim of providing information is to give women choices about how to protect themselves and their children and where to go for help. The first option will usually be to signpost the woman to a specialist IPV organisation. Contact details for national support services can be found in 'Further Reading and Information'. It may also be a local service depending on the woman's individual needs. For example, for women who do not speak English, or have safe access to the Internet or a phone. It is important that the midwife giving the information is trained to do so, aware of key sources of information or local services and considers the safety of the woman and her children as part of the process.

4. Do NOT give advice on what to do – it is her decision, and she will have real reasons behind it.

5. Support her in whatever decision she makes.

6. Keep detailed records that can only be accessed by relevant professionals. Do NOT document these discussions in a woman's hand-held notes.

7. Arrange a follow-up appointment and any follow-up referrals that may be helpful (see 'Further Reading and Information' for a list of these resources and ensure you are aware of local support services and advocacy groups). Discuss these with the woman.

RECOMMENDATIONS FOR FUTURE UK MATERNITY SERVICES

The review by Marmot et al. (2008) of social determinants of health encourages the development of partnerships, with those affected by complex social factors working with their health providers. Central to this approach is empowerment through putting in place effective mechanisms that give those affected a real say in decisions that affect their lives, and that recognise their fundamental human rights. These values are echoed in recent maternity service policies and guidelines, encouraging women-centred, individualised care, with a focus on choice and continuity of carer. Research on maternal and infant outcomes of women with complex social factors, including IPV, has described how community-based antenatal care and continuity of care improves access and engagement with services and clinical outcomes, including preterm birth and low birth weight (Rayment-Jones et al., 2021, 2023a). When women experience continuity of care, they are more likely to disclose sensitive issues such as IPV due to increased opportunity and trust (Rayment-Jones et al., 2023).

CHILDHOOD SEXUAL ABUSE: AN OVERVIEW

Women who access maternity services whilst experiencing IPV are more likely than other women to have also experienced CSA. Seng et al. (2008) found that women were three times more likely to be abused as an adult if they had been abused as a child. More recently, the Office for National Statistics (ONS) in the UK has revealed that 51% of those who experience abuse as children go on to experience IPV as adults (ONS, 2017). CSA casts a long shadow and unlike those experiencing IPV, survivors may not be in present danger and have obvious injuries, the physical and psychological impact can last a lifetime (Hughes et al., 2017). The term 'non-recent abuse' is therefore a more accurate reflection of survivors' lived experience than the often-used 'historic abuse'. This is how one research participant described her on-going experience:

> It is something that I carry around with me like… a little bag… it is part of me. I can't make it go away…so it's just sort of encompassed as part of the person that I am (Sam).

(Montgomery, 2012)

It must be remembered that some women in the maternity system will be pregnant by the perpetrator.

DEFINING CHILDHOOD SEXUAL ABUSE

CSA can be defined as "forcing or enticing a child or young person to take part in sexual activities, not necessarily involving a high level of violence, whether or not the child is aware of what is happening" (HM Government, 2018). Table 17.5 shows the list of activities that may constitute CSA and illustrates that CSA does not necessarily involve contact.

Children are commonly abused by people known to them, family members, acquaintances or people outside those immediate circles but in positions of trust or authority. In a National Society for the Prevention of Cruelty to Children (NSPCC) report, it was identified that nearly 66% of contact sexual abuse was perpetrated by under-18s against other children or young adults. Of concern is the fact that when children had experienced contact abuse by a peer, no one else knew in nearly 83% of cases compared with 34% of cases when contact abuse had been perpetrated by an adult. Although most perpetrators are male (Radford et al., 2011), it is increasingly recognised that women also sexually abuse children.

PREVALENCE AND EFFECTS ON HEALTH

There is no source in England and Wales that provides prevalence figures for abuse in childhood. Determining prevalence from the literature is complicated by variations in whether young people aged 16–18 are included and whether the definition encompasses both contact and non-contact abuse. Furthermore, it can take a long time for children to disclose abuse and for some, traumatic memories are buried deep and do not surface for many years. It is generally recognised that approximately 20% of females experience CSA (Pereda et al., 2009). This figure was broadly

Table 17.5 Defining sexual abuse

Contact	Includes:
	• Assault by penetration (e.g. rape or oral sex)
	• Non-penetrative acts such as masturbation, kissing, rubbing and touching outside of clothing
Non-contact	Includes:
	• Involving children in looking at, or in the production of, sexual images
	• Watching sexual activities
	• Encouraging children to behave in sexually inappropriate ways
	• Grooming a child in preparation for abuse (including via the Internet)

Source: Adapted from HM Government (2018).

corroborated in an international meta-analysis including studies from 16 countries that reported a pooled prevalence of 24% (Pan et al., 2021).

As with victims of IPV, those with a history of CSA are likely to have significant health issues. Adverse childhood experiences (ACEs) (see Table 17.6), including CSA, significantly increase the risk of conditions in adults that are major global public health challenges. The risk increases for those with multiple ACEs (Hughes et al., 2017). Conditions include cancer, cardiovascular and respiratory disease, diabetes, depression, and anxiety. Those who have experienced ACE are also more likely to be smokers, have problematic alcohol use and take illicit drugs (Hughes et al., 2017).

Mental health-related causes currently account for nearly 40% of the maternal deaths that happen from six weeks to a year after birth in the UK and Ireland (Knight et al., 2023). Suicide is the leading cause of direct deaths during this period. Overall, 7% of the women who died in the latest MBRRACE report had a known history of abuse as a child. This information was missing for 40% of the women (Knight et al., 2023). The multiple disadvantages, that is a significant factor among the women who died include both IPV and CSA.

Survivors of CSA are regular users of health services but frequently do not disclose their history of abuse to healthcare professionals. They are a silent, hidden population within the maternity system (Montgomery et al., 2015a) and this can create challenges for those providing their care.

CHILDHOOD SEXUAL ABUSE AND PREGNANCY

In their systematic review on ACE and adverse pregnancy outcomes, Mamum et al. (2023) found an association with pre-term birth, low birth weight, gestational diabetes, and antenatal depression. However, Brunton and Dryer (2021), in their systematic review which focuses specifically on CSA and pregnancy outcomes, were more cautious. Although they agreed the evidence suggests that those with a history of CSA are probably more likely to have adverse experiences, their conclusions were tentative due to variability in the way abuse was operationalised and measured in studies. What is clear is that many aspects of pregnancy and birth can replicate survivors' experiences of abuse and be traumatising (Montgomery et al., 2015b). The intimate aspects of care, like vaginal examinations, can of course be

Table 17.6 Adverse childhood experiences

- Physical abuse
- Sexual Abuse
- Emotional Abuse
- Living with someone who abused drugs
- Living with someone who abused alcohol
- Exposure to domestic violence
- Living with someone who has gone to prison
- Living with someone with serious mental illness
- Losing a parent through divorce, death, or abandonment

Source: Adapted from Huges et al. (2017).

difficult, but it is not necessarily these aspects that are particularly challenging. For some, pregnancy itself can be triggering because the baby is taking over their body. Survivors often feel guilt and shame about their childhood history. Fear of judgement prevents disclosure (Montgomery et al., 2015a). From the perspective of the midwife caring for them, there may be little to distinguish them from many other clients.

IDENTIFYING CHILDHOOD SEXUAL ABUSE

NICE guidelines for Antenatal Care (2021) recommend enquiry for IPV, but do not mention CSA. They recommended that women are asked about previous or current mental health concerns. Although screening for CSA occurs elsewhere (e.g., the Netherlands and the United States), there is little evidence to show that it improves outcomes (Ades et al., 2019). Seng et al. (2008) discovered that less than 27% of the women with histories of CSA identified in a research setting were identified by clinical screening. It requires a great deal of trust for women to disclose abuse, not least because once they have revealed their history, they potentially lose control over what happens to the information about a very private aspect of their life. It may be that asking a direct question is not helpful in relation to experience of CSA. However, indicating that it is an appropriate topic of conversation should they wish to discuss it is very important. Explaining to women that for some pregnancy can trigger unexpected memories or feelings from childhood and that they are welcome to discuss it if that happens to them may provide an opening if a woman would like to talk. Ultimately, the decision as to whether to disclose and control of the information must stay with the woman.

Few healthcare professionals cover caring for women who have experienced CSA during their undergraduate or post qualifying education and often feel anxious about broaching the subject (Montgomery & Chang, 2023). Personalised care following the woman's lead is needed. Recognising discomfort, providing the opportunity to talk, and responding in a way that avoids re-traumatisation is important (Law et al., 2021). If a woman does disclose, a trauma-informed approach is essential. This includes listening carefully, letting her know that she is believed, acknowledging the harm experienced and the courage disclosure must have taken (The Survivors Trust, n.d.). It is also important that the decision as to what happens to the information rests with the woman – unless they indicate that there may be a current safeguarding issue. Some will want the information to be recorded in their medical records so that they do not have to repeat the disclosure every time they see someone new. Others will prefer to decide on an individual basis who they trust with the information and will not therefore want it to be documented.

CARING FOR WOMEN WITH A HISTORY OF CSA

Whether or not the abuse is disclosed, it is important that they experience sensitive care during the perinatal period. Unlike those suffering from IPV, there are no usually outward signs to alert midwives to the issue of CSA. Once IPV has been recognised, there is a clear pathway for midwives to follow; however, there is less explicit guidance available for midwives caring for women when they suspect CSA. As midwives may not realise that they are caring for a woman who experienced CSA, 'universal precautions' (Coles & Jones, 2009) are needed. This means that all women are treated in a manner that minimises the risk of trauma for those affected and are treated with dignity and respect. What is helpful or unhelpful will depend on the woman, how they are at that time, their relationship with those providing care, their attitude, and the context (Montgomery et al., 2015a).

Feeling safe is important for those who experienced non-recent CSA. However, for the latter group of women, 'feeling safe' means not being reminded of their abuse (Montgomery, 2013). Unfortunately, even when midwifery care is provided in a sensitive manner, there are many ways in which pregnancy, birth and maternity care can be reminiscent of abuse. Sometimes, this is due to the similarity of bodily sensations experienced, or the vulnerability felt during intimate examinations. Sometimes, less immediately obvious situations can trigger memories for women such as hearing footsteps outside the room and wondering who it is and what it means for them (Montgomery et al., 2015b). These situations may not be predicted by the women themselves, which adds an extra layer of complexity in caring for them. As recognised by Garratt (2011, p189), 'the most useful guide to providing appropriate care for a woman with a history of abuse is the woman herself'. This is sound advice that empowers the woman, and was echoed by a survivor in the study by Montgomery and Chang (2023):

> It's going back to this 'oh we've done our training; we know what you as a survivor want' and actually they need to just ask.

(p. 5)

Although women report feeling violated again by their experience of childbirth, it can also be a healing process. Control is pivotal in determining how women experience their maternity care (Montgomery, 2013). Sensitive care, in which women get to know and trust those caring for them are viewed as partners in their care and during which midwives both listen to them and hear the messages they are trying to convey, can help a woman to change her perception of herself and appreciate the good her body can do.

PRACTICE POINTS

- Women may not respond to a direct question about abuse but need to know they can talk about it if they want to.
- Recognise and respond sensitively to a woman's distress even if she does not want to name abuse.
- Control is of paramount importance for these women.

SUMMARY

- Both IPV and CSA are complex issues which severely impact on women's physical and mental health.
- Midwives are in a unique position to identify IPV due to the nature of antenatal care and the known increased incidence of abuse in pregnancy.
- Inquiry should only take place in a safe and private environment when a woman is on her own.
- Women should be given information on how to access support and protect themselves and their children in a safe way.
- Women want to 'feel safe' and for those with a history of CSA this means not being reminded of their abuse.
- A trauma-informed approach will facilitate provision responsive, personalised care to all.

REFERENCES

Ades, V., Goddard, B., & Ayala, S. P. (2019). Caring for long term health needs in women with a history of sexual trauma. *BMJ, 367,* l5825. https://doi.org/10.1136/bmj.l5825

Aizer, A. (2011). Poverty, violence, and health: The impact of domestic violence during pregnancy on newborn health. *Journal of Human Resources, 46*(3), 518–538. https://doi.org/10.1353/jhr.2011.0024

Barron, J. (2014). Sources of referral and support for domestic violence. In S. Bewley & J. Welch (Eds.), *ABC of Domestic and Sexual Violence* (pp. 41–45). Chichester: Wiley.

Bonomi, A. E., Anderson, M. L., Rivara, F. P., & Thompson, R. S. (2009). Health care utilization and costs associated with physical and nonphysical-only intimate partner violence. *Health Services Research, 44*(3), 1052–1067. https://doi.org/10.1111/j.1475-6773.2009.00955.x

Brunton, R., & Dryer, R. (2021). Child sexual abuse and pregnancy: A systematic review of the literature. *Child Abuse and Neglect, 111,* 104802. https://doi.org/10.1016/j.chiabu.2020.104802

Bullock, L., Bloom, T., Davis, J., Kilburn, E., & Curry, M. A. (2006). Abuse disclosure in privately and medicaid-funded pregnant women. *Journal of Midwifery and Women's Health, 51*(5), 361–369. https://doi.org/10.1016/j.jmwh.2006.02.012

Campbell, J., Matoff-Stepp, S., Velez, M. L., Cox, H. H., & Laughon, K. (2021). Pregnancy-associated deaths from homicide, suicide, and drug overdose: Review of research and the intersection with intimate partner violence. *Journal of Women's Health, 30*(2), 236–244. https://doi.org/10.1089/jwh.2020.8875

Chang, J. C., Decker, M. R., Moracco, K. E., Martin, S. L., Petersen, R., & Frasier, P. Y. (2005). Asking about intimate partner violence: Advice from female survivors to health care providers. *Patient Education and Counseling, 59*(2), 141–147. https://doi.org/10.1016/j.pec.2004.10.008

Coker, A. L., Smith, P. H., Mckeown, R. E., & King, M. J. (2000) Frequency & correlates of intimate partner violence by type. *Am J Public Health, 90*(4), 553–559.

Coles, J., & Jones, K. (2009). Universal precautions: Perinatal touch and examination after childhood sexual abuse. *Birth, 36*(3), 230–236. https://doi.org/10.1111/j.1523-536X.2009.00327.x

Cook, J., & Bewley, S. (2008). Acknowledging a persistent truth: Domestic violence in pregnancy. *Journal of the Royal Society of Medicine, 101*(7), 358–363. https://doi.org/10.1258/jrsm.2008.080002

Decker, M. R., Holliday, C. N., Hameeduddin, Z., Shah, R., Miller, J., Dantzler, J., & Goodmark, L. (2019). "You do not think of me as a human being": Race and gender inequities intersect to discourage police reporting of violence against women. *Journal of Urban Health, 96*(5), 772–783. https://doi.org/10.1007/s11524-019-00359-z

Department of Health & Social Care. (2022). *Women's Health Strategy for England August 2022* (publishing.service.gov.uk). Women's Health Strategy for England - GOV.UK (www.gov.uk)

Ellsberg, M., Jansen, H. A. F. M., Heise, L., Watts, C. H., & Garcia-Moreno, C. (2008). Intimate partner violence and women's physical and mental health in the WHO multi-country study on women's health and domestic violence: An observational study. *The Lancet, 371*(9619), 1165–1172. https://doi.org/10.1016/S0140-6736(08)60522-X

Evans, M. L., Lindauer, M., & Farrell, M. E. (2020). A pandemic within a pandemic – Intimate partner violence during COVID-19. *New England Journal of Medicine, 383*(24), 2302–2304. https://doi.org/10.1056/nejmp2024046

Garcia-Moreno, C., Jansen, H. A., Ellsberg, M., Heise, L., & Watts, C. H. (2006). Prevalence of intimate partner violence: Findings from the WHO multi-country study on women's health and domestic violence. *The Lancet, 368*(9543), 1260–1269. https://doi.org/10.1016/S0140-6736(06)69523-8

Garratt, L. (2011). *Survivors of Childhood Sexual Abuse and Midwifery Practice.* Oxford: Radcliffe Publishing.

Garthe, R. C., Hidalgo, M. A., Hereth, J., Garofalo, R., Reisner, S. L., Mimiaga, M. J., & Kuhns, L. (2018). Prevalence and risk correlates of intimate partner violence among a multisite cohort of young transgender women. *LGBT Health, 5*(6), 333. https://doi.org/10.1089/lgbt.2018.0034

Hegarty, K., McKibbin, G., Hameed, M., Koziol-McLain, J., Feder, G., Tarzia, L., & Hooker, L. (2020). Health practitioners' readiness to address domestic violence and abuse: A qualitative meta-synthesis. *PLoS One, 15*(6), e0234067. https://doi.org/10.1371/journal.pone.0234067

Hegarty K, Taft A, Feder G. Violence between intimate partners: working with the whole family. BMJ. 2008 Aug 4;337:a839. doi: 10.1136/bmj.a839. PMID: 18678595.

Heise, L., & Garcia-Moreno, C. (2002). Violence by intimate partners. In E. Krug, L. Dahlberg, J. Mercy, A. Zwi, & R. Lozano (Eds.), *World Report on Violence and Health* (pp. 87–121). WHO.

HM Government. (2018) *Working Together to Safeguard Children: A Guide to Inter-Agency Working to Safeguard and Promote the Welfare of Children.* London: Crown Copyright.

Hughes, K., Bellis, M. A., Hardcastle, K. A., Sethi, D., Butchart, A., Mikton, C., Jones, L., & Dunne, M. P. (2017). The effect of multiple adverse childhood experiences on health: a systematic review and meta-analysis. *The Lancet Public Health, 2*(8), e356–e366. https://doi.org/10.1016/S2468-2667(17)30118-4

Knight, M., Bunch, K., Felker, A., Patel, R., Kotnis, R., Kenyon, S., & Kurinczuk, J. J. (2023). *Saving Lives, Improving Mothers' Care Maternal, Newborn and Infant Clinical Outcome Review Programme*. www.hqip.org.uk/national-programmes.

Knight, M., Bunch, K., Tuffnell, D., Patel, R., Shakespeare, J., Kotnis, R., Kenyon, S., & Kurinczuk, J. J. (2021). *Saving Lives, Improving Mothers' Care Maternal, Newborn and Infant Clinical Outcome Review Programme*. www.hqip.org.uk/national-programmes.

Law, C., Wolfenden, L., Sperlich, M., & Taylor, J. (2021). *A Good Practice Guide to Support Trauma-Informed Care in the Perinatal Period* (J. Seng & T. Julie (Eds.)). https://www.england.nhs.uk/publication/a-good-practice-guide-to-support-implementation-of-trauma-informed-care-in-the-perinatal-period/

Marmot, M., Friel, S., Bell, R., Houweling, T. A., & Taylor, S. (2008). Closing the gap in a generation: Health equity through action on the social determinants of health. *The Lancet, 372*(9650), 1661–1669. https://doi.org/10.1016/S0140-6736(08)61690-6

McLean, G., & Gonzalez Bocinski, S. (2017). *The Economic Cost of Intimate Partner Violence, Sexual Assault, and Stalking*, Fact Sheet, Institute of Women's Policy Research.

Montgomery, E. (2012). *Voicing the Silence: The Maternity Care Experiences of Women Who Were Sexually Abused in Childhood*. Midwives. 2015 Spring;18:36. PMID: 25958452

Montgomery, E. (2013). Feeling safe: A metasynthesis of the maternity care needs of women who were sexually abused in childhood. *Birth, 40*(2), 88. https://doi.org/10.1111/birt.12043

Montgomery, E., & Chang, Y. S. (2023). 'What do I do?' A study to inform development of an e-resource for maternity healthcare professionals and students caring for people with lived experience of childhood sexual abuse. *Midwifery, 125*, 103780. https://doi.org/10.1016/j.midw.2023.103780

Montgomery, E., Pope, C., & Rogers, J. (2015a). A feminist narrative study of the maternity care experiences of women who were sexually abused in childhood. *Midwifery, 31*(1), 54–60. https://doi.org/10.1016/j.midw.2014.05.010

Montgomery, E., Pope, C., & Rogers, J. (2015b). The re-enactment of childhood sexual abuse in maternity care: A qualitative study. *BMC Pregnancy and Childbirth, 15*(1). https://doi.org/10.1186/s12884-015-0626-9

NICE. (2010). *Pregnancy and Complex Social Factors: A Model for Service Provision for Pregnant Women with Complex Social Factors Clinical guideline*. www.nice.org.uk/guidance/cg110

NICE. (2021). *Antenatal Care NICE Guideline*. www.nice.org.uk/guidance/ng201

Office for National Statistics. (2017, September 27). *People Who Were Abused as Children are More Likely to be Abused as an Adult*. People who were abused as children are more likely to be abused as an adult - Office for National Statistics (ons.gov.uk)

Pan, Y., Lin, X., Liu, J., Zhang, S., Zeng, X., Chen, F., & Wu, J. (2021). Prevalence of Childhood Sexual Abuse Among Women Using the Childhood Trauma Questionnaire: A Worldwide Meta-Analysis. Trauma, Violence, & Abuse, 22(5), 1181–1191. https://doi.org/10.1177/1524838020912867

Pence, E., & Paymar, M. (1993). *Education Groups for Men Who Batter. The Duluth Model*. New York: Springer.

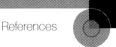
Pereda, N., Guilera, G., Forns, M., & Gómez-Benito, J. (2009). The prevalence of child sexual abuse in community and student samples: A meta-analysis. *Clinical Psychology Review*, *29*(4), 328–338. https://doi.org/10.1016/j.cpr.2009.02.007

Pinheiro, Paulo S. de M. S., & UN. Independent Expert for the United Nations Study on Violence against Children. (2006). *World Report on Violence against Children*. UN.

Pires de Almeida, C., Sá, E., Cunha, F., & Pires, E. P. (2013). Violence during pregnancy and its effects on mother-baby relationship during pregnancy. *Journal of Reproductive and Infant Psychology*, *31*(4), 370–380. https://doi.org/10.1080/02646838.2013.822058

Radford, L., Corral, S., Bradley, C., Fisher, H., Bassett, C., Howat, N., & Collishaw, S. (2011). *Child Abuse and Neglect in the UK Today*. Child abuse and neglect in the UK today | NSPCC Learning

Rayment-Jones, H., Dalrymple, K., Harris, J., Harden, A., Parslow, E., Georgi, T., & Sandall, J. (2021). Project20: Does continuity of care and community-based antenatal care improve maternal and neonatal birth outcomes for women with social risk factors? A prospective, observational study. *PLoS ONE*, *16*(5), e0250947. https://doi.org/10.1371/journal.pone.0250947

Rayment-Jones, H., Dalrymple, K., Harris, J. M., Harden, A., Parslow, E., Georgi, T., & Sandall, J. (2023a). Project20: Maternity care mechanisms that improve access and engagement for women with social risk factors in the UK – A mixed-methods, realist evaluation. *BMJ Open*, *13*(2), e064291. https://doi.org/10.1136/bmjopen-2022-064291

Rayment-Jones, H., Harris, J., Harden, A., Khan, Z., & Sandall, J. (2019). How do women with social risk factors experience United Kingdom maternity care? A realist synthesis. *Birth*, *46*(3), 461–474. https://doi.org/10.1111/birt.12446

Rayment-Jones, H., Harris, J., Harden, A., Turienzo, C. F., & Sandall, J. (2023). Project20: Maternity care mechanisms that improve (or exacerbate) health inequalities. A realist evaluation. *Women and Birth*, *36*(3), e314–e327. https://doi.org/10.1016/j.wombi.2022.11.006

Román-Gálvez RM, Martín-Peláez S, Fernández-Félix BM, Zamora J, Khan KS, Bueno-Cavanillas A. Worldwide Prevalence of Intimate Partner Violence in Pregnancy. A Systematic Review and Meta-Analysis. Front Public Health. 2021 Aug 30;9:738459. doi: 10.3389/fpubh.2021.738459. PMID: 34527656; PMCID: PMC8435609

Sardinha, L. M., & Catalán, H. E. N. (2018). Attitudes towards domestic violence in 49 low- and middle-income countries: A gendered analysis of prevalence and countrylevel correlates. *PLoS One*, *13*(10). https://doi.org/10.1371/journal.pone.0206101

Sardinha, L., Maheu-Giroux, M., Stöckl, H., Meyer, S. R., & García-Moreno, C. (2022). Global, regional, and national prevalence estimates of physical or sexual, or both, intimate partner violence against women in 2018. *Lancet*, *399*(10327), 803–813. https://doi.org/10.1016/S0140-6736(21)02664-7

Seng, J. S., Sperlich, M., & Low, L. K. (2008). Mental health, demographic, and risk behavior profiles of pregnant survivors of childhood and adult abuse. *Journal of Midwifery and Women's Health*, *53*(6), 511–521. https://doi.org/10.1016/j.jmwh.2008.04.013

Sohal, A., & Johnson, M. (2014). Identifying domestic violence and abuse. In S. Bewley & J. Welch (Eds.), *ABC of Domestic and Sexual Violence* (pp. 30–36). Wiley Blackwell.

The Survivors Trust. (n.d.). *What To Do When Someone Tells You They Have Been Raped or Sexually Abused*. UK: How To Support A Survivor - The Survivors Trust – Rape & Sexual Abuse Services.

United Nations. (2023). *What Is Domestic Abuse*. COVID-19 Response. Retrieved 19 November 2023, from https://www.un.org/en/coronavirus/what-is-domestic-abuse

World Health Organisation. (2012). *Understanding and Addressing Violence Against Women*. Understanding and addressing violence against women: overview (who.int)

World Health Organisation. (2021). *Addressing Violence against Women in Health and Multisectoral Policies: A Global Status Report*. ddressing violence against women in health and multisectoral policies: a global status report (who.int

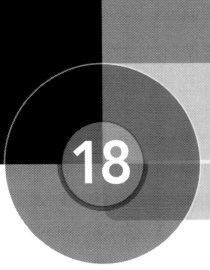

Vaccinations and Pregnancy

SAM BASSETT

INTRODUCTION

Vaccines and vaccination programmes play an important part public health and health promotion. Maintaining the health of the population, improving lives and helping protect those who are the most at risk in Society. Midwives play a central part in the vaccination programmes both for the pregnant woman or pregnant person and for their fetus and neonate.

This chapter will review the history of the vaccines, how they work and explore the main vaccines recommended in pregnancy.

WHAT ARE VACCINES AND HOW DO THEY WORK?

A vaccine is a biological substance produced to ensure active acquired immunity to a certain infectious disease. Typically, these are prepared from the causative agent of the disease which are weakened forms of the microbe, its toxins or surface proteins. In this way, a vaccine trains our immune system to fight a particular pathogen, such as a virus, bacteria or toxin. With the immune system creating antibodies to fight off the vaccine and then storing this information away in case it meets that disease again in the future (Federman, 2014).

There are two types of vaccines.

- Prophylactic – preventing and improving the effects of any future infection.
- Therapeutic – fighting a disease that has already occurred.

However, it is important to note that vaccines cannot guarantee immediate and life-long immunity for everyone. If the body is not exposed to the pathogen or vaccine

DOI: 10.4324/9781003350071-18

again for a long time, it can 'forget' how to make the antibodies and may not fully fight off the infection. Booster vaccines are required to keep the immune system primed, however who needs them and when can vary.

HISTORY OF VACCINES

Although the world's first vaccine (against smallpox) is attributed to the English Physician Edward Jenner in 1796, the practice of immunisation can be dated back further to the Eastern world with some sources suggesting that these practices were taking place as early as 200 BCE. With the first written evidence found in the 17th century in China and the smearing of cowpox on breaks in the skin by Buddhist monks to gain immunity against smallpox. This immunising procedure called 'inoculation' then travelled west through the Ottoman Empire, with Lady Mary Wortley Montagu in 1721, while observing the practice in Turkey, brought smallpox inoculation to Europe by asking for her daughters to be inoculated against smallpox.

Work by Benjamen Jesty in 1774 on the protection against smallpox by the bovine cowpox infection was expanded on by Jenner, who serving as a surgeon/apothecary apprentice noticed that many of the diary workers in rural areas never contracted the more fatal smallpox if they had already caught cowpox. In 1796, he inoculated 8-year-old James Phillips with pus collected from a cowpox sore on the hand of a milkmaid, then two months later testing Phillips resistance in the same manner. Phillips remains in perfect health. In 1798, Jenner coined the term 'vaccine', taken from the Latin word for cow, – 'Vacca'.

Jenner's success was met with both great enthusiasm and bitter opposition on scientific and ideological grounds. With philosophers such as Immanuel Kant and the clergy opposing vaccinations mainly because of poorly trained practitioners carrying out Jenner's procedure without fully understanding it and as a result spreading the disease rather than containing it. Nonetheless, when applied well Jenner's methods were highly successful and were implemented across Europe. With Napoleon Bonaparte in 1805 ordering the vaccination of his whole army and the Spanish government striving to bring vaccination to the Spanish Empire including the Americas, Philippines, Macao, and China. In 1840, the British government passed laws to vaccinate the entire population for free.

Louis Pasteur spearheaded vaccinations by introducing vaccines for chicken Cholera and anthrax in the 1872 and Rabies in 1885. Followed in 1894 by Dr Anna Wessels Williams the discovery of Diphtheria vaccine. In 1918, the Spanish flu pandemic, which killed an estimated 20–50 million people worldwide, made an influenza vaccine a worldwide priority. However, it wasn't until the invention of the electron microscope in 1930s which allowed the visualisation of viruses that further progress could be made. Paving the way for vaccines for yellow fever, pertussis, influenza, polio, Hepatitis B, measles, mumps, rubella, and pneumococcal pneumonia in the 1900s (Figure 18.1).

The creation of the World Health Organization (WHO) in 1948 led to a reframing of public health as a global problem. This led to worldwide vaccination eradication programmes. The first being the Intensified Smallpox eradication programme in 1966, aimed at eradicating smallpox in more than 30 countries, reaching its goal 14 years later in 1980 (Fenner et al., 1988). Many lessons were learnt in this process including:

- the need to establish measurable objectives and evaluate progress and performance.
- to establish procedures for quality control both of vaccines and performance.
- to recruit and support the best possible personnel.
- to ensure an on-going programme of problem-orientated research which can co-ordinate activities and resolve apparently illogical observations.

(Henderson, 1987)

These were put into action with the WHO Global Polio Eradication Initiative launched in 1988 and although not completely as successful as the smallpox programme polio case numbers have decreased by 99%. Polio now survives only among the world's poorest and most marginalised communities in three countries: Afghanistan, Nigeria, and Pakistan.

Successful vaccination programmes continued with the meningitis vaccine programme in 2016, which within its first five years has nearly eliminated serogroup A meningococcal disease within the meningitis belt countries of Africa; the malaria vaccine pilot implementation launched in 2019 in Ghana, Malawi, and Kenya; Ebola vaccine in 2019 with a stockpile established in 2021 to ensure coverage for any future outbreak; and the fast development and widespread vaccination against COVID-19 across continents in 2020. However, whilst an unprecedented success, unfortunately, the COVID-19 vaccine programme has also highlighted vast inequalities. As of January 2023, nearly 70% of the global population has received at least one dose but this only equates to just one-quarter of people in low-income countries (Bergen et al., 2023).

Other vaccination programmes although initially successful have seen a resurgence of their diseases due to a decline in uptake. A case in point here is Pertussis (whooping cough) where cases hit an all-time low in 1976. With so few cases, families started to delay or refuse vaccines altogether due to a misunderstanding of the safety and effectiveness with these outweighing fears of the disease itself (Fullen et al., 2020). This pattern has unfortunately repeated itself regarding MMR with a worrying recent 30-fold upsurge of measles cases in 2023 in the WHO European region (WHO, 2023). This encompasses the UK in 2024, despite the UK being declared as measles free in 2016. The reasons for this are complex including:

- influential misleading information such as the 1998 claim by Andrew Wakefield that the MMR vaccine was linked with autism, a theory now widely discredited.
- parents not realising that the NHS was still offering MMR vaccinations during the COVID-19 pandemic.
- reduced transmission of measles during the COVID-19 pandemic.
- parents having issues accessing appointments or being swayed by anti-vaccine theory conspiracy theories.

(Torracinta et al., 2021)

UK Health
Security
Agency

Historical vaccine development and introduction of routine vaccine programmes in the UK

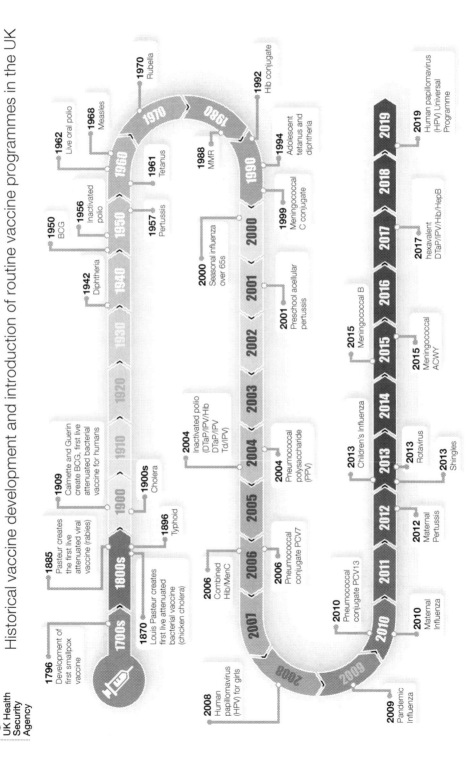

Figure 18.1 Flowchart of the history of vaccine development and British routine vaccine programmes.

Source: UK Health Security Agency. Contains public sector information licensed under the open government licence V3.0

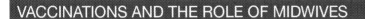

VACCINATIONS AND THE ROLE OF MIDWIVES

Midwives by the very nature of their role are integral in the provision of maternal and newborn health care (UNFPA, 2021). Pregnancy is known to increase health-seeking behaviours and as a result, midwifery care is a key focus of public health policy for governments. Therefore, midwives have an important role in counselling and educating women and their families and the wider community in general on promoting vaccination in pregnancy and for the newborn (Homer et al., 2022). The available evidence reflects this with the uptake of vaccines in pregnancy directly related to positive recommendations from healthcare providers (including midwives) as well as direct access to the vaccine (McHugh et al., 2021; Ralph et al., 2022).

However, despite this at a global level, it is known that many healthcare workers do not recommend some vaccines such as influenza to pregnant women (Yuen & Tarrant, 2014). Perhaps more worrying despite being seen as best placed to provide information/advice regarding vaccinations, it has been shown that midwives are more likely to express safety concerns than any other health care professional and as such are less likely to recommend for infections such as influenza and pertussis (Qiu et al., 2021).

The potential rationale for this is complex but much appears to rest with education. Although health promotion is recognised as a core role of a midwife specific routine training to support the education women receive to support vaccination remains at best limited (Homer et al., 2022). Much of what does exist appears to centre around vaccine information provision rather than communication skills leading to recommendation/persuasion (Kaufman et al., 2019). With some midwives going as far to say that vaccination recommendation is a doctor's professional responsibility rather than theirs (Lehner et al., 2021). However, another Australian study using an online survey of 300 midwives showed that most midwives did support maternal (influenza 83%, pertussis 90.5%) and childhood immunisation (85.8%) with two-thirds wanting further training in this area (Frawley et al., 2020). Education of midwives is therefore key to ensure midwives are vaccine ready. This was illustrated clearly in a pertussis programme in the UK where midwives received additional training and attended influenzas and pertussis clinics throughout the influenza season as well as providing vaccinations to women who were inpatients on antenatal, labour, and post-natal wards resulting in highly successful 70% uptake of pertussis (Green et al., 2017).

There are several interventions known to support the uptake of vaccinations in pregnancy (Table 18.1). One approach is looking at effective factors using three psychological propositions (Brewer et al., 2017). The first proposition relates to 'thoughts and feelings' which recognises that vaccination is an individual decision. As such, midwives must ascertain how women view the disease itself. How confident they feel about the vaccination, exploring their views around its effectiveness and safety concerns, and the role this has in their final motivation to have the vaccine.

The second proposition relates to 'social processes' and how these motivate an individual to be vaccinated. This can include the role of a woman's social networks and the perceived social norms about vaccination as well as the relationship between the woman and their midwife. The final proposition relates to 'facilitating

Table 18.1 Structured approaches for midwives to address vaccination concerns

Approaches	Components
EASE Approach (Brewer et al., 2017)	• **Elicit** main concerns. • **Acknowledge** without judgement. • **Share** commitment to vaccine. • **Explain** the science.
Ask Acknowledge Advise Approach (Henrikson et al., 2015)	• **Ask** for concerns. • **Acknowledge** concerns without judgement. • **Advise**/educate about disease and vaccine benefits and risks, recommend vaccine, end with a plan of action
CASE approach (Public Health Live, 2010)	• **Corroborate**: acknowledge concerns without judgement • **About me**: describe own vaccination expertise. • **Science**: explain the relevant scientific findings • **Explain/Advise**: explain why science suggests and recommends vaccination.

vaccination directly' by leveraging, but not trying to change, what women think and feel. This relates to having systems and processes in place that make it easy to access vaccination services and harder to forget. Including interventions that facilitate action (through reminders, prompts and primes), reducing barriers (increasing availability of transport, provision of childcare, scheduling clinic opening times to suit, one-stop clinics) and providing incentives (offering reward). A recent literature review of 157 publications and 117 documents looking at vaccination programmes

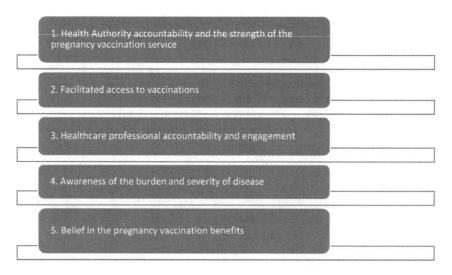

1. Health Authority accountability and the strength of the pregnancy vaccination service

2. Facilitated access to vaccinations

3. Healthcare professional accountability and engagement

4. Awareness of the burden and severity of disease

5. Belief in the pregnancy vaccination benefits

Figure 18.2 Five Pillar framework of key components needed to increase vaccine uptake in pregnancy.

Source: Adapted from Baïssa et al. (2021).

in the UK, the United States, and Spain built on these principles further suggesting a five-pillar framework to describe key components needed to increase vaccination uptake in pregnancy (Baïssas et al., 2021) (Figure 18.2).

VACCINES AND PREGNANCY

VACCINATIONS NOT USUALLY ADVISED IN PREGNANCY

During pregnancy, live vaccines are not usually advised and women are advised to wait until after their baby is born before being vaccinated. The rationale being a potential risk that the baby could become infected. However, it is worthy of note here that there is no evidence of live vaccines resulting in birth defects (Laris-González et al., 2020).

Live vaccines include:

- BCG (vaccination against tuberculosis)
- MMR (measles, mumps, and rubella)
- Oral polio (which forms part of the Hexavalent 6-in-1 vaccine given to infants)
- Oral typhoid
- Yellow fever

TRAVEL VACCINES IN PREGNANCY

When pregnant, it is advised that women avoid visiting countries, or areas, where travel vaccinations are required. However, this is not always possible and as a result women are advised to talk with a midwife and/or GP for further advice. This discussion will centre around a risk/benefit approach as if a high risk of infection is likely it is considered safer, for both mother and baby, to have the vaccine than travel unprotected.

A case in point here is yellow fever, an epidemic-prone virus spread to humans by the bites of infected mosquitos. The incubation period is typically around three to six days with many people experiencing no symptoms. Common symptoms that do occur include fever, muscle pain, headache, loss of appetite, nausea and vomiting. However, a small percentage of people will enter a second more toxic phase within 24 hours of recovery from initial symptoms. Resulting in high fever, liver damage, and jaundice (hence the name yellow fever), renal failure and uncontrolled bleeding, and disseminated intravascular coagulation. Over half of those entering this stage will die within seven to ten days (Gaythorpe et al., 2021). Due to ethics, few studies have investigated the safety of yellow fever vaccination in pregnancy but a large retrospective cohort study of U.S. military women on active duty ($n = 196,802$ pregnancies and 160,706 singleton infants) for whom yellow fever vaccination is mandatory before assignment to endemic areas did not appear to be associated with adverse outcomes with just a tenuous association between pre-conception yellow fever vaccine exposure and birth defects that warrants further investigation (Hall et al., 2020). Therefore, using a risk/benefit analysis, although a live vaccine, the advice would be to vaccinate.

VACCINES RECOMMENDED IN PREGNANCY

Currently the UK government recommends that pregnant women receive three vaccines.

- Pertussis– from week 16 of pregnancy
- Flu Vaccine – at any stage of pregnancy, especially during flu season (September to March)
- COVID-10 vaccine – at any stage of pregnancy, especially during flu season (September to March)

PERTUSSIS

Pertussis is a serious infectious disease affecting all age groups. Dating back to the Middle Ages it is highly contagious. The bacterium that causes pertussis, Bordetella pertussis, was first isolated in 1906 and is spread through contact with airborne droplets. Once in the respiratory tract the bacterium attaches to the cilia of the epithelial cells where it produces toxins that paralyse the cilia, causing inflammation and subsequently impaired clearing of pulmonary secretions (Kuchar et al., 2016).

The incubation period commonly lasts between seven and ten days with the clinical course of the disease divided into three stages: catarrhal, paroxysmal, and convalescent. The first catarrhal stage shows many signs and symptoms of the common cold including a slow onset of a runny nose, sneezing, low grade fever and a mild occasional cough. However, instead of improving over the next one to two weeks, the paroxysmal stage begins, which leads to the diagnosis of pertussis. During this stage, the individual is prone to bursts of numerous rapid coughs as they try to expel thick mucus from their tracheobronchial tree. This results in a long inspiratory effort accompanied by the characteristic high-pitched whoop. These paroxysmal attacks occur more frequently at night with the individual likely to become cyanotic, appear very ill and distressed (especially children) with vomiting and exhaustion following. Serious complications can include secondary bacterial pneumonia, seizures, encephalopathy, and even death. Minor complications can include otitis media, anorexia, dehydration, and from increased pressure due to paroxysms pneumothorax, epistaxis, hernias, and on occasions subdural haematomas (Havers et al., 2021).

Once common a childhood disease and a major cause of childhood mortality right up until the 20th century. Pertussis became part of the routine childhood vaccination in Britain in 1957, offered to babies initially at three months and then extended in 1990 to two, three and four months with a fourth dose introduced in the pre-school booster since 2001 (Amirthalingam et al., 2013). There is no whooping cough only vaccine, so it is given as part of Boostrix IPV, which also protects against polio, diphtheria, and tetanus. It is not a live vaccine and side effects if any are usually mild and can include swelling, redness or tenderness lasting a few days at the injection site, high temperature, nausea and loss of appetite, tiredness, and headache.

The programme was a resounding success with cases dropping from 122,000 (and 374 deaths) in 1956 to just 20,400 cases (and 24 deaths) in 1970 (PHE, 2016). However, in 1974 doctors from Great Ormond Street published a paper suggesting a link between the vaccine and brain damage (Kulenkampff et al., 1974). The resulting media attention and public debate led to a rapid reduction in the uptake of the vaccine, which only abated in the mid-1980s after the final court cases brought by parents against the government collapsed and public confidence began to increase (Baker, 2003).

In April 2012, the UK Health protection agency in response to a rise in antici-pated cases declared a national outbreak of pertussis. Following further increases and deaths in young infants in October 2012, the Department of Health launched what was at first intended to be a temporary vaccination programme for pregnant women. However, given its success the programme was extended and continues to the present day with the aim to vaccinate all pregnant women between 16 and 32 weeks even if they have had the vaccine before. As such, typically the vaccine is offered to women after their 20-week scan. It can be given after 32 weeks but as the body needs time to make antibodies to be passed on to the fetus it may not offer the same level of protection to the baby until they receive their first vaccination at two months of age (PHE, 2018). If women do not have the vaccine in pregnancy, it is still recommended in the first two months following birth as it offers what is known as a cocooning effect against pertussis by immunising their parents, and if possible, the extended family (Marchal et al., 2022). Included in cocooning is the recommendation that healthcare workers are vaccinated and if they haven't been vaccinated against pertussis within the last five years, they are eligible through occupational health services.

Published data from the UK vaccination programme shows that the programme has been highly successful with babies born to mothers vaccinated at least a week before birth having a 91% reduced risk of becoming ill with pertussis in the first weeks of life (Amirthalingam et al., 2013). There is no evidence of the vaccine being a risk to pregnant women, the pregnancy, or the baby confirmed by a large obser-vational cohort study carried out in 2014. This study comprised of 20,074 vaccinated women reported that there were no risks to pregnancy in relation to preterm birth, stillbirth, pre-eclampsia, haemorrhage, fetal distress, uterine rupture, placenta, or vasa previa, caesarean delivery, low birth weight, or neonatal renal failure with over-all maternal and neonatal outcomes no different to women that were unvaccinated.

INFLUENZA

Influenza (flu) is another highly infectious airborne disease, spread via tiny droplets when people with flu cough, sneeze or talk or less often via direct transmission when people touch a surface or object that has the flu virus then touching their own mouth nose or eyes. It has a range of symptoms from mild to severe which can include fever (although not always), cough, sore throat, runny or stuffy nose, muscle or body aches, headaches, fatigue, on occasion diarrhoea and vomiting and in the worst-case outcome death. Unlike pertussis the influenza virus comprises of four types: A, B, C, and D. Influenza A, B, and C can be spread human to human, animal to human (i.e. swine, avian) and human to animal. However, influenza D primarily affects cattle with some spillover to other animals such as pigs but is not known to cause human infections. Influenza A and B are known to cause seasonal epidemics every year in what is commonly know as Flu season – December to April. With Influenzas A virus being particularly prevalent and known to cause global flu pandemics. In contrast, Influenza C virus infections tend to cause mild illness (Barberis et al., 2016).

Dating back to the 1500s with the first pandemic occurring in 1,580 and decimating populations in Asia, Russia, Europe, Northwest Africa, and subsequently the Americas (Barberis et al., 2016) and being responsible for the deaths of between 20 and 50 million people during the 'Spanish Influenza' pandemic in 1918–1919.

During the Spanish flu, pandemic work started on a vaccine but it wasn't until the mid-1930s that the first clinical trials were undertaken with the first licence granted in 1942. However, the success of the vaccine has been hampered by the viruses ever changing mutations. This is known as 'antigenic drift' and consists of small mutations to the genes of the virus that lead to changes in the surface proteins (antigens) of the virus. As a result, even if the individual has had that strain of virus before the body's immune system doesn't recognise the antigens and therefore an immune response is not initiated, including the production of antibodies to fight the infection. As a result, any flu vaccine needs to be updated each year and this is determined based on the most frequent three to four strains isolated in the previous season during continuous surveillance by WHO. Side effects are usually again very mild and can include pain or soreness at the injection, a slightly raised pyrexia and an aching body. These can lead to the misconception that the flu vaccine gives you flu but the vaccine is not live, so this is not the case.

Pregnant women are at higher risk of having severe influenza during pregnancy compared to non-pregnant women due to physiological and immunological changes that occur in pregnancy. Severe complications are also higher, especially regarding cardiopulmonary and admissions to hospital requiring intensive care are higher particularly in second and third trimesters (Regan & Munoz, 2021). During the H1N1 pandemic in 2009, a UK cohort study for UKOSS highlighted maternal risk factors included obesity, asthma, multiparity, black or other ethnic minority groups and smoking particularly in those age under 25 (Yates et al., 2010). There is strong evidence that influenza influences the unborn baby with the inflammatory response leading to four times the risk of being born prematurely and to have a low birth weight or even to stillbirth or neonatal death in the first week of life (ANZIC, 2009).

In 2005, the WHO recommended flu vaccination for all pregnant women, and due to the severity of 2009 H1N1 pandemic infections among pregnant women, they became the highest priority group for inclusion (Baïssas et al., 2021). As a result, the vaccine is recommended for all pregnant women in the UK and although best given in the flu season can be given at any stage of pregnancy and is often done so alongside the pertussis vaccine. As the most prevalent strain of flu in the previous year is used to compile the next years, vaccine annual vaccinations are key. A study reported that only 69% of midwives ($n = 266$) agreed with the policy of vaccinating all pregnant women with doubts around necessity (34%), safety (25%) and effectiveness (10%) (Ishola et al., 2013). Despite there being robust evidence that the vaccine is not a risk to pregnant women, the pregnancy or the baby (Sheffield et al., 2012: Kharbanda et al., 2017).

COVID-19

The outbreak of the infectious respiratory disease COVID-19 in 2020 triggered one of the deadliest pandemics in modern history. Where exactly the virus originated from remains hotly debated with Wuhan city in China still largely considered the place of origin. However, it is also probable that the virus had been present in China well before the Wuhan epidemic explosion (Platto et al., 2020). Coronaviruses are in fact a large group of viruses that have crown-like thorns on their surface. With the Latin word 'corona' meaning crown or halo. First discovered in 1964 in Glasgow, they are commensals that live in respiratory secretions of the nasopharynx. There are many types of coronaviruses, seven of which include human pathogens, including 229E responsible for the common cold, MERS-CoV which causes a Middle East Respiratory syndrome (MERS outbreak 2012), and SARS-CoV, which causes severe respiratory syndrome (SARS outbreak China 2003). In 2019, scientists identified a novel coronavirus, which they originally named SARS-Cov-2 but is better known now as COVID-19. 'CO' standing for corona, VI for virus, D for disease, and 19 for the year it was first discovered. On 11 March 2020, the WHO declared the COVID-19 outbreak a worldwide pandemic.

Within COVID-19, the spike proteins which cover the coronavirus bind to angiotensin converting enzyme 2 (ACE2) allowing the virus to inject its RNA and replicate many more copies and release them into the alveolus. The host cell is destroyed in the process and the new coronavirus infect the neighbouring cells. As ACE2 is found within all endothelium, the virus rapidly spreads to all body organs causing multiple signs and symptoms with the most common, including cough, sore throat, fever, diarrhoea, headache, muscle or joint pain, fatigue, and a loss of smell and taste (Struyf et al., 2022). Since the start of the pandemic worldwide, there have been 774,771,942 cases reported to the WHO and over 7,035,337 deaths with 230,626 of these occurring in the UK (Official UK Coronavirus dashboard, 2023, WHO COVID-19 dashboard, n.d.).

The only hope of mitigation of the pandemic was through vaccination and the world came together to rapidly work on vaccine development the likes of which had never been witnessed before. With the UK becoming the first country to approve a COVID-19 vaccine in December 2020 (Kashte et al., 2021). With vulnerable individuals including the elderly, immunosuppressed, those with pre-existing morbidities and those from racially diverse communities being targeted early on within the vaccination programme. Pregnancy was an exclusion criterion in early clinical trials. However, evidence amassed quickly confirming that the benefits clearly outweighed the risks which included higher rates of several adverse maternal outcomes such as increased ICU admission, increased invasive ventilation, and significantly higher rates of death with pregnancy identified as an independent risk factor for severe COVID-19 (Badell et al., 2022).

Routine vaccination in pregnancy was finally recommended in the UK in April 2021. However, at first, there was a real issue with vaccination hesitancy from both the women themselves and perhaps more worryingly from midwives, who were in the position to recommend. A UKOSS report from 1st February 2021 to 30th September 2021 illustrated the urgency of this, reporting that out of 1,714 pregnant women that were admitted to hospital with symptomatic COVID-19, 98.1% were unvaccinated, 1.5% had one dose and 0.4% two doses. Of the 235 admitted to ICU only, 3 had received a single vaccine dose and none had received both (Engjom et al., 2022).

Those from racially diverse communities were known to have been disproportionally affected by COVID-19, initial evidence also showed a lower uptake of the vaccine particularly amongst black females of reproductive age with unfounded concerns including potential future fertility (Odejinmi et al., 2022). This finding also applied to midwives of black ethnicities who were found to be four times less likely to have received a COVID-19 vaccine compared to white colleagues.

Large-scale education and reinforcement initiatives from various organisation bodies – NHS, RCM, RCOG – followed with very much the ethos of ensuring every contact counts with the following initiatives:

- Support all GPs, practice nurses, midwives and obstetricians to advise women on vaccination in pregnancy at every antenatal contact.
- Ensure information and materials are available for women in all antenatal and primary care settings.
- Encourage all maternity staff to receive the protection offered by vaccination.

Robust observational evidence has also substantially grown regarding the safety of COVID-19 vaccination again showing that the vaccine is not a risk to pregnant women, the pregnancy, the baby or future fertility (Badell et al., 2022)

SUMMARY

- Vaccines and vaccinations are not new.
- Vaccines improve the lives of women, their babies, families, and wider communities.
- Midwives play a vital health promotion role, but their own personal views can impact on that role and the uptake of vaccines by their clients.

REFERENCES

Amirthalingam, G., Gupta, S., & Campbell, H. (2013). Pertussis immunisation and control in England and from, 1957 to 2012: A historical review. *Euro Surveillance*. 18(38), pii=20587. Available from: https://www.eurosurveillance.org/images/dynamic/EE/V18N38/art20587.pdf

ANZIC Influenza Investigators. (2010). Critical illness due to 2009 A/H1N1 influenza in pregnant and postpartum women: Population-based cohort study. *British Medical Journal*. 340, c1279. https://doi.org/10.1136/bmj.c1279

Badell, M. L., Dude, C. M., Rasmussen, S. A., & Jamieson, D. J. (2022). COVID-19 vaccination in pregnancy. *British Medical Journal*. 378, e069741. https://doi.org/10.1136/bmj-2021-069741

Baïssas, T., Boisnard, F., Cuesta Esteve, I, Garcia Sánchez, M., Jones, C. E., de Fougerolles, T. R., et al (2021). Vaccination in pregnancy against pertussis and seasonal influenza: key learnings and components from high-performing vaccine programmes in three countries: the United Kingdom, the United States and Spain. *BMC Public Health*. 21(1), 2182. https://doi.org/10.1186/s12889-021-12198-2

Baker, J. P (2003). The pertussis vaccine controversy in Great Britain (2003) 1974–1986. *Vaccine*. 21(25–26), 4003–4010. https://doi.org/10.1016/s0264-410x(03)00302-5.

Barberis, I., Myles, P., Ault, S. K., Bragazzi, N. L., & Martini, M. (2016). History and evolution of influenza control through vaccination: From the first monovalent vaccine to universal vaccines. *Journal of Preventive Medicine and Hygiene*. 57(3), E115–E120.

Bergen, N., Johns, N. E., Chang Blanc, D., & Hosseinpoor, A. R. (2023). Within-country inequality in COVID-19 vaccination coverage: A scoping review of academic literature. *Vaccines (Basel).* 11(3), 517. https://doi.org/10.3390/vaccines11030517

Brewer, N. T., Chapman, G. B., Rothman, A. J., Leask, J., & Kempe, A. (2017). Increasing vaccination: Putting psychological science into action. *Psychological Science Public Interest.*, 18(3), 149–207. https://doi.org/10.1177/1529100618760521

Engjom, H., van den Akher, T., Aabakke, A., Ayras, O., et al (2022). Severe COVID-19 in pregnancy is almost exclusively limited to unvaccinated women – Time for policies to change. *Lancet Regional Health – Europe.* 13,100313. https://doi.org/10.1016/j.lanepe.2022,100313

Federman, R. S. (2014) Understanding vaccines: A public imperative. *Yale Journal of Biology and Medicine.* 87(4), 417–422.

Fenner, F., et al., (1988) *Smallpox and its Eradication.* Geneva: WHO.

Frawley, J. E., McKenzie, K., Sinclair, L., Cummins, A., Wardle, J., & Hall, H. (2020). Midwives' knowledge, attitudes and confidence in discussing maternal and childhood immunisation with parents: A national study. *Vaccine.* 38(2), 366–371. https://doi.org/10.1016/j.vaccine.2019.10.006

Fullen, A. R., Yount, K. S., Dubey, P., & Deora, R. (2020). Whoop! There it is: The surprising resurgence of pertussis. *PLoS Pathogens.* 16(7), e1008625. https://doi.org/10.1371/journal.ppat.1008625

Gaythorpe, K., Hamlet, A., Jean, K., Garkauskas Ramos, D., Cibrelus, L., Garske, T., & Ferguson, N. (2021) The global burden of yellow fever. *eLife.* 10, e64670. https://doi.org/10.7554/eLife.64670

Green, D., Labriola, G., Smeaton, L., & Falconer, M. (2017). Prevention of neonatal whooping cough in England: The essential role of the midwife. *British Journal of Midwifery.* 25(4), 224–228. https://doi.org/10.12968/bjom.2017.25.4.224

Hall, C., Khodr, Z. G., Chang, R. N., Bukowinski, A. T., Gumbs, G. R., & Conlin, A. M. (2020). Safety of yellow fever vaccination in pregnancy: Findings from a cohort of active duty US military women. *Journal of Travel Medicine.* 27(6), taaa138. https://doi.org/10.1093/jtm/taaa138

Havers, F., Moro, P., Hairiri, S., & Skoff, T. (2021). Perussis. In *The pink book. Epidemology and prevention of vaccine-preventable diseases.* Centres for disease Control and prevention. Chapter 16: Pertussis | Pink Book | CDC Available from https://www.cdc.gov/vaccines/pubs/pinkbook/pert.html

Henderson, D. A. (1987). Principle and lessons from the smallpox eradication programme. *Bulletin of the World Health Organisation.* 65(4), 535–546. Available from PMC2491023.pdf (who.int).

Henrikson, N. B., Opel, D. J., Grothaus, L., Nelson, J., Scrol, A., & Dunn J, et al. (2015). Physician communication training and parental vaccine hesitancy: A randomized trial. *Pediatrics.* 136, 70–79. https://doi.org/10.1542/peds.2014-3199

Homer CSE, Javid N, Wilton K, Bradfield Z. Vaccination in pregnancy: The role of the midwife. Front Glob Womens Health. 2022 Oct 24;3:929173. doi: 10.3389/fgwh.2022.929173. PMID: 36353468; PMCID: PMC9637860

Ishola, D. A. Jr., Permalloo, N., Cordery, R. J., & Anderson, S. R. (2013). Midwives' influenza vaccine uptake and their views on vaccination of pregnant women. *Journal of Public Health (Oxford).* 35(4), 570–577. https://doi.org/10.1093/pubmed/fds109.

Kashte, S., Gulbake, A., El-Amin Iii, S. F., & Gupta, A. (2021). COVID-19 vaccines: Rapid development, implications, challenges and future prospects. *Human Cell*. 34(3), 711–733. https://doi.org/10.1007/s13577-021-00512-4

Kaufman, J., Attwell, K., Hauck, Y., Omer, S. B., & Danchin, M. (2019). Vaccine discussions in pregnancy: interviews with midwives to inform design of an intervention to promote uptake of maternal and childhood vaccines. *Human Vaccines Immunotherapeutics*. 15(11), 2534–2543. https://doi.org/10.1080/21645515.2019.1607131

Kharbanda, E. O., Vazquez-Benitez, G., Romitti, P. A., Naleway, A. L., et al (2017). Vaccine safety datalink. First trimester influenza vaccination and risks for major structural birth defects in offspring. *Journal of Pediatrics*. 187, 234–239.e4. https://doi.org/10.1016/j.jpeds.2017.04.039

Kuchar, E., Karlikowska-Skwarnik, M., Han, S., & Nitsch-Osuch, A. (2016). Pertussis: History of the disease and current prevention failure. *Advances in Experimental Medicine and Biology*. 934, 77–82. https://doi.org/10.1007/5584_2016_21

Kulenkampff, M., Schwartzman, J. S., & Wilson, J. (1974). Neurological complications of pertussis inoculation. *Archives of Disease Childhood*. 49(1), 46–49. https://doi.org/10.1136%2Fadc.49.1.46

Laris-González, A., Bernal-Serrano, D., Jarde, A., & Kampmann, B. (2020). Safety of administering live vaccines during pregnancy: A systematic review and meta-analysis of pregnancy outcomes. *Vaccines*. 8(1), 124. https://www.mdpi.com/2076-393X/8/1/124

Lehner, L., Gribi, J., Hoffmann, K., Paul, K. T., & Kutalek, R. (2021). Beyond the "information deficit model" – understanding vaccine-hesitant attitudes of midwives in Austria: A qualitative study. *BMC Public Health*. 21(1), 1671. https://doi.org/10.1186/s12889-021-11710-y

Marchal C, Belhassen M, Guiso N, Jacoud F, Cohen R, Le Pannerer M, Verdier R. Cocooning strategy: Pertussis vaccination coverage rate of parents with a new-born in 2016 and 2017 in France. Front Pediatr. 2022 Oct 18;10:988674. doi: 10.3389/fped.2022.988674. PMID: 36330369; PMCID: PMC9624187

McHugh L, O'Grady KF, Nolan T, Richmond PC, Wood N, Marshall HS, Lambert SB, Chatfield MD, Perrett KP, Binks P, Binks MJ, Andrews RM. National predictors of influenza vaccine uptake in pregnancy: the FluMum prospective cohort study, Australia, 2012-2015. Aust N Z J Public Health. 2021 Oct;45(5):455–461. doi: 10.1111/1753-6405.13130. Epub 2021 Aug 19. PMID: 34411398.

Odejinmi, F., Mallick, R., Neophytou, C., & Mondeh, K,m et al. (2022). COVID-19 vaccine hesitancy: A midwifery survey into attitudes towards the COVID-19 vaccine. *BMC Public Health*. 22, 1219. https://bmcpublichealth.biomedcentral.com/articles/10.1186/s12889-022-13540-y

Official UK Coronavirus Dashboard. (n.d.) https://coronavirus.data.gov.uk/details/deaths (accessed 14 December 2023). COVID-19: track coronavirus cases - GOV.UK (www.gov.uk)

Platto, S., Xue, T., Carafoli, E. (2020). COVID-19: An announced pandemic. *Cell Death Diseases*. 11, 799–812. https://doi.org/10.1038/s41419-020-02995-9Public Health England (PHE). (2016). *Pertussis Notifications. England and Wales 1940–2003*. Available at https://www.ncbi.nlm.nih.gov/books/NBK545994/figure/ch5.fig1/

Public Health England (PHE). (2018). *Pertussis Brief for Healthcare Professionals*.Gov. UK. Assets publishing.

Public Health Live! (2010, December 9). *Making the Case for vaccine safety: A new model for communicating with parents* [video recording]. School of Public Health, University at Albany, State University of New York. Available from https://vimeo.com/36486181

Ralph, K. M., Dorey. R. B., Rowe, R., & Jones, C. E. (2022). Improving uptake of vaccines in pregnancy: A service evaluation of an antenatal vaccination clinic at a tertiary hospital in the UK. *Midwifery*. 105, 103222. https://doi.org/10.1016/j.midw.2021.103222

Regan, A. K., & Munoz, F. M. (2021). Efficacy and safety of influenza vaccination during pregnancy: Realizing the potential of maternal influenza immunization. *Expert Review Vaccines*. 20(6), 649–660. https://doi.org/10.1080/14760584.2021.1915138

Sheffield, J. S., Greer, L. G., Rogers, V. L., Roberts, S. W., Lytle, H., McIntire, D. D., Wendel, G. D. Jr. (2012). Effect of influenza vaccination in the first trimester of pregnancy. *Obstetrics Gynecology*. 120(3), 532–537. https://doi.org/10.1097/AOG.0b013e318263a278

Struyf, T., Deeks, J. J., Dinnes, J., Takwoingi, Y., Davenport, C., Leeflang, M. M. G., et al. (2022). Cochrane COVID-19 diagnostic test accuracy group. Signs and symptoms to determine if a patient presenting in primary care or hospital outpatient settings has COVID-19. *Cochrane Database of Systematic Reviews*. 5, CD013665. https://doi.org/10.1002/14651858.CD013665.pub3

Torracinta, L., Tanner, R., & Vanderslott, S. (2021). MMR vaccine attitude and uptake research in the United Kingdom: A critical review. *Vaccines (Basel)*. 9(4), 402. https://doi.org/10.3390/vaccines9040402

UNFPA. (2021). *The State of the World's Midwifery*. New York: United Nations Population Fund. Available from https://www.unfpa.org/publications/sowmy-2021

Qiu, X., Bailey, H., & Thorne, C. (2021). Barriers and facilitators associated with vaccine acceptance and uptake among pregnant women in high income countries: A mini-review. *Frontiers Immunology*. 12, 626717. COVID-19: track coronavirus cases - GOV.UK (www.gov.uk)

WHO COVID-19 dashboard. (n.d.). *COVID-19 deaths* | WHO COVID-19 dashboard (accessed 8 March 2024).

World Health Organisation (WHO). (2023). A 30-fold rise of measles cases in 2023 in the WHO European Region warrants urgent action. New release 14th December 2023

Yates, L., Pierce, M., Stephens, S., Mill, A. C., Spark, P., & Kurinczuk, J. J., et al. (2010). Influenza A/H1N1v in pregnancy: An investigation of the characteristics and management of affected women and the relationship to pregnancy outcomes for mother and infant. *Health Technology Assessment*. 14(34), 109–182. https://doi.org/10.3310/hta14340-02

Yuen, C. Y., & Tarrant, M. (2014). Determinants of uptake of influenza vaccination among pregnant women – A systematic review. *Vaccine*. 32(36), 4602–4613. https://doi.org/10.1016/j.vaccine.2014.06.067

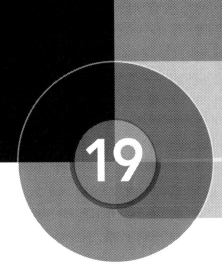

The Displaced or Migrant Client

19

MARIA GARCIA DE FRUTOS AND
OCTAVIA WISEMAN

INTRODUCTION

This chapter will explore the personal and structural issues faced by migrant women and birthing people attending for maternity care in the UK. We will clarify different kinds of 'legal status' and how this, along with charging policies, impacts migrants' access to care and their maternal and neonatal outcomes. Improving equity of access and outcomes in maternity services is an important public health issue and this chapter will also detail migrant women's rights, and what midwives can do to support them. Throughout this chapter, when we refer to *migrants*, we include refugees, asylum seekers, undocumented migrant and any other displaced population. UK Monetary figures are current as of 2023.

Migration is a worldwide phenomenon. The numbers of people who have been forcibly displaced globally continue to increase as a result of climate-relate challenges, armed conflict, poverty, and global political instability. In mid-2022, UNHCR estimates that around 103 million people are forcibly displaced worldwide. During global crisis, women and girls are worst affected, making up to 50% of any refugee, displaced or stateless population (UNHCR, 2022). Migration occurs both within and outside national borders and has numerous impacts on individual health, as well as on local health systems and health policy response. In recent years, migration has been a dominant topic of political agendas and anti-migration policies and sentiments have increased across the world. However, the protection of sexual and reproductive health rights and availability of sexual and reproductive health services is endorsed within international and human rights law. Lokugamage et al. (2022) remind us that Western medicine was established at a time characterised by patriarchy, racism, and Euro-centrism which pathologised women's bodies – especially black and brown women's bodies. This can affect our clinical care as well as our training and attitudes as midwives. Indigenous and non-European groups are under-represented in the research which underpins our clinical practice which means that 'standard' biochemical and haematological markers are mostly based on research on white populations. At the same time, the lived experiences of these groups have been marginalised and women from Black, Asian, and ethnic minority groups are more likely to report not being listened to by health care professionals (HCPs) (NHS Race and Health Observatory, 2023). As well as facing multiple risk factors, migrant women face intersectional discrimination which compounds oppression and impacts on health outcomes (Selvarajah et al., 2022).

To respond to the needs of those displaced, midwives and other HCPs need to be aware of a range of issues related to public health, migration policy, and health systems, as well as key health concerns which those displaced faced at different points in their maternity journeys.

DEFINITIONS

Migrants in the UK are not a homogeneous group, nor are they treated as such by maternity services. Although many may encounter similar biases and barriers to NHS care, it is helpful to understand how the different 'status' of migrants affects their right to maternity care (Gov.UK 2014, 2020, 2023). See a summary of their entitlements in Table 19.1.

ASYLUM SEEKERS

Migrants who have arrived in the UK (through formal or informal routes) apply for asylum in the UK based on 'a well-founded fear of being persecuted for reasons of race, religion, nationality, membership of a particular social group, or political opinion' (UN Convention Relating to the Status of Refugees 1951, Article 1). Gender-related violence, of particular relevance in maternity, comes under 'membership of a particular group'. While their claim is being processed, asylum seekers are entitled to free maternity care but do not have the right to work or claim benefits. Instead they are supported by the UK Border Agency (UKBA) Section 95 support (2023) and can choose from the following:

- *Subsistence only:* Currently this is £47.39 per week and a travel voucher
- *Subsistence and accommodation:* Accommodation is provided, as well as all meals, plus £9.59 per week. Accepting this option may involve dispersal to other areas of the country with little warning.

Pregnant asylum seekers are entitled to an additional £3 per week during pregnancy and for every child under three years, and to a one-off maternity grant of £300 after 32/40.

REFUGEES

At the end of their application, asylum seekers may be granted *Refugee Status or Humanitarian Protection for five years*, after which they can apply for 'Indefinite Leave to Remain' and 12 months later, they can apply for British Citizenship, which includes sitting the 'Life in the UK Test'. Indefinite Leave to Remain gives migrants to free NHS maternity care, benefits and the right to work. Another positive outcome of an asylum claim can be *Discretionary Leave to Stay* which comes with the same rights, but at the end of this period, they need to reapply for asylum.

REFUSED ASYLUM SEEKERS

Asylum seekers have the right to appeal a negative decision, and once an appeal has been lodged they will be considered 'asylum seekers' again until a decision is made (this entitles them to free maternity care). They may reach a point where they are considered 'Appeals Rights Exhausted' (ARE). At this point, they will become 'no recourse to public funds' (see below). UKBA may also seek to repatriate them. However, they do have the right to submit a fresh claim for asylum on compassionate grounds (i.e. a life-threatening medical condition and new evidence or a change in the political situation in their country of origin).

NO RECOURSE TO PUBLIC FUNDS

This group is referred to using a range of (often derogatory) terms, including 'overseas visitors', 'illegal migrants', 'undocumented migrants', economic migrants', and 'health tourists'. It is difficult to estimate the number of migrants in the UK with no recourse to public funds as they live, by definition, under the radar. This group may have arrived in the UK by formal routes on tourist, student or spousal visas who have 'overstayed' or been unable to regularise their status. This group also includes women who have arrived through informal routes (e.g. boats across the Channel) but who do not have the right to claim asylum, for example if they are fleeing poverty rather than persecution. It also includes refused asylum seekers who have not been returned to their country of origin.

Women and pregnant people with no recourse to public funds have access to free primary care and A&E, and have access to maternity care as this is considered 'urgent and immediately necessary care', but women will be subsequently be charged 150% of the national tariff. Trusts are required to check chargeable status of anybody presenting for care. Where payment is due, they have a legal obligation to pursue any such debts, including using debt collectors, and are required to report any unpaid debt above £1,000 to the Home Office.

A summary of what all pregnant women/birthing people are entitled to, regardless of their status, can be found in Table 19.2.

MIGRANTS WITH VISAS

One challenge to understanding migrant's 'entitlement' to free maternity care is that there are a wide range of different visas available to migrants and new schemes are launched in response to political events (i.e., the Ukrainian war or 'Settled Status'

The Displaced or Migrant Client

Table 19.1 Summary of migrant's entitlements based on their legal status in the UK

Status	Has the right to primary and A&E NHS care	Has the right NHS maternity care	Has the right to work	Has the right to social support, housing, education	Notes
Asylum Seeker	YES	YES – free	NO	NO	Support ceases once their case is resolved.
Refugee	YES	YES – free	YES	YES	Same rights has British citizen
No recourse to public funds	YES	YES – but will be charged	NO	NO	
Pregnant migrants on Visas >6 months	YES	YES – free	Depends on the visa	NO	Have to pay the Health Surcharge
Minors under 18 years	YES	YES – free	NO	YES – education, social support	Right to citizenship depends on parents' status

for Europeans living in the UK before Brexit). Those applying for temporary leave to remain for more than six months who are not otherwise exempt must pay a £624 Health Surcharge to cover the cost of any NHS treatment.

BABIES AND MINORS UNDER 18

Babies born in the UK have the right to free NHS care, free education and social services support but do not have the right to British citizenship unless at the time of their birth one of their parents is British or legally settled in the UK.

One-third of asylum applications in the UK are made by women, but they are more likely to be initially refused compared to men (87%). This may be because women find it harder to document persecution: gender violence is more likely to happen in the private rather than public realm so they rarely have prison or police records, articles about them, or scars from torture. Nevertheless, half of the appeals lodged by women are successful. Whether the outcome of an asylum claim is positive or negative, UKBA support will cease within 21 days which can lead to destitution – even for those who have been granted refugee status, this is rarely long enough to establish housing and benefits.

MIGRANT AND DISPLACED POPULATIONS: AN OVERVIEW OF THE UK CONTEXT

In 2021, people born outside of the UK made up an estimated 14.5% (9.6 million) of the UK's population. Compared to the UK born, migrants are more likely to be aged 26 to 64. In 2019, about 53% of the foreign-born population were women and girls. Migrants are much more likely to live in some parts of the UK than others. In the year ending June 2021, about half of the UK's foreign-born population (48% in total) were either in London (35% – 3,346,000) or the South East (13% – 1,286,000) (Migration Observatory, 2022).

WHY IS IT IMPORTANT TO DISCUSS MIGRANT COMMUNITIES' HEALTH?

First, migration is a key political issue not only in the UK but globally. Second, the MBRRACE-UK report (Knight et al., 2022) state that Black, Asian and women born outside of the UK have higher mortality rates than their British counterparts, which includes a four times higher rate in black women and a worrying increase in still-birth and neonatal death among their babies. Furthermore, a confidential enquiry into maternal health estimated that a quarter of women who died were born outside the UK, of which 46% were not UK citizens (Knight et al., 2016). Third, migrants are among the most vulnerable and excluded people in the UK; however, their maternal and child health outcomes can be improved by midwives who are in a position to make a difference. Reducing inequalities in health has long been part of the midwifery profession's goals and standards, as stated in the government's Better Births review (NHS England, 2016), and in the Nursing and Midwifery Council's

Code (NMC, 2018). Migrant health is not only a public and human rights concern, it is also recognised as a key factor for integration into society, yet migrant sexual and reproductive health issues present some of the most important and still unmet, public health challenges. In the UK, the subject of immigration appears high on the political agenda and policies that limit health care access have become more prevalent. Current law and regulations related to maternity care and NHS charges for undocumented migrants are part of this (Garcia de Frutos, 2020). For further information, see Chapter 5.

NHS CHARGING FOR MATERNITY CARE IN ENGLAND

The UK and the overseas NHS visitors charging regulation system for maternity care The Immigration Act 2014 restricted free NHS care to those who have resided in the UK for five years or more. Those who do not meet the residence requirement, but hold a visa, must pay the 'immigration health surcharge' of £400 per year. *Overseas Visitors* must pay 150% of the face-value cost (NHS rate). In 2017, an amendment to the Immigration Act 2014 meant patients were required to give evidence of eligibility, sometimes up front. Consequently, NHS providers are now legally obliged to establish a patient's residential status and where appropriate recover the cost of the treatment (Shahvisi & Finnerty, 2019). To date, NHS Trusts are required to inform the Home Office about patients who have an outstanding debt of more than £500 to the NHS for over two months. This can impact on future immigration applications. Previous restrictions to accessing health care in the UK have contributed to an increase in social and health inequalities that affect the most vulnerable migrant populations (Poduval et al., 2015) and act as a deterrent from accessing necessary maternity care (Feldman, 2021). The introduction of these changes ignores ongoing concerns expressed by medical professionals, researchers and UK organisations about the increasing restrictions of access to health care by migrants, asserting not only ethical and public health reasons but also that it is more cost effective to provide continuous health care. Eligibility labels and the imposition of charges are incompatible with midwives' ability to provide appropriate and timely care, including interprofessional and specialist support (Feldman et al., 2019).

WHAT ARE THE IMPLICATIONS OF THE LAW AND REGULATIONS FOR UNDOCUMENTED MIGRANTS?

Maternity care cannot be denied as it is considered 'immediately necessary', however, it is not free for women who are not 'ordinarily residents' in the UK. The charges vary and range from £4000 to £7000 for prenatal, intrapartum, and postnatal care — up to 150% higher than the regular NHS tariff. Abortion services are chargeable and range between £900 and £1,400 (Shahvisi & Finnerty, 2019). Family planning is free of charge (Department of Health and Social Care, 2021); however, women may either not be aware of this or be fearful of accessing institutions.

Health inequalities that could be avoided but are not are unjust. It is a matter of social justice (Marmot, 2017). There is a vast amount of evidence that confirms facilitating access to maternity and abortion care plays an important role in maternal and child health outcomes.

HEALTH OUTCOMES AND CHALLENGES IN ACCESSING MATERNITY SERVICES IN THE UK

MBRRACE-UK reports show that year after year, women in deprived communities including those born outside of the UK have poorer sexual and reproductive health (SRH)outcomes compared to women born in the UK. In addition, they face multiple barriers when accessing health care services such as, fear of deportation, NHS charges, lack of information, support, and trust in the midwife and other HCPs (Poduval et al., 2015, Shortall et al., 2015, Juárez et al., 2019, Nellums et al., 2020).

Migrants' SRH is complex and takes a socioecological approach to allow for the interplay between individual (micro) factors and environmental factors (Orcutt et al., 2021). Multiple factors have been identified as contributing to poor sexual and reproductive outcomes in displaced communities, such as:

- poor access to healthcare in the country of origin
- untreated existing or new health conditions occurring during the journey
- malnutrition
- exposure to violence
- engagement in dangerous activities as a means of securing food and or protection (sex industry, including exploitation through trafficking)
- increased rate of forced marriage/child marriage
- unmet contraception needs
- unsafe abortion
- language barriers
- fear of reporting sexual abuse due to stigma
- structural racism

In addition, migrants face complex challenges when accessing NHS maternity care services

- Fear of deportation
- Unknown health systems
- Language barriers
- Lack of funds
- Lack of documentation
- Unstable accommodation

Identified risks for maternal and child health outcomes:

- Late booking
- Delays in accessing antenatal care
- Missing antenatal screenings
- Missed diagnosis
- Less antenatal appointments than recommended

Qualitative data has found that refugee women want to feel safe in the maternity system and in their communities. In addition to fair and equal access and treatment in maternity care (Evans et al., 2022). Midwives, and other HCPs, would benefit from additional training to understand how the wider issues described above and those related to the negative discourses around migration, and use this knowledge in practice when caring for women to help them feel safe.

CARING FOR MIGRANT WOMEN: THE MIDWIFE'S ROLE

Midwives have a well-documented public health role (Marshall et al., 2019) which is embedded in the NMC Code and includes an obligation to advocate for the women they care for.

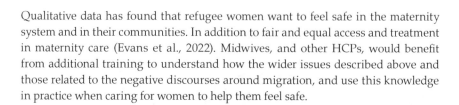

The Nursing and Midwifery Council's Code (2018)

1.5 – Respect and uphold people's human rights

3.4 – Act as an advocate for the vulnerable, challenging poor practice and discriminatory attitudes and behaviour relating to their care

5.1 – Respect a person's right to privacy in all aspects of their care

5.4 – Share necessary information with other healthcare professionals and agencies 'only' when the interests of patient safety and public protection override the need for confidentiality

7.2 – Take reasonable steps to meet people's language and communication needs

7.3 – Use a range of verbal and non-verbal communication methods, and consider cultural sensitivities, to better understand and respond to people's personal and health needs

20.4 – Keep to the laws of the country in which you are practising

20.5 – Treat people in a way that does not take advantage of their vulnerability or cause them upset or distress.

Source: NMC Code (2018).

Maternity care is not 'one-size-fits-all'. The code clarifies that midwives are expected to actively challenge discriminatory attitudes, show respect for all women and develop personalised plans to meet women's individual medical, social, emotional, and communication needs. The key concepts which should guide maternity care for migrant women and birthing people, and vulnerable populations generally, are discussed below.

When considering care pathways for a vulnerable group, the first step for commissioners and managers is to understand their local population, and to consult with them in order to understand their needs and preferences (NHS, 2018). Services should be designed to avoid stigma and bias. Information about your local population can be gathered through local Healthwatch and the Fingertips data service, and this should be followed by a co-production process involving your local Maternity Voices Partnership and other charities/stakeholders. A number of tools are available to support involving service users in healthcare design and carrying out equalities impact assessments.

BOOKING APPOINTMENT

While migrant women are not a homogeneous group, they are more likely to have complex social, medical and mental health histories. Special care should be taken during the booking appointment to explore previous trauma, social isolation, housing needs and health history as well as migration status and personal preferences to safeguard their emotional and cultural safety.

CARE-PLANNING

Migrant women may be wary of figures of authority which can affect disclosure (Feldman, 2021), so consideration of confidentiality and dignity are especially important. Relational models of care increase trust and minimise the need for complex histories to be repeated. Continuity of carer has been shown to improve maternal and neonatal outcomes, with the greatest impact seen in vulnerable groups (Rayment-Jones et al., 2015; Sandall et al., 2016 – see Case Study 19.1). Models of care which build social support, such as group antenatal care (Hunter et al., 2018), may be appropriate for migrant women who are isolated. Specialist teams (such as those specialising in asylum seekers and refugees) can enable midwives to integrate clinical care with expertise in the social issues facing this group, although services should be mindful of women feeling stigmatised by such services. Poorly designed care pathways can result in harm for vulnerable people (Pollard & Howard, 2021). Midwives should follow the four principles of trauma-informed care (NHSE, 2021):

- Recognition and compassion
- Communication and collaboration 1
- Consistency and continuity
- Recognising diversity and facilitating

Case Study 19.1: Continuity of Care

Background: The Lambeth Early Action Partnership (LEAP), funded by the National Lottery Community Fund as part of its A Better Start initiative, utilises a public health approach to improve outcomes for families. Given the markedly higher maternal and neonatal mortality and morbidity risk for women living in the LEAP area (Lambeth South London), investing in enhanced pregnancy care became a priority.

Intervention: LEAP worked with the local NHS Trust (Guy's and St. Thomas') to commission a Midwifery Continuity of Care (MCoC) team targeting pregnant people in the LEAP area with Black or other minority ethnicity and/or social risk factors. A named midwife provides longer and more frequent appointments, delivering continuity of care across the antenatal, intrapartum and postnatal period. The team was based in a local children's centre, benefitting from referral pathways to wider sources of support, including infant feeding and enhanced domestic abuse.

Outcomes: Over 600 LEAP babies have been born since the service began in 2018. Ninety per cent of clients live in areas of highest deprivation, and

62% identify their ethnicity as non-white. This intervention showed significant reductions in pre-term birth rates and caesarean births compared with clients who received traditional midwifery care. Hundred per cent of clients reported that they trusted staff and felt like they understood their needs (Hadebe et al. 2021).

SIGNPOSTING

Migrant women may be unfamiliar with NHS processes, the role of midwives and health visitors, wider services and their rights under UK law (i.e., their right to have time off work to attend maternity care, or make informed choices). Midwives should clarify care pathways and signpost migrant women to external sources of support such as Children's Centres, Community hubs, advocacy groups such as Maternity Action and Birthrights, and local charities (see Case Study 19.2).

Case Study 19.2: Community Volunteer Programmme

Background: Auntie Pam's was created in 2009 to provide a community-based resource in Kirklees to support pregnant women/birthing people, parents and children, funded by Public Health at Kirklees Council working closely with the local MVP to address poor maternal health outcomes and behaviours.

Intervention: Auntie Pam's trains volunteers from the local community who speak a range of languages (Urdu, Arabic, and Kurdish) who offer a time-rich, person-centred service, giving clients the chance to identify and talk through their issues, prioritise their own needs, solutions and goals. They also provide a baby bank, baby weighing facilities, and a drop-in information service covering housing, benefits, domestic violence, healthy eating, mental health, baby feeding support and smoking cessation.

Outcomes: Eighty per cent of their clients come from the lowest 30% deprivation decile, many of whom are migrants, refugees and asylum seekers. Auntie Pam's have achieved the lowest rate smoking at time of delivery rates in Kirklees in the last ten years. They use social marketing techniques and co-production to maintain and evaluate the service and their 'whole-life' approach addresses the fact that if an individual struggles with money, relationships or housing, they are less likely to identify poor health behaviours as a priority for change. For more information, see www.auntiepams.org.uk

Activity: (1) How can midwives support women's wider social needs? (2) What local services near you can work with maternity services to provide additional support for migrant women?

FINANCIAL SUPPORT

Women on benefits should be supported to apply for the Healthy Start food card and the Sure Start Maternity Grant (this is aimed at primiparas, but can also be claimed by multiparas if it is their first baby in the UK). All women on low income, regardless of status, can apply for an HC1 Form which can help with costs, including travel to hospital appointments (asylum-seekers will be given an HC2 Form by the Home Office, covering the same support).

WOMEN WITH LIMITED ENGLISH PROFICIENCY (LEP)

The NICE Guideline for Pregnancy and Complex Factors (2010) specifies that interpreting services should always be used for women with limited English proficiency (LEP) and midwives should not rely on friends or family to interpret. Where women speak limited English, midwives should check their understanding and offer to use interpreters. Additional, or longer, appointments may be needed (NICE, 2010). Meeting women with LEP's communication needs includes consideration of how they can access to parent education and collating reputable sources of information about pregnancy in a range of local languages. Research has shown that women with LEP prefer to receive care from somebody who speaks their own language, rather than through interpreters (Rayment-Jones et al., 2021), so consideration should be given to making better use of multi-lingual staff where available or working with volunteer doulas who speak local languages.

NO ACCESS TO PUBLIC FUNDS

Women and birthing people without access to public funds experience both emotional and financial challenges due to being charged for care. Midwives can provide continuity of care to build trust, explaining the importance of attending all their appointments and providing reassurance that they have a right to receive maternity care regardless of their ability to pay. Midwives can help women navigate what can be a frightening situation, encouraging them to engage with the Foreign Visitor's Department to arrange an affordable repayment schedule in order to avoid aggressive debt collection or their debt being reported to the Home Office. Midwives cannot offer immigration advice, but can signpost women to organisations such as Maternity Action, Doctors without Borders, Praxis or Citizen's Advice.

GENDER-BASED VIOLENCE

Migrant women without recourse who disclose that they have been subject to gender-based violence (FGM, sexual violence, domestic violence, trafficking) may not be aware that they can apply for asylum which will entitle them to receive Section 95 support and free maternity care while their case is being considered. They should be referred to local services and the British Red Cross for support (British Red Cross, 2023).

ASYLUM-SEEKERS

Asylum-seekers are regularly dispersed from one part of the country to another with little notice. For pregnant asylum-seekers, already at risk of premature birth and poor outcomes, dispersal represents additional risk as it may separate them from their support system, impact continuity of carer and result in the loss of important information about her pregnancy. Midwives have a role in advocating for asylum-seekers if they are threatened with dispersal. Changes to the woman's medical status (i.e., developing pre-eclampsia; a diagnosis of HIV or Tuberculosis; mental health treatment) could have a material impact on a woman's asylum claim. Templates for letters of support can be found on the Maternity Action website and these are taken into consideration when dispersal decisions are made. Pregnant women should not be dispersed six weeks before or after their due date, but where dispersal does occur, the midwife should ensure effective handover of care (Refugee Council, 2021; UK Visas and Immigration, 2016).

CULTURAL SAFETY

When caring for migrant women, midwives must consider clinical issues such as the accuracy of identifying APGAR scores, pulse oximeters, jaundice, mastitis, and cyanosis on dark skin (useful resources include Mukwende et al., 2020, NHS Race and Health Observatory, 2023; NHSE Cultural Competency training). However, focusing on physiological differences can lead to pathologising Black and Brown women's bodies, preventing them receiving high quality care which responds to their individual needs NHS Race and Health Observatory, 2023). Midwives must explore their own internalised bias (discover this with the Harvard test – see resources) and guard against stereotyping. Cultural safety does not mean understanding everything about a particular culture or ethnicity: it means understanding colonial legacies and historic power imbalances, and within that context ensuring that you provide individualised, person-centred care grounded in respect. What does the person sitting in front of you want and need? Using inclusive language and listening to women's voices, respecting their unique identity, is a key tool of decolonisation and addressing oppression (Lokuamage et al., 2022).

Table 19.2 Entitlements of all pregnant migrant women/birthing people, regardless of legal status

- Pregnant migrant women and their babies are more vulnerable to adverse outcomes.
- Migrant women's legal status may vary.
- Migrant women cannot be denied maternity care in the UK, regardless of their ability to pay, but some may be charged for their care.
- Midwives have a professional obligation to consider a woman's status, her needs and preferences when developing personalised care plans.
- Midwives cannot offer immigration advice but can signpost migrant women to relevant organizations and write letters of support.
- Midwives should provide continuity of care and additional appointments or interpreters as required.

Migrant communities face multiple complexities when they arrive in a new country. Research has found that women and families from migrant backgrounds suffer poorer maternal and child health outcomes. Midwives play a key role in public health and working towards improving equity as a means to reduce health inequalities. Maternity health care professionals need to understand what all migrant women are entitled to (Table19.2) and keep up to date with latest guidance and recommendations to provide kind, high quality, competent, and safe care.

SUMMARY

This chapter has explored the impact on the health of clients whose status to stay depends on the asylum process and their access to maternity care and the following are key points for learning:

Key Learning Points

- Pregnant migrant women and their babies are more vulnerable to adverse outcomes.
- Migrant women's legal status may vary.
- Migrant women cannot be denied maternity care in the UK, regardless of their ability to pay, but some may be charged for their care.
- Midwives have a professional obligation to consider a woman's status, her needs and preferences when developing personalised care plans.
- Midwives cannot offer immigration advice but can signpost migrant women to relevant organisations and write letters of support.
- Midwives should provide continuity of care and additional appointments or interpreters as required.

REFERENCES

British Red Cross. (2023). *Sexual and Gender-Based Violence: Strengthening Protection for Migrant, Refugee and Asylum-Seeking Women.* Available from: Sexual and gender-based violence | British Red Cross [accessed 20 October 2023]

Department of Health and Social Care. (2021). *Upfront Charging Operational Framework to Support Identification and Charging of Overseas Visitors.* https://www.gov.uk/government/publications/overseas-nhs-visitors-framework-to-support-identification-and-upfront-charging/upfront-charging-operational-framework-to-support-identification-and-charging-of-overseas-visitors

Evans, M., et al. (2022, September). What refugee women want from maternity care: A qualitative study. *British Journal of Midwifery*, 30(9). Maria first name, ISSN 9print) 0969-4900. British Journal Of Midwifery - What refugee women want from maternity care: a qualitative study

Feldman, R. (2021). NHS charging for maternity care in England: Its impact on migrant women. *Critical Social Policy*, 41(2), 447–467.

Feldman, R., Hardwick, J., & Malzoni, R. (2019). *Duty of Care? The Impact on Midwives of NHS Charging for Maternity Care.* London: Maternity Action, 2019. Available from: https://www.maternityaction.org.uk/wp-content/uploads/DUTY-OF-CARE-with-cover-for-upload.pdf

Garcia de Frutos, M. (2020, March). Maternal global health matters, reflections from a local perspective. *MIDIRS Midwifery Digest*, 30(1), 123–127.

Gov.UK. (2014). *NHS Entitlements: Migrant Health Guide* (updated 2023). Available NHS entitlements: migrant health guide – GOV.UK, www.gov.uk [accessed 20 October 2023]

Gov.UK. (2020). *New Immigration System: What You Need to Know* (updated 2023). Available New immigration system: what you need to know – GOV.UK, www.gov.uk [accessed 20 October 2023]

Gov.Uk. (2023). *Seek Protection or Asylum: Claiming Asylum as a Refugee, the Asylum Process and Support*. Available Seek protection or asylum – GOV.UK, www.gov.uk [accessed 20 October 2023]

Hadebe, R., Seed, P. T., Essien, D., et al. (2021). Can birth outcome inequality be reduced using targeted caseload midwifery in a deprived diverse inner city population? A retrospective cohort study. *BMJ Open*, 11, e049991. https://doi.org/10.1136/bmjopen-2021–049991

Hunter, L., Da Motta, G., McCourt, C., Wiseman, O., Rayment, J., Haora, P., Wiggins, M., & Harden, A. (2018). Better together: A qualitative exploration of women's perceptions and experiences of group antenatal care. *Women and Birth*. 32(4), 336–345. https://doi.org/10.1016/j.wombi.2018.09.001

Juárez, S., Honkaniemi, H., Dunlavy, A., et al. (2019). Effects of non health-targeted policies on migrant health: A systematic review and meta-analysis. *The Lancet Global Health*, 7(4), e420–e435. http://doi.org/10.1016/S2214-109X(18)30560-6

Knight, M., Bunch, K., Patel, R., Shakespeare, J., Kotnis, R., Kenyon, S., & Kurinczuk, J. J., (Eds.) on behalf of MBRRACE-UK. (2022). *Saving Lives, Improving Mothers' Care Core Report – Lessons Learned to Inform Maternity Care from the UK and Ireland Confidential Enquiries into Maternal Deaths and Morbidity 2018–20*. Oxford: National Perinatal Epidemiology Unit, University of Oxford.

Knight, M., Nair, M., Tuffnell, D., et al., eds. on behalf of MBRRACEUK. (2016). *Saving Lives, Improving Mothers' Care. Surveillance of Maternal Deaths in the Uk 2012–14 and Lessons Learned to Inform Maternity Care from the UK and Ireland Confidential Enquiries*. zliamt.pdf (hqip.org.uk)

Lokugamage, A. U., Robinson, N., & Pathberiya, S. D. C., et al. (2022). Respectful maternity care in the UK using a decolonial lens. *SN Social Science*, 2, 267. https://doi.org/10.1007/s43545-022-00576-5

Marmot, M. (2017). Social justice, epidemiology and health inequalities. *European Journal of Epidemiology*, 32(7), 537–546.

Marshall, J., Baston, H., & Hall, J. (2019). *Midwifery Essentials: Public Health* (1st ed., vol. 7). London: Elsevier.

Mukwende, M., Tamonv, P., & Turner, M. (2020). *Mind the Gap: A Handbook of Clinical Signs in Black and Brown Skin*. London: St. George's University of London. Available from: Mind the Gap — Black & brown skin, blackandbrownskin.co.uk

National Institute of Health and Care Excellence (NICE). (2010). *Pregnancy and Complex Social Factors: A Model for Service Provision for Pregnant Women with Complex Social Factors. Guideline CG110*. Available from: http://www.nice.org.uk/guidance/cg110/chapter/1-guidance

Nellums LB, Powis J, Jones L, Miller A, Rustage K, Russell N, Friedland JS, Hargreaves S. "It's a life you're playing with": A qualitative study on experiences of NHS maternity services among undocumented migrant women in England. Soc Sci Med. 2021 Feb;270:113610. doi: 10.1016/j.socscimed.2020.113610. Epub 2020 Dec 14. PMID: 33383485; PMCID: PMC7895812.

NHS England. (2016). *Better Births. Improving Outcomes of Maternity Services in England. A Five Year Forward View for Maternity Care.* London: NHS England. Available from: NHS England » Better Births: Improving outcomes of maternity services in England – A Five Year Forward View for maternity care

NHS. (2018). *Effective Co-production Through Local Maternity Voices Partnerships (MVPs).* Available from: mat-mvp-coproduction-052018.pdf; nationalmaternityvoices.org.uk [accessed 20 October 2023]

NHS England. (2021). *A Good Practice Guide to Support Implementation of Trauma-Informed Care in the Perinatal Period.* Available from: NHS England » A good practice guide to support implementation of trauma-informed care in the perinatal period [accessed 20 October 23]

NHS Race and Health Observatory. (2023). *Review of Neonatal Assessment and Practice in Black, Asian, and Minority Ethnic Newborns.* Available from: RHO-Neonatal-Assessment-Report.pdf, nhsrho.org

Nursing and Midwifery Council (NMC). (2018). *The Code.* Available from: https://www.nmc.org.uk/globalassets/sitedocuments/nmc-publications/nmc-code.pdf

Orcutt, M., Shortall, C., Walpole, S., Abbara, A., Garry, S., Issa, R., Zumla, A., & Abubakar, I. (Eds.). (2021). *Handbook of Refugee Health: for Healthcare Professionals and Humanitarians Providing Care to Forced Migrants* (1st ed.). CRC Press. https://doi.org/10.1201/9780429464874

Poduval, S., Howard, N., Jones, L., et al. (2015). Experiences among undocumented migrants accessing primary care in the United Kingdom: A qualitative study. *International Journal of Health Services: Planning, Administration, Evaluation,* 45(2), 320–333.

Pollard, T., & Howard, N. (2021). Mental healthcare for asylum-seekers and refugees residing in the United Kingdom: A scoping review of policies, barriers, and enablers. *International Journal of Mental Health System,* 15, 60. https://doi.org/10.1186/s13033-021-00473-z

Rayment-Jones, H., Harris, J., Harden, A., et al. (2021). Project20: interpreter services for pregnant women with social risk factors in England: What works, for whom, in what circumstances, and how? *International Journal of Equity Health,* 20, 233. https://doi.org/10.1186/s12939-021-01570-8

Rayment-Jones H, Murrells T, Sandall J. An investigation of the relationship between the caseload model of midwifery for socially disadvantaged women and childbirth outcomes using routine data--a retrospective, observational study. Midwifery. 2015 Apr;31(4):409-17. doi: 10.1016/j.midw.2015.01.003. Epub 2015 Jan 14. PMID: 25661044

Refugee Council. (2021). *Maternity Care in the UK for Women on Asylum Support.* Available from: Maternity-care-in-the-UK-for-women-on-asylum-support-read-version_July_2021.pdf; refugeecouncil.org.uk [accessed 19 April 2023]

Sandall, J., Soltani, H., Gates, S., Shennan, A., & Devane D. (2016). Midwife-led continuity models versus other models of care for childbearing women. *Cochrane Database of Systematic Reviews,* 4, CD004667. https://doi.org/10.1002/14651858.CD004667.pub5

Selvarajah, S., Maioli, S.C., Deivanayagam, T.A., de Morais Sato, P., Devakumar, D., Kim, S-S. et al. (2022). Racism, xenophobia, and discrimination: mapping pathways to health outcomes. *Lancet*, 400(10368), P2109–2124. https://doi.org/10.1016/S0140-6736(22)02484-9

Shahvisi, A., & Finnerty, F. (2019). Why is it unethical to charge migrant women for pregnancy care in the national health service. *Journal of Medical Ethics*, 45(8), 489–496. https://doi.org/10.1136/medethics-2018-105224

Shortall, C., McMorran, J., Taylor, K., et al. (2015). *Experiences of Pregnant Migrant Women Receiving Ante/Peri and Postnatal Care in the UK: A Longitudinal Follow-up Study of Doctors of the World's London Drop-in Clinic Attendees.* https://b.3cdn.net/droftheworld/08303864eb97b2d304_lam6brw4c.pdf

The Migrant Observatory. (2022). *Migrants in the UK: An Overview.* Oxford University. Available from: Migrants in the UK: An Overview - Migration Observatory - The Migration Observatory, ox.ac.uk [accessed 20 October 2023]

The Migration Observatory. University of Oxford. (2022). Available from: https://migrationobservatory.ox.ac.uk/resources/briefings/migrants-in-the-uk-an-overview/a

UK Visas and Immigration. (2016). *New Healthcare Needs and Pregnancy Dispersal Policy.* Available from: new_Healthcare_Needs_and_Pregnancy_Dispersal_Policy_EXTERNAL_v3_0.pdf (publishing.service.gov.uk) [Accessed 3 December 2022].

UNHCR. (2022). *Refugee Statistics.* Available from: https://www.unhcr.org/refugee-statistics/

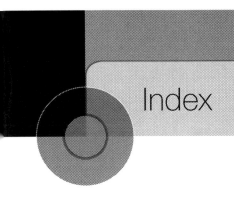

Index

Note: **Bold** page numbers refer to tables and *italic* page numbers refer to figures.

Printed in the United States
by Baker & Taylor Publisher Services